Rural Nursing

DATE DUE

Charlene A. Winters, PhD, APRN-BC, is an Associate Professor in the College of Nursing at Montana State University–Bozeman, Missoula Campus. She serves as Project Director for the Clinical Nurse Leader graduate option. Dr. Winters teaches the rural health course in the graduate program. Her research interests are illness uncertainty, adaptation and chronic illness self-management, and rural nursing theory development. She is an active member of the American Association of Critical Care Nurses, the Western Institute of Nursing, the Montana Association of Clinical Nurse Specialists, Sigma Theta Tau International, the Rural Nurse Organization, the Council for the Advancement of Nursing Science, and is a charter member of the International Council of Nursing—Rural and Remote Nurses Network. Dr. Winters holds a doctorate in nursing from Rush University, Chicago, Illinois, and bachelor and master of science degrees in nursing from California State University, Long Beach.

Helen J. Lee, PhD, RN, is Professor Emeritus in the College of Nursing, Montana State University–Bozeman, Missoula Campus. She holds a BSN and Master of Nursing from Montana State College, Bozeman and a PhD in nursing from the University of Texas at Austin. Her research interests are rural, gerontological, and end-of-life issues, rural nursing theory development, and the variables of hardiness, perception of health, and mobility. Her memberships include the American Nurses' Association, the Oncology Nursing Society, the National Rural Health Association, the Rural Nurse Organization, the Western Institute of Nursing, the Zeta Upsilon Chapter of Sigma Theta Tau International, and she is a charter member of the International Council of Nursing—Rural and Remote Nurses Network.

Rural Nursing

Concepts, Theory, and Practice
3rd Edition

CHARLENE A. WINTERS, PhD, APRN-BC
HELEN J. LEE, PhD, RN

EDITORS

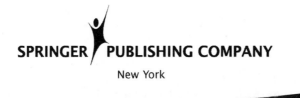

SPRINGER **PUBLISHING COMPANY**

New York

Copyright © 2010 Springer Publishing Company, LLC.

Springer Publishing Company, LLC
11 West 42nd Street
New York, NY 10036
www.springerpub.com

Acquisitions Editor: Margaret Zuccarini
Project Manager: Mary Zemaitis
Cover Designer: David Levy
Composition: Publication Services, Inc.

Ebook ISBN: 978-08261-0457-1

12 13 / 5 4 3

Library of Congress Cataloging-in-Publication Data

Library of Congress Cataloging-in-Publication Data

Rural nursing : concepts, theory, and practice / Charlene A. Winters, Helen J. Lee, editors. -- 3rd ed.
    p. ; cm.
Includes bibliographical references and index.
ISBN 978-0-8261-0456-4 (softcover)
1. Rural nursing. I. Winters, Charlene A. II. Lee, Helen J., PhD.
[DNLM: 1. Community Health Nursing. 2. Rural Health Services. 3. Rural Health. 4. Rural Population. WY 106 R9484 2010]
RT120.R87C66 2010
610.73'43--dc22

                                                                2009028245

Printed in the United States of America by the Hamilton Printing Company

To our research colleagues Elizabeth H. "Betty" Thomlinson (deceased 2004) and Marlene A. Reimer (deceased 2005). We enjoyed knowing them, working with them, and we miss them.

Contents

Contributors

Ronda L. Bales, MN, RN, FNP
Adjunct Assistant Professor
Montana State University–Bozeman
College of Nursing, Billings Campus
Billings, MT

Mary Bliesmer, DNSc, MPH, RN
Professor
Minnesota State University–Mankato
College of Allied Health & Nursing
School of Nursing
Mankato, MN

Robin Boland, MN, RN, FNP-C
Clinical Telehealth Nurse Specialist
REACH Montana Telehealth Network
Benefis Healthcare
Great Falls, MT

Victoria Brogoitti, BS
Director
Union County Commission on Children & Families
La Grande, OR

Janice A. Buehler, PhD, RN
Associate Professor (retired)
Montana State University–Bozeman
College of Nursing, Billings Campus
Billings, MT

Patricia Butterfield, PhD, RN, FAAN
Professor and Dean
Washington State University
College of Nursing
Spokane, WA

Patricia A. Earle, PhD, RN
Associate Professor (retired)
Minnesota State University–Mankato
College of Allied Health & Nursing
School of Nursing
Mankato, MN

Dana S. Edge, PhD, RN
Associate Professor
School of Nursing, Queen's University
Kingston, Ontario, Canada

Sandra Eggenberger, PhD, RN
Associate Professor
Minnesota State University–Mankato
College of Allied Health & Nursing
School of Nursing
Mankato, MN

Nancy Findholt, PhD, RN
Associate Professor
Oregon Health & Science University
School of Nursing
La Grande, OR

Desley Hegney, PhD, RN
Professor
The University of Queensland and the University of Southern Queensland
Chair, Rural and Remote Area Nursing; and
Director, The Centre for Rural and Remote Area Health in Tawoomba
Toowong, Queensland, Australia

Lori Hendrickx, EdD, RN, CCRN
Associate Professor
South Dakota State University–Brookings
College of Nursing
Brookings, SD

Wade G. Hill, PhD, RN
Associate Professor
Montana State University–Bozeman
College of Nursing, Bozeman Campus
Bozeman, MT

Patricia Holkup, PhD, RN
Associate Professor
Montana State University–Bozeman
College of Nursing, Missoula Campus
Missoula, MT

Bette Ide, PhD, RN
Professor
University of North Dakota
College of Nursing
Great Forks, ND

Linda Jerofke, PhD
Assistant Professor
Eastern Oregon University
School of Nursing
La Grande, OR

Brenda D. Koessl, MN, RN, FNP
Director of Nursing
Frances Mahon Deaconess Hospital
Glasgow, MT

Norma Krumwiede, EdD, RN
Associate Professor
Minnesota State University–Mankato
College of Allied Health & Nursing
School of Nursing
Mankato, MN

Judith Kulig, DNSc, RN
Professor
University of Lethbridge
School of Health Sciences
Lethbridge, Alberta, Canada

Sandra K. Kuntz, PhD, RN
Assistant Professor
Montana State University–Bozeman
College of Nursing, Missoula Campus
Missoula, MT

Helen J. Lee, PhD, RN
Professor Emeritus and Campus Director, Missoula Campus (retired)
Montana State University–Bozeman
College of Nursing, Missoula Campus
Missoula, MT

Jacqueline Left Hand Bull, BA
Administrative Officer
Aberdeen Area Tribal Chairmen's Health Board
Rapid City, SD

Beverly D. Leipert, PhD, RN
Associate Professor & Chair, Rural Women's Health Research
University of Western Ontario
Faculty of Health Sciences & Faculty of Medicine and Dentistry
London, Ontario, Canada

Kathleen Ann Long, PhD, APRN, FAAN
Dean
University of Florida
College of Nursing
Gainesville, FL

Janis M. Majerus-Wegerhoff, MN, RN
Calgary, Alberta, Canada

Maureen Malone, MN, RN
Public Health Nurse (retired)
Indian Health Service
Hardin, MT

Meg K. McDonagh, RN, MN, ENC(C)
Senior Instructor
University of Calgary
Faculty of Nursing
Calgary, Alberta, Canada

Sonja J. Meiers, PhD, RN
Associate Professor and Director, Graduate Programs
Minnesota State University–Mankato
College of Allied Health & Nursing
School of Nursing
Mankato, MN

Yvonne Michael, ScD
Assistant Professor
Oregon Health & Science University
Dept. of Public Health & Preventive Medicine
Portland, OR

Elizabeth Nichols, DNS, RN, FAAN
Dean and Professor (retired)
Montana State University–Bozeman
College of Nursing, Bozeman Campus
Bozeman, MT

Chad O'Lynn, PhD, RN, CNRN
Assistant Professor
University of Portland
School of Nursing
Portland, OR

Susan J. Raph, MN, RN, CNAA, BC
Campus Director and Assistant Professor
Montana State University–Bozeman
College of Nursing, Great Falls Campus
Great Falls, MT

Marlene A. Reimer, RN, PhD, CNN(C) (deceased)
Professor
University of Calgary
Faculty of Nursing
Calgary, Alberta, Canada

Melanie Reynolds, MPH
Health Officer, Supervisor
Public Health System Improvement and Training Section
Lewis & Clark City-County Health Dept.
Helena, MT

T. Kim Rodehorst, PhD, RN
Associate Professor
University of Nebraska Medical Center
College of Nursing
Scottsbluff, NE

Kathryn (Kay) Ayres Rosenthal, PhD, RN
Director of Nursing, Harmony Foundation Inc.
Director, Options for Healthy Living Inc.
Estes Park, CO

Emily Matt Salois, MSW, ACS
Montana State University–Bozeman
College of Nursing, Missoula Campus
Missoula, MT

Jane Ellis Scharff, MN, RN
Campus Director and Assistant Professor
Montana State University–Bozeman
College of Nursing, Billings Campus
Billings, MT

Jean Shreffler-Grant, PhD, RN
Campus Director and Associate Professor
Montana State University–Bozeman
College of Nursing, Missoula Campus
Missoula, MT

Jane Smilie, MPH
Administrator
Montana Dept. of Public Health & Human Services
Public Health & Safety Division
Helena, MT

Mary Beth Flanders Stepans, PhD, RN
Assistant Executive Director, Practice and Education Consultant
Wyoming State Board of Nursing
Cheyenne, WY

Therese Sullivan, PhD, RN
Associate Professor (retired)
Montana State University–Bozeman
College of Nursing, Bozeman Campus
Helena, MT

Elizabeth H. Thomlinson, RN, PhD (deceased)
Associate Professor and Associate Dean, Undergraduate Programs
University of Calgary
Faculty of Nursing
Calgary, Alberta, Canada

Linda Troyer, MN, FNP, RN
Big Horn Hospice
Hardin, MT

Clarann Weinert, SC, PhD, RN, FAAN
Sister of Charity (Cincinnati OH); Professor
Montana State University–Bozeman
College of Nursing, Bozeman Campus
Bozeman, MT

Katharine S. West, MPH, MSN, RN, CNS
Nurse Clinical Systems Project Manager
Southern California Permanente Medical Group
Covina, CA

Susan L. Wilhelm, PhD, RNC
Assistant Professor
University of Nebraska Medical Center
College of Nursing
Scottsbluff, NE

Charlene A. Winters, PhD, APRN-BC
Associate Professor
Montana State University–Bozeman
College of Nursing, Missoula Campus
Missoula, MT

Foreword

It is a great honor to have been invited by Dr. Charlene Winters and Dr. Helen Lee to write the foreword for *Rural Nursing*, the third edition. In reflecting on the history and development of the rural nursing phenomenon, I note the role faculty and graduates connected with Montana State University–Bozeman (MSU) have played for more than three decades.

Initially, in the mid-1970s, Dr. Anna Shannon, former Dean of the College of Nursing at Montana State, developed a master's degree program focusing on nursing in the rural environment. At that time Dr. Helen Lee was a nursing instructor at MSU and I was fortunate to be a student in the program. Subsequently, Dr. Lee wrote a chapter that discussed definitions of "rural" for a text that I edited on rural nursing (Sage, 1991). Several years later Dr. Lee edited *Conceptual Basis for Rural Nursing* (Springer, 1998), highlighting scholarly findings from MSU nursing faculty and students and primarily focusing on the intermountain region of the United States. Dr. Lee's *Rural Nursing: Concepts, Theory, and Practice, 2nd Edition*, co-authored by Dr. Charlene Winters, expanded on the concepts for an evolving theory for rural nursing; and, included perspectives from Canada and beyond the intermountain region.

The third edition of *Rural Nursing: Concepts, Theory, and Practice* by Dr. Winters and Dr. Lee has an even greater scope—geographically and contentwise. While seminal chapters from the two previous texts are updated herein, along with the Canadian perspective, information from Australian experts is included. Other timely topics focus on health disparities, public health issues, evidence-based practice, childhood obesity, challenges confronting male caregivers, community-based participatory research within tribal communities, and complementary therapy. The authors of the various chapters are leaders in rural nursing, and for me, reinforce the MSU connection among many of them. This extended text on rural nursing is definitely a significant contribution to the knowledge base on a phenomenon that is of significant importance to nurse educators, researchers, policy makers, and clinicians.

Angeline Bushy, PhD, RN, FAAN
Professor & Bert Fish Chair
Community Health Nursing
University of Central Florida
College of Nursing

Preface

The third edition of *Rural Nursing: Concepts, Theory, and Practice* will provide nurses with a broad understanding of the characteristics of health care in rural settings and what is required for effective nursing practice in this context. The book had its genesis in a small working group at Montana State University–Bozeman, which has been developing a theoretical model of the practice of rural nursing for more than 30 years. This expanded edition contains information of interest to all nurses whose practices are primarily in rural settings, those who are preparing nurses for this type of practice, as well as those conducting research with rural populations. The unique characteristics of this environment are explored in this text.

Several differences exist between the second edition of *Rural Nursing: Concepts, Theory, and Practice* and this edition. New chapters were added to the third edition on male care giving, complementary therapy, evidence-based practice, community resiliency, childhood obesity, and gaining access to Native American communities for the purposes of conducting research. Many chapters retained from the second edition were updated with references to the latest literature or newly collected data. The third edition continues our tradition of branching out to colleagues from around the world by including chapters written by Montana State University–Bozeman College of Nursing faculty, graduate students, and former faculty, as well as colleagues throughout the United States, Canada, and Australia.

As with the first and second editions, we are reporting on the continuing quest to provide a theory structure, the "seeking of patterns which [are helping and those that] ultimately will help rural nurses provide better care for persons in rural communities" (Lee, 1998, p. xxi). Part I contains the seminal article on the rural nursing theory base, followed by two chapters in which the authors examine the rural theory base and report on the exploration of rural nursing theory in a comparison research study. Part II includes chapters about the perspectives of rural persons, and Part III focuses on rural dwellers and their response to illness. Part IV begins with the seminal article about rural nursing practice and follows with reports of studies conducted with nurses in differing rural nurse practice settings. Part V contains chapters devoted to rural public health and Native American communities. Part VI, the final section, contains two chapters: in the first the authors outline implications for rural nursing education, practice, and policy, and in the second, the authors provide an updated analysis of the key concepts first introduced in the first edition.

Several factors led to the publication of the third edition of this text. The first was our continued involvement in teaching the Rural Health Nursing course at Montana State University–Bozeman. The second is our ongoing interest in rural nursing, rural health issues, and the development of rural nursing theory. The third was our positive experience of working with the editorial staff from Springer Publishing and the many authors from a variety of rural settings who contributed to the second edition. We hope our readers find the third edition thought-provoking, and we look forward to the comments and critique from our rural nursing colleagues.

Charlene A. Winters
Helen J. Lee

REFERENCE

Lee, H. J. (1998). Preface. In H. J. Lee (Ed.), *Conceptual basis for rural nursing*. New York: Springer Publishing.

We express our appreciation to the students who participated in our research endeavors, and to the participants who shared their perceptions in the studies reported within the contents of this text. We also thank the contributors for their time and effort in preparing manuscripts.

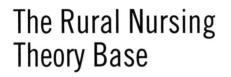

The Rural Nursing Theory Base

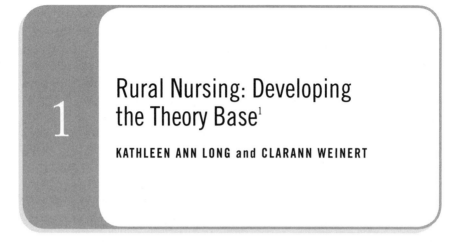

Rural Nursing: Developing the Theory Base[1]

KATHLEEN ANN LONG and CLARANN WEINERT

A logger suffering from "heart lock" does not have a cardiovascular abnormality. He is suffering from a work-related anxiety disorder and can be assisted by an emergency room nurse who accurately assesses his needs and responds with effective communication and a supportive interpersonal relationship. A farmer who has lost his finger in a grain thresher several hours earlier does not have time during the harvesting season for a discussion of occupational safety. He will cope with his injury assisted by a clinic nurse who can adjust the timing of his antibiotic doses to fit with his work schedule in the fields.

Many health care needs of rural dwellers cannot be adequately addressed by the application of nursing models developed in urban or suburban areas but require unique approaches emphasizing the special needs of this population. Although nurses are significant, and frequently the sole, health care providers for people living in rural areas, little has been written to guide the practice of rural nursing. The literature provides vignettes and individual descriptions, but there is a need for an integrated, theoretical approach to rural nursing.

Rural nursing is defined as the provision of health care by professional nurses to persons living in sparsely populated areas. Over the past 8 years, graduate students and faculty members at the Montana State University College of Nursing have worked toward developing a theory

3

base for rural nursing. Theory development has used primarily a retroductive approach, and data have been collected and refined using a combination of qualitative and quantitative methods. The experiences of rural residents and rural nurses have guided the identification of key concepts relevant to rural nursing. The goal of the theory-building process has been to identify commonalities and differences in nursing practice across all rural areas and the common and unique elements of rural nursing in relation to nursing overall. The implications of developing a theory of rural nursing for practice have been examined as a part of the ongoing process.

The theory-building process was initiated in the late 1970s. At that time, literature and research related to rural health care were limited and focused primarily on the problem of retaining physicians in rural areas and providing assessments of rural health care needs and prescriptions for rural health care services based on models and experiences from urban and suburban areas (Coward, 1977; Flax, Wagenfeld, Ivens, & Weiss, 1979). The unique health problems and health care needs of extremely sparsely populated states, such as Montana, had not been addressed from the perspective of the rural consumer. No organized theoretical base for guiding rural health care practice in general, or rural nursing in particular, existed.

QUALITATIVE DATA

The target population for qualitative data collection was the people of Montana. Montana, the fourth largest state in the United States, is an extremely sparsely populated state, with nearly 800,000 people and an average population density of approximately five persons per square mile. One-half of the counties in Montana have three or fewer persons per square mile, with six of those counties having less than one person per square mile. There is only one metropolitan center in the state; it is a city of nearly 70,000 people, with a surrounding area that constitutes a center of approximately 100,000 (*Population Profiles*, 1985).

Qualitative data were collected through ethnographic study by Montana State University College of Nursing graduate students. These data provided the initial ideas about health and health care in Montana. Since general propositions about rural health and rural health care did not exist, the gathering of concrete data was the first step toward subsequent development of more general theoretical propositions.

Graduate students used ethnographic techniques as described by Spradley (1979) to gather information from individuals, families, and health care providers. Interview sites were selected by students on the basis of specific interest and convenience. During a 6-year period, data were gathered from approximately 25 locations. In general, each student worked in depth in one community, collecting data from 10 to 20 informants over a period of at least 1 year. Data were gathered primarily from persons in ranching and farming areas and from towns of less than 2,500 persons. In some instances, student interest led to extensive interviews with specific rural subgroups, such as men in the logging industry or older residents in a rural town (Weinert & Long, 1987). Open-ended interview questions were developed using Spradley's guidelines. The questions emphasized seeking the informants' views without superimposing the cultural biases of the interviewer. The opening question in the interview was, "What is health to you . . . from your viewpoint? . . . your definition?" Interviewers used standard probes and a standard format of questions regarding health beliefs and health care preferences.

Spradley (1979) indicated that the goal of ethnographic study is to "build a systematic understanding of all human cultures from the perspective of those who have learned them" (p. 10). The goal of data collection in Montana was to learn about the culture of rural Montanans from rural Montanans. Emphasis in the cultural learning process was on understanding health beliefs, values, and practices. Rigdon, Clayton, and Diamond (1987) have noted that understanding the meaning that persons attach to subjective experiences is an important aspect of nursing knowledge. The ethnographic approach captured the meanings that rural dwellers ascribe to the subjective states of health and illness and facilitated the development of a rich database.

As the database developed, the following definitions and assumptions were accepted as a foundation for theory development. Rural was defined as meaning sparsely populated. Within this context, states such as Montana, which are sparsely populated overall, are viewed as rural throughout, despite the existence of some population centers within them. Further, based on this definition, rural regions or areas can be identified within otherwise heavily populated states. The assumption is made that, to some degree, health care needs are different in rural areas from that of urban areas. Also, all rural areas are viewed as having some common health care needs. Finally, the assumption is made that urban models are not appropriate to, or adequate for, meeting health care needs in rural areas.

Retroductive Theory Generation

Faculty work groups were developed to examine and organize the qualitative data. The work groups involved three to five nursing faculty members, each with rural nursing experience, but with varied backgrounds and expertise. Thus, a work group included experts from various clinical areas, as well as persons with direct experience either in small rural hospitals or in larger, metropolitan centers within rural states. Standard ethnographic content analysis (Spradley, 1979) was used to sort and categorize the ethnographic data. Groups worked toward consensus about the meaning and organization of specific data. Recurring themes were identified, and these were viewed as having relevance and importance for the rural informants in relation to their views of health.

A retroductive approach, as originally described by Hanson (1958), was used to examine the initial ethnographic data and build the theory base. Specific concepts and relational statements were derived from the data, and more general propositions were induced from these statements. The new propositions were then used to develop additional specific statements which could be supported by existing data or which were categorized for later testing. The retroductive approach was literally a "back and forth" process that permitted persons familiar with the data to move between the data and beginning-level theoretical propositions. The process was orderly and consistent and required group consensus about data interpretation and the relevance of derived propositions. The retroductive process continued in work groups over several years as additional ethnographic data were gathered. Consultants participated at key points in the process, in order to raise questions, add insights, and critically evaluate the group's theory-building approach. Walker and Avant (1983) have noted that the retroductive process "adds considerably to the body of theoretical knowledge. It is, in fact, the way theory develops in the 'real world'" (p. 176).

QUANTITATIVE DATA

Following several years of ethnographic study, the faculty members involved in theory development wished to enrich the qualitative database by collecting relevant quantitative data. Kleinman (1983) stated,

"Qualitative description, taken together with various quantitative measures, can be a standardized research method for assessing validity. It is especially valuable in studying social and cultural significance, e.g. illness beliefs interaction norms, social gain, ethnic help seeking, and treatment responses" (p. 543). Hinds and Young (1987) noted, "The combination of different methodologies within a single study promotes the likelihood of uncovering multiple dimensions of a phenomenon's empirical reality" (p. 195).

A survey developed by Weinert in 1983 attempted to validate some of the rural health concepts that had emerged from the ethnographic data. These concepts were health status and health beliefs, isolation and distance, self-reliance, and informal health care systems. Survey instruments with established psychometric properties were selected to measure the specific concepts of interest. A mail questionnaire completed by the respondents included the Beck Depression Inventory (Beck, 1967) and the Trait Anxiety Scale (Spielberger, Gorsuch, & Lushene, 1970) to tap mental health status, and the General Health Perception Scale (Davies & Ware, 1981) to measure physical health status and health beliefs. A background information form assessed demographic variables, including length of residence and geographic locale. The Personal Resource Questionnaire (Brandt & Weinert, 1981) assessed use of informal systems for support and health care.

The convenience sample of survey participants was located through the Agricultural Extension Service, social groups, and informal networks. All participants lived in Montana, completed the questionnaires in their homes, and returned them by mail to the researcher. The 62 survey participants were middle-class Whites, with an average of 13.5 years of education and a mean age of 61.3 years, who had lived in Montana an average of 45.6 years. The survey sample consisted of 40 women and 22 men residing in one of 13 sparsely populated Montana counties. The most populated county has a population density of 5.9 persons per square mile and one town of nearly 6,000 people. In the most sparsely populated county, there is one town of 600 people and an average population density of 0.5 persons per square mile.

Findings from the quantitative study were used throughout the theory development process to support or refute concept descriptions and relational statements derived from the ethnographic data. Survey findings are discussed in the following section as they relate to key concepts and relational statements.

REFINING THE BUILDING BLOCKS OF THEORY

To order the data and foster the formation of relational statements, an organizational scheme for theory development was adopted. Using the paradigm first described by Yura and Torres (1975) and later by Fawcett (1984), ethnographic data were categorized under the four major dimensions of nursing theory: person, health, environment, and nursing. The data were then ordered from the more general to the more specific. This process led to the identification of constructs, concepts, variables, and indicators.

An example helps to illustrate this process. Ethnographic data had been gathered from "gypo" loggers. These men are independent logging contractors from northwestern Montana who work in rugged isolated areas, usually living in trailers or tents while working. Examples of quotes from these loggers and their associates as found in the data are: A logger states, "We worry about the here and now"; a local physician says, "Loggers enter the health care system during times of crisis only"; the public health nurse in the area says, "Loggers don't want to hear about health care problems; they don't return until the next accident."

Table 1.1 shows the scheme used to organize these data. The concepts "present time" orientation and crisis orientation to health are identified. These are placed under the person dimension. In this example, the constructs are not fully developed, but are viewed as psychological,

Table 1.1

DATA ORDERING SCHEME

COMPONENT	EXAMPLES
Dimension	Psychological/sociocultural
Concept	"Present time" orientation Crisis orientation to health
Variable	Definitions of time Definitions of crisis
Indicators	Hours, minutes, days Seasons, work seasons Number of injuries Number of illnesses

sociocultural, or both. The important variables identified thus far are definitions of time and of crisis. Possible indicators are measures of time, such as hours or seasons, and measures of crisis, such as numbers of illnesses or injuries.

Key Concepts

In the process of data organization it was noted that some concepts appeared repeatedly in ethnographic data collected in several different areas of the state. In addition, aspects of several of these concepts were supported by the quantitative survey data (Weinert, 1983). Using Walker and Avant's (1983) model of concept synthesis, these concepts were identified as key concepts in relation to understanding rural health needs and rural nursing practice. These key concepts are as follows: work beliefs and health beliefs, isolation and distance, self-reliance, lack of anonymity, outsider/insider, and old-timer/newcomer.

As key concepts in this theory, work beliefs and health beliefs are viewed as different in rural dwellers as contrasted with urban or suburban residents. These two sets of beliefs appear to be closely interrelated among rural persons. Work, or the fulfilling of one's usual functions, is of primary importance. Health is assessed by rural people in relation to work role and work activities, and health needs are usually secondary to work needs.

The related concepts of isolation and distance are identified as important in understanding rural health and nursing. Specifically, they help in understanding health care-seeking behavior. Quantitative survey data indicated that rural informants who lived outside of towns traveled a distance of almost 23 miles, on average, for emergency health care and over 50 miles for routine health care. Despite these distances, ethnographic data indicated that rural dwellers tended to see health services as accessible and did not view themselves as isolated.

Self-reliance and independence of rural persons are also seen as key concepts. The desire to do for oneself and care for oneself was strong among the rural persons interviewed and has important ramifications in relation to the provision of health care.

Two key concept areas, lack of anonymity and outsider/insider, have particular relevance for the practice of rural nursing. Lack of anonymity, a hallmark of small towns and surrounding sparsely populated areas, implies a limited ability for rural persons to have private areas of their lives. Rural nurses almost always reported being known to their patients as neighbors, part of a given family, members of a certain church, and so on. Similarly, these nurses usually know their patients in several different social and personal relationships beyond the nurse–patient relationship. The old-timer/newcomer concept, or the related concept of outsider/insider, is relevant in terms of the acceptance of nurses and of all health care providers in rural communities. The ethnographic data indicated that these concepts were used by rural dwellers in organizing their view of the social environment and in guiding their interactions and relationships. Survey data revealed that those who had lived in Montana over 10 years, but less than 20, still considered themselves to be "newcomers" and expected to be viewed as such by those in their community (Weinert & Long, 1987).

Relational Statements

In an effort to move from a purely descriptive theory to a beginning level explanatory one, some initial relational statements were generated from the qualitative data and were supported by the quantitative data that had been collected thus far. The statements are in the early stages of testing.

The first statement is that rural dwellers define health primarily as the ability to work, to be productive, to do usual tasks. The ethnographic data indicate that rural persons place little emphasis on the comfort, cosmetic, and life-prolonging aspects of health. One is viewed as healthy when able to function and be productive in one's work role. Specifically, rural residents indicated that pain was tolerated, often for extended periods, so long as it did not interfere with the ability to function. The General Health Perception Scale indicated that rural survey participants reported experiencing less pain than an age-comparable urban sample (Weinert & Long, 1987). Further, scores on the Beck Depression Inventory and the Trait Anxiety Scale (Weinert, 1983) revealed that they experienced less anxiety and less depression.

The second statement is that rural dwellers are self-reliant and resist accepting help or services from those seen as "outsiders" or from agencies seen as national or regional "welfare" programs. A corollary to this statement is that help, including needed health care, is usually sought through an informal rather than a formal system. Ethnographic data supported both the second statement and its corollary. Numerous references were found showing, for example, a preference for "the 'old doc' who knows us" over the new specialist who was unfamiliar. Data from the Personal Resource Questionnaire (Weinert, 1983) indicated that rural dwellers relied primarily on family, relatives, and close friends for help and support. Further, the rural survey respondents reported using health care professionals and formal human service agencies much less frequently than did comparable urban respondents in previous studies.

A third statement is that health care providers in rural areas must deal with a lack of anonymity and much greater role diffusion than providers in urban or suburban settings. This statement has marked significance for rural nursing practice. Although limited ethnographic and survey data have been collected from rural nurses thus far, some emerging themes have been identified. In addition to identifying a sense of isolation from professional peers, rural nurses emphasize their lack of anonymity and a sense of role diffusion. There is an inability to keep separate the activities and the behaviors of the individual nurse's various roles. In a small town, for example, the nurse's behavior as a wife, a mother, and a church attendee are all significantly related to her effectiveness as a health care professional in that community. Further, in their professional role, nurses reported experiencing role diffusion. Nurses are expected to perform a variety of diverse and unrelated tasks. On a single shift, a nurse may work in obstetrics delivering a baby, care for a dying patient on the medical-surgical unit, and initiate care of a trauma patient in the emergency room. Likewise, on evening shift or weekends, a nurse may be required to carry out tasks reserved for the pharmacist or dietitian on the day shift.

RELATIONSHIP OF CONCEPTS AND STATEMENTS TO THE LARGER BODY OF NURSING KNOWLEDGE

How people define health and illness has a direct impact on how they seek and use health care services and is a key concept in understanding client behavior and in planning intervention.

Definition of Health

The rural Montana dwellers primarily define health as the ability to work and to be productive. The work of other researchers supports the finding that residents of sparsely populated areas view health in terms of ability to work and to remain productive. Ross (1982), a nurse anthropologist, studied the health perceptions of women living in the Lake District along the coast of Nova Scotia. She conducted in-depth interviews with 60 women of both British and French backgrounds in small coastal fishing communities. Similar to the rural dwellers in Montana, these women described good health as being "able to do what you want to do" and to be "able to work." Lee's (1987) recent work in Montana supports earlier findings on which the rural nursing theory was built. She found that work and health practices were closely related among farmers and ranchers; health is viewed as a functional state in relation to work. Scharff's (1987) interviews with nurses practicing in small rural hospitals in eastern Washington, northern Idaho, and western Montana indicated that they viewed the health needs of rural people as overlapping those of people living in urban situations in many instances. The nurse informants, however, noted that rural people equate health with the ability to work or function in their daily activities. Rural people were viewed as delaying health care until they were very ill, thus often needing hospitalization at the point of seeking care.

Self-Reliance

The statement derived from the Montana data that "rural dwellers resist accepting help from outsiders or strangers" has been supported in data from research in rural Maryland (Salisbury State College, 1986). People living in the rural eastern shore area were described as highly resistant to care from persons viewed as outsiders, and rural shore residents often refused to go "across the bridge" to Baltimore to seek health care, even though this was a trip of less than 100 miles and would allow access to sophisticated, specialized treatment. Like the rural people in Montana, these Maryland residents sought health care information and assistance from local, and often informal, sources. The self-reliance of rural persons and their resistance to outside help were also reported by Counts and Boil (1987) in relation to residents of the Appalachian area. Self-reliance was noted as a major feature that must be considered in planning nursing care services for this population.

The rural Nova Scotia women studied by Ross (1982) indicated informal personal networks of family, friends, and neighbors as important sources of health information who also provided the physical, financial, emotional, and social support that contributes to well-being. When these women were asked what connection there was between health and the availability of hospitals, doctors, and other medical care, 42% indicated that it was the individual's responsibility for health knowledge and care; 25% thought professionals were useful to a certain point in providing advice and services such as routine physical exams; 19% indicated that these services were for sick persons, not healthy persons; and 9% felt the formal health care system had no relationship to health (Ross, p. 311). One woman commented, "Health is not a topic to discuss with doctors and nurses" (Ross, p. 309).

Rural Nursing

The Montana data and the theory derived from it indicate that nurses and other health care providers in rural areas must deal with a lack of anonymity. Nurses are known in a variety of roles to their patients, and in turn, know their patients in a variety of roles. Most of the nurses interviewed by Scharff (1987) felt that by knowing their patients personally they could give better care. Other nurses, however, noted that providing professional care for family or friends can be a frightening experience. Nurses indicated that there was no anonymity for them in the rural community, which at times was reassuring, and at other times, constricting (Scharff).

The concept of role diffusion in the rural hospital setting was very apparent in Scharff's (1987) work. She reported that a rural hospital nurse must be a jack-of-all-trades who often practices within the realm of numerous other health care disciplines, including respiratory therapy, laboratory technology, dietetics, pharmacy, social work, psychology, and medicine. Examples of the intersections between rural nursing and other disciplines include doing EKGs, performing arterial punctures, running blood gas machines, drawing blood, setting up cultures, going to the pharmacy to pour drugs, going to the local drugstore to get medications for patients, ordering x-rays and medications, delivering babies, directing the actions of physicians, and cooking meals when the cook gets snowed in. As Scharff noted, some of these functions are carried out by urban nurses practicing in particular settings such as a trauma center or an intensive care unit. Rural nurses, however, are usually not circumscribed by assignment to a particular unit or department and are expected to function in multiple roles, even within one work shift.

This generalist work role and the lack of anonymity of rural nurses are substantiated by findings and descriptions from several other rural areas of the United States (Biegel, 1983; St. Clair, Pickard, & Harlow, 1986). A study of nurses in rural Texas noted, "Nurses play roles as nurse, friend, neighbor, citizen, and family member" within a community; further, rural nurses in their work roles were described as needing to be "all things to all people" (St. Clair et al., 1986, p. 28).

Generalizability

The issue of a situation or locale-specific theory and its relationship to the larger body of nursing knowledge needs serious consideration. The work of Scharff (1987) indicated that the core of rural nursing is not different from urban nursing. The intersections, however, those "meeting points at which nursing extends its practice into the domains of other professions"; the dimensions, that is, the "philosophy, responsibilities, functions, roles, and skills"; and the boundaries, which "respond to new and growing needs and demands from society" (American Nurses Association, 1980), appear to be very distinct for rural nursing practice.

Questions still remain as to how generalizable findings from Montana residents are to other rural populations. Clearly, there is a need for more organized and rigorous data collection in relation to rural nursing before these questions can be answered. A sound theory base for rural practice requires continued research, conducted across diverse rural settings.

IMPLICATIONS FOR NURSING PRACTICE

The findings from the Montana research about people living in sparsely populated areas have implications for nursing practice in rural areas. Since work is of major importance to rural people, health care must fit within work schedules. Health care programs or clinics that conflict with the rural economic cycle, such as haying or calving, will not be used. Since health is defined as the ability to work, health promotion must address the work issue. For example, health education related to cardiovascular disease should highlight strategies for preventing conditions that involve long-term disability, such as stroke. These aspects will be more meaningful to rural dwellers than preventive aspects that emphasize a longer, more comfortable life.

The self-reliance of rural dwellers has specific nursing implications. Rural people will often delay seeking health care until they are gravely ill or incapacitated. Nursing approaches need to address two distinct aspects: nonjudgmental intervention for those who have delayed treatment and a strong emphasis on preventive health teaching. If the nurse can provide adequate health knowledge, the rural dweller's desire for self-reliance may lead to health-promotion behaviors. With a good information base, rural people can make appropriate decisions about self-care versus the need for professional intervention.

Health care services must be tailored to suit the preferences of rural persons for family and community help during periods of illness. Nurses can provide instruction, support, and relief to family members and neighbors, who are often the primary care providers for sick and disabled persons.

The formal health care system needs to fit into the informal helping system in rural areas. A long-term community resident, such as the drugstore proprietor, can be assisted in providing accurate advice to residents through the provision of reference materials and a telephone backup system. One can anticipate greater acceptance and use by rural residents of an updated but old and trusted health care resource, rather than a new professional but "outsider" service (Weinert & Long, 1987).

Nurses who enter rural communities must allow for extended periods prior to acceptance. Involvement in diverse community activities, such as civic organizations and recreational clubs, may assist the nurse in being known and accepted as a person. In rural communities, acceptance as a health care professional is often tied to personal acceptance. Thus it appears that rural communities are not appropriate practice settings for nurses who prefer to maintain entirely separate professional and personal lives.

The stresses that appear to affect nurses in rural practice settings have particular importance. Rural nurses see themselves as cut off from the professional mainstream. They are often in situations where there is no collegial support to assist in defining an appropriate practice role and its boundaries. The educational preparation of those who wish to practice in rural settings needs to emphasize not only generalist skills, but also a strong base in change theory and leadership techniques. Nurses in rural practice need a sound orientation to techniques for accessing diverse sources of current information. If the closest library is several hundred miles away, for example, can all arrangements for interlibrary loan and access to material via telephone, bus, or mail be arranged? Networks that link together nurses practicing in distant rural sites are particularly useful, both for information exchange and for mutual support.

SUMMARY

It is becoming increasingly clear that rural dwellers have distinct definitions of health. Their health care needs require approaches that differ significantly from urban and suburban populations. Subcultural values, norms, and beliefs play key roles in how rural people define health and from whom they seek advice and care. These values and beliefs, combined with the realities of rural living—such as weather, distance, and isolation—markedly affect the practice of nursing in rural settings. Additional ethnographic and quantitative data are needed to further define both the common and the locale-specific conditions and characteristics of rural populations. Continued research can provide a more solid base for the nursing theory that is required to guide practice and the delivery of health care to rural populations.

ACKNOWLEDGMENTS

Qualitative data collected and analyzed by Montana State University College of Nursing graduate students and faculty form the basis for a substantial portion of this paper. Ethnographic data collection and analysis was supported, in part, by a U.S. Department of Health and Human Services, Division of Nursing, Advanced Training Grant to the Montana State University College of Nursing (#1816001649AI). The project that provided the survey data was funded by a Montana State University Faculty Research/Creativity Grant. This article is based partially on a paper presented at the Western Society for Research in Nursing Conference, Tempe, AZ, May 1987.

NOTE

1. From "Rural Nursing: Developing the Theory Base," by K. A. Long and C. Weinert, 1989, *Scholarly Inquiry for Nursing Practice: An International Journal, 3*, pp. 113–127. Copyright 1989 by Springer Publishing Company. Reprinted with permission.

REFERENCES

American Nurses Association. (1980). *Nursing. A social policy statement* (No. NP-63 20M 9/82R). Kansas City, MO: Author.

Beck, A. (1967). *Depression: Causes and treatment.* Philadelphia: University of Pennsylvania Press.

Biegel, A. (1983). Toward a definition of rural nursing. *Home Health Care Nursing, 1,* 45–46.

Brandt, P., & Weinert, C. (1981). The PRQ: A social support measure. *Nursing Research, 30,* 277–280.

Counts, M., & Boyle, J. (1987). Nursing, health and policy within a community context. *Advances in Nursing Science, 9,* 12–23.

Coward, R. (1977). Delivering social services in small towns and rural communities. In R. Coward (Ed.), *Rural families across the life span: Implications for community programming* (pp. 1–17). West Lafayette: Indiana Cooperative Extension Services.

Davies, A., & Ware, J. (1981). *Measuring health perceptions in the health insurance experiment.* Santa Monica, CA: Rand.

Fawcett, J. (1984). *Analysis and evaluation of conceptual models of nursing.* Philadelphia: F. A. Davis.

Flax, J., Wagenfeld, M., Ivens, R., & Weiss, R. (1979). *Mental health and rural America: An overview, and annotated bibliography.* Rockville, MD: U.S. Government Printing Office.

Hanson, N. (1958). *Patterns of discovery.* Cambridge: Cambridge University Press.

Hinds, P., & Young, K. (1987). A triangulation of methods and paradigms to study nurse-given wellness care. *Nursing Research, 36,* 195–198.

Kleinman, A. (1983). The cultural meanings and social uses of illness: A role for medical anthropology and clinically oriented social science in the development of primary care theory and research. *Journal of Family Practice, 16,* 539–545.

Lee, H. (1987). *Relationship of hardiness and current life events to perceived health and rural adults.* Manuscript submitted for publication.

Population profiles of Montana counties: 1980. (1985). Bozeman: Montana State University Center for Data Systems and Analysis.

Rigdon, I., Clayton, B., & Diamond, M. (1987). Toward a theory of helpfulness for the elderly bereaved: An invitation to a new life. *Advances in Nursing Science, 9,* 32–43.

Ross, H. (1982). Women and wellness: Defining, attaining, and maintaining health in Eastern Canada. *Dissertation Abstracts International, 42,* DEO 82–12624.

Salisbury State College. (1986, June). *Discussion of Salisbury State College rural health findings.* Presented at the Contemporary Issues in Rural Health Conference, Salisbury, MD.

Scharff, J. (1987). *The nature and scope of rural nursing: Distinctive characteristics.* Unpublished master's thesis, Montana State University–Bozeman.

Spielberger, C., Gorsuch, R., & Lushene, R. (1970). *STAI manual for the State-Trait Anxiety Questionnaire.* Palo Alto, CA: Consulting Psychologist.

Spradley, J. (1979). *The ethnographic interview.* New York: Holt, Rinehart, & Winston.

St. Clair, C., Pickard, M., & Harlow, K. (1986). Continuing education for self actualization: Building a plan for rural nurses. *Journal of Continuing Education in Nursing, 17,* 27–31.

Walker, L., & Avant, K. (1983). *Strategies for theory construction in nursing.* Norwalk, CT: Appleton-Century-Crofts.

Weinert, C. (1983). [Social support: Rural people in their new middle years]. Unpublished raw data.

Weinert, C., & Long, K. (1987). Understanding the health care needs of rural families. *Journal of Family Relations, 36,* 450–455.

Yura, H., & Torres, G. (1975). *Today's conceptual frameworks with the baccalaureate nursing programs* (NLN Pub. No. 15–1558, pp. 17–75). New York: NLN.

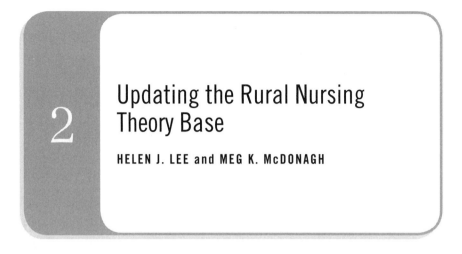

Updating the Rural Nursing Theory Base

2

HELEN J. LEE and MEG K. McDONAGH

We have four purposes for this chapter. First, we present a brief historical perspective of the rural nursing theory development. It is followed by
a summary of the rural nursing theory structure explicated by Long and
Weinert in 1989. Then, we present a review of the literature supporting or refuting the viability of the theoretical statements and concepts.
Based on the findings from the literature review, we propose changes in
the theoretical structure of the rural nursing theory and make suggestions for future work.

HISTORICAL PERSPECTIVES

"Sparsely Populated Areas: Toward Nursing Theory" was the title of
a Western Council on Higher Education for Nursing (now Western
Institute of Nursing) symposium presented in 1982 by Montana State
University–Bozeman. Organized by faculty member, Jacqueline Taylor
(1982), the symposium was introduced to its audience by the Dean of
the School of Nursing, Anna Shannon. In her introductory remarks,
Dean Shannon (1982) stated that the presentation to the council members would demonstrate to its audience how a school could "maximize
its resources, provide opportunities for faculty and student research and
contribute . . . to the development of an empirically based theory of

19

rural nursing" (pp. 70–71). She noted the lack of literature and research about rural nursing plus the placement of little emphasis on the context of environment within nursing theories.

The symposium included faculty and graduate students' studies about (a) the beliefs and practices of Crow Indian women, Hmong refugees, and Hutterite colony members; (b) sodium in drinking water and adolescent blood pressure; and (c) the role of distance in home dialysis adjustment. Concluding remarks, given by faculty member Ruth Ludeman, included the information that a plan for theory construction and testing was in place using *retroduction,* a process involving both inductive and deductive reasoning. Theory development activity continued at Montana State University–Bozeman College of Nursing resulting in the subsequent publication of the initial theoretical article titled "Rural Nursing: Developing the Theory Base" (Long & Weinert, 1989).

THE RURAL NURSING THEORY STRUCTURE

"Many disciplines exist to generate, test, and apply theories that will improve the quality of people's lives" (Fawcett, 1999, p. 1). The quality of the lives of rural persons and the lack of empirical studies about their health care was of concern to Montana State University–Bozeman nursing researchers. A middle-range theory emerged from a recognized need of rural nurses for a practice framework that acknowledges the unique perceptions of rural persons and the generalist experience of nurses who practice in rural settings. Prior to the development of the theory, it was assumed that nursing care of rural persons was similar to the care of persons living in urban environments.

The resulting descriptive theory is the "most basic type of middle range theory" (Fawcett, 1999, p. 15). It emerged from observations gathered through qualitative and quantitative descriptive studies conducted in the sparsely populated rural setting of Montana. It describes specific characteristics and observations made of rural persons seeking health care and their health care providers. The published theory contains several key concepts and three theoretical statements (Long & Weinert, 1989).

The first statement is descriptive and states that "rural dwellers define health primarily as the ability to work, to be productive, to do usual tasks" (Long & Weinert, 1989, p. 120). Key concepts associated with this statement are *work beliefs* and *health beliefs.*

The second statement is relational and proposes that "rural dwellers are self-reliant and resist accepting help or services from those seen as 'outsiders' or from agencies seen as national or regional 'welfare' programs" (Long & Weinert, 1989, p. 120). Rural persons prefer to seek health care from *insiders,* persons with whom they were familiar. Additional key concepts pertaining to this statement are *old-timer* and *newcomer.* A corollary to the second statement is "that help, including needed medical care, is usually sought through an informal rather than a formal system" (p. 120).

The third statement is relational and focuses on health care providers; it indicates that *lack of anonymity* and *role diffusion* is experienced more acutely among rural providers than among providers in urban or suburban settings. Lack of anonymity also applies to the recipients of health care in rural areas as all persons in that environment have a "limited ability . . . to have private areas of their lives" (Long & Weinert, 1989, p. 119).

In addition to the above three statements, an understanding of the concepts "isolation" and "distance" is important in the health care-seeking behavior of rural residents. The concept of *isolation* refers to separation from or being placed alone (Lee, Hollis, & McClain, 1998). *Distance* is measurable time, physical distance between places, and personal perception of that space (Henson, Sadler, & Walton, 1998). Qualitative data upon which the theoretical work was based indicated that rural residents did not feel isolated despite the fact that they averaged 23 miles of travel to their nearest emergency room and over 50 miles to their primary health care source (Long & Weinert, 1989).

RELATED NURSING LITERATURE

The content of Long and Weinert's (1989) rural nursing theory article was and is widely quoted in nursing literature, including community health and rural nursing texts, and in presentations given about rural nursing. However, a rural nursing literature review conducted in 2003 and 2008 contained few citations that specifically focused on health perceptions and needs of rural persons. We located three qualitative studies through conference proceedings, the contents of which were subsequently published (Bales, Winters, & Lee, 2006; Lee & Winters, 2004; Thomlinson, McDonagh, Reimer, Crooks, & Lees, 2004). Other sources included two nursing master's theses (Bales, 2006; Moran, 2005), a study that focused on the health care meanings, values, and practices of Anglo-American males in the rural American midwest (Sellers, Poduska, Propp, & White, 1999), a study exploring rurality and health in midlife women (Thurston & Meadows, 2003), and a study examining the health information seeking experiences of rural women in Ontario, Canada (Wathen & Harris, 2006, 2007). We also located several journal articles, mostly qualitative rural research, that included rural concepts found in this rural nursing theory. In the following sections, each theoretical statement is followed by findings from the literature supporting or refuting the statement.

Theoretical Statement #1 (Descriptive)

"... [R]ural dwellers define health primarily as the ability to work, to be productive, to do usual tasks" (Long & Weinert, 1989, p. 120).

Four qualitative studies conducted in the United States (one with rural men aged 25–49 years, one with rural men and women aged 28–63 years, and two with older rural persons aged 60–85) examined health perceptions. Three provided support for the above descriptive statement that defines health as being able to carry out important functions (Niemoller, Ide, & Nichols, 2000; Pierce, 2001; Sellers et al., 1999). In the fourth study, Averill (2002) found that definitions of health varied across her southwest United States sample that included older, more recent retirees, and Hispanic elders. The older retirees from mining and ranching communities viewed health in a similar manner to the original qualitative theory development samples while more recent retirees focused on strategies to remain healthy—proper diet, regular exercise, and regular health exams. The Hispanic elders in Averill's sample frequently mentioned incorporating home remedies and herbal preparations into their health maintenance practices.

Participants in the six health perceptions and needs studies (Bales, 2006; Bales et al., 2006; Lee & Winters, 2004; Moran, 2005; Thomlinson et al., 2004; Winters, Thomlinson, O'Lynn, et al., 2006b) conducted in the United States and Canada were more likely to define health holistically. Lee and Winters found that for rural persons working in service occupations, being able to function included being physically, mentally, and emotionally fit. Participants in a study conducted by Bales et al. thought that being healthy meant being mentally and physically active, eating well, and having an overall sense of well-being. Thomlinson and her colleagues interpreted their participants' responses by saying that health was a "holistic relationship between the physical, mental, social and spiritual aspects of one's life" (p. 261).This same view of health was echoed by Canadian middle-aged women in Thurston and Meadows' (2003) study.

Australian women in de la Rue and Coulson's (2003) study, ages 73–87, equated health with not being ill. They knew maintenance of their health was influenced by their geographical location and their desire to remain living on the land.

Summary

The literature both supports and refutes the first theoretical statement. Support appears in studies of rural male adults and of older persons and retirees from the extractive industries (mining, farming). Lack of support for the functional definition of health emerges from a variety of settings and from differing rural samples. It may be that age, the rural environmental setting, the influence of the work ethic, and culture are factors in defining health (de la Rue & Coulson, 2003). Potentially, younger rural participants may be influenced by increased media exposure and its emphasis on health promotion and use of preventive health practices. In addition, health care providers may be expanding their view of health beyond the illness care model and sharing this with their clients.

Theoretical Statement #2 (Relational)

" . . . [R]ural dwellers are self-reliant and resist accepting help or services from those seen as 'outsiders' or from agencies seen as national or regional 'welfare' programs" (Long & Weinert, 1989, p. 120).

The attribute of self-reliance dominates the literature about rural persons and their health-seeking behaviors (Davis & Magilvy, 2000; Jirojwong & MacLennan, 2002; Lee & Winters, 2004; Niemoller et al., 2000; Sellers et al., 1999; Thomlinson et al., 2004; Wathen & Harris, 2006, 2007; Winters et al., 2006b). Care was sought by rural residents after first "consulting books" (Jirojwong & MacLennan, p. 251) and trying "to deal with an illness themselves" (Thomlinson et al., p. 262). Because of the presence of chronic illnesses, older adults were knowledgeable about medical resources (physicians, physician's assistants, and nurse practitioners) in nearby areas (Niemoller et al.; Pierce, 2001; Roberto & Reynolds, 2001), and, if available, would use them "to achieve their desired level of independence" (Niemoller et al., p. 39). However, if the desired resources were not available, these same older adults stated they would "manage" (p. 39).

Canadian women (age range 20–82) in the study conducted by Wathen and Harris (2006) shared differing strategies when faced with an urgent health situation. Some would visit a hospital emergency room while others would self-medicate and wait until the next morning to contact their family doctor. Decision making was influenced by their perception of the knowledge and skills of available professional practitioners and, in some situations, by the results of previous interactions with regard to managing their chronic illnesses. In addition, decisions were affected by the distances they needed to travel, especially during the winter.

Corollary to Relational Statement #2

"... [H]elp, including needed health care, is usually sought through an informal rather than a formal system" (Long & Weinert, 1989, p. 120).

The literature revealed a variety of findings related to the relational statement corollary. Bales (2006) found that mothers living in frontier settings in the United States would seek advice from family, friends, and neighbors and would initiate self-care activities if health care situations were not considered serious. However, if the illness or injury was gauged as serious, professional health care was immediately accessed no matter the distance involved. Bypassing the informal for the formal system because of the seriousness of the illness or injury also was found in studies conducted by Buehler, Malone, and Majerus (1998) and Thomlinson et al. (2004).

Participants in two Canadian studies (Thomlinson et al., 2004; Wathen & Harris, 2006, 2007) indicated that family, friends, and neighbors were cited as a major source of support, particularly during the information gathering phase (Wathen & Harris, 2006). Those particularly valued were persons who held a health care professional role or had experienced a disease or illness firsthand (Wathen & Harris). Although older rural women in the United States study conducted by Pierce (2001) stated they were eager to help neighbors and the less fortunate, they also shared their reluctance to tell family and neighbors about their needs unless really necessary.

Help gained through accessing informal knowledge via the media, popular magazines, books, libraries, and the Internet was cited in three studies (Roberto & Reynolds, 2001; Thomlinson et al., 2004; Wathen & Harris, 2007). A sample of older women living in the United States actively sought information about living with their osteoporosis (Roberto

& Reynolds); members of Canadian samples stated that they frequently made use of formal information sources through libraries, books, and computers (Thomlinson et al.; Wathen & Harris).

Summary

The second theoretical statement and its corollary is both sustained and refuted by the findings in the literature. Self-reliance remains a characteristic attribute of rural persons and influences the way they respond to illness or injury and their subsequent care-seeking behaviors. The informal system (family, friends, and neighbors) is still frequently used as a resource. However, the rural cultural barrier to accessing care through formal resources appears to be changing. The accessibility of knowledge through a variety of sources and the need to have information about health and the chronic illnesses they are experiencing may be beginning to remove the cultural barrier of approaching "outsiders" for health and medical care. In part, this may be occurring because desired health information can now be obtained through use of computers while maintaining anonymity. Prior to the current age of information technology, maintaining anonymity while seeking health information was not an option.

Theoretical Statement #3 (Relational)

"... [H]ealth care providers in rural areas must deal with a lack of anonymity and much greater role diffusion than providers in urban or suburban settings" (Long & Weinert, 1989, p. 120).

The findings for the two concepts forming this relational statement—lack of anonymity and role diffusion—are sustained in the literature about health care providers from Australia, New Zealand, and the United States. In relation to the lack of anonymity, authors stated that "in close knit communities . . . news travels fast" (Lau, Kumar, & Thomas, 2002, p. 10) and that "social life realities in small communities frequently blur professional boundaries" (Blue & Fitzgerald, 2002, p. 319–320). Social factors pertaining to practice in rural communities include privacy issues for both the professional and the clients for whom they give care (Lau et al.). Health care practitioners in rural environments who are known by their clients may find that older women prefer receiving professional care from a familiar person (Courtney, Tong, & Walsh, 2000; Pierce, 2001), whereas middle-aged women will prefer to go elsewhere for care because of that familiarity (Brown, Young, & Byles, 1999; Lee & Winters, 2004). Lee and Winters found this particularly true for women's health care and mental health.

Role diffusion was found in studies conducted with psychiatrists and nurses in Australia (Lau et al., 2002) and by Rosenthal (1996) in her study of rural nursing in America. Hegney (1997) described role diffusion in her study of Australian rural nursing practice as the generalist and extended practice role. Role diffusion was evident in the practice of hospice nurses in New Zealand (McConigley, Kristjanson, & Morgan, 2000). The reality in sparsely populated areas is that with fewer persons to perform the multiple tasks, more tasks must be undertaken by the individuals who choose to practice in those areas.

Summary

The third theoretical statement about lack of anonymity and role diffusion is well supported in the available literature. The concept of familiarity, the antonym of lack of anonymity, can be a facilitator or a barrier to seeking health and illness care from local health care practitioners. Familiarity is a distinguishing feature of rural nursing that allows rural nurses a special knowledge of those for whom they provide care within their communities (Hegney, 1997).

The lack of anonymity that health care providers experience in rural communities is in itself a paradox. On the one hand, it is often the familiarity and knowing of community members and the lack of anonymity that draws health care professionals to rural areas. Yet, it is often the same attribute of rural practice that can later drive them away.

The review of the literature pertaining to the descriptive middle-range rural nursing theory base revealed a variety of findings. The rural residents' definition of health in the first descriptive statement is changing from that of a functional nature to a more holistic view that includes physical, mental, social, and spiritual aspects. The self-reliance of rural residents in the second relational statement is broadly supported; however, the resistance to seeking help from those seen as "outsiders" is changing. The third relational statement pertaining to health care providers and their lack of anonymity and role diffusion is supported. The findings for the concept of distance in the original rural theory development work are not supported. This literature appraisal of the rural nursing theory base structure supports a need for change.

THE REVISED RURAL NURSING THEORY STRUCTURE

Based on the review of the literature, Lee and McDonagh (2006) recommended the following revisions to the first two theoretical statements originally proposed by Long and Weinert in 1989.

Theoretical Statement #1 (Descriptive)

"Rural residents define health as being able to do what they want to do; it is a way of life and a state of mind; there is a goal of maintaining balance in all aspect of their lives" (Lee & McDonagh, 2006, p. 314).

"Older rural residents and those with ties to extractive industries are more likely to define health in a functional manner—to work, to be productive, and to do usual tasks" (Lee & McDonagh, p. 314).

Essential to understanding rural persons' motivation for illness treatment, health maintenance, and health promotion is knowledge of their health perceptions (Long, 1993). The above replacement statements provide a broader view of the health perceptions being found with more recent research with rural individuals, families, and communities. They reflect both the earlier emphasis on role performance that is evident among older residents and those employed in primary industries and the expanded view of health perception definitions elicited from other individuals living in rural communities.

Theoretical Statement #2 (Relational)

"Rural residents are self-reliant and make decisions to seek care for illness, sickness, or injury depending on their self-assessment of the severity of their present health condition and of the resources needed and available" (Lee & McDonagh, 2006, p. 315).

"Rural residents with infants and children who experience illness, sickness, or injury will seek care more quickly than for themselves" (Lee & McDonagh, 2006, p. 315).

These theoretical statements refer to the health-seeking behaviors of rural residents. Key concepts from the 1989 model included self-reliance, seeking care from insiders, and the use of the informal system. Research findings continue to assert that self-reliance is a key characteristic identified in the management of health care situations by rural persons. However, changes were seen in the health-seeking behaviors of these residents as they seek advice and care from insiders and outsiders and also make use of both informal and formal systems of care.

Additional concepts emerged from the comparative research about rural persons' health behaviors: *health-seeking behaviors* and *choice* (Winters et al., 2006b). *Health-seeking behaviors*, defined as "conscious behaviors designed to promote healthy relationships among physical, mental, social and spiritual aspects of one's life so that life balance is maintained," includes three subthemes: symptom–action–time-line process (SATL) (Buehler et al., 1998), resources, and self-reliance.

Conscious *choice* is made in at least two domains of rural persons' lives. The first is the choice to live in a rural environment; the second is in accessing health care resources. Choosing to live in a rural environment is closely associated with the concept of place (see discussion later in this paper).

Theoretical Statement #3 (Relational)

Health care providers continue to experience lack of anonymity and role diffusion. Because the original statement was well supported by the literature review, no changes are recommended.

FUTURE DIRECTION

Exploration of the literature regarding rural health perceptions and needs revealed many new avenues for future exploration. Themes of *distance* and *resources* were identified repeatedly in the literature reviewed. Newly proposed concepts emerging from the literature review included *health-seeking behaviors, choice, environmental context,* and *social capital.* Each of these concepts is addressed in the following sections.

Distance

Although *distance* was not part of any of the three theoretical statements making up the rural nursing theory base, the content of the rural literature we accessed for this review frequently touched on the concept. In the seminal article by Long and Weinert (1989), the participants included in the multiple studies tended to see health services as accessible and did not view themselves as isolated. Canadian authors MacLeod, Browne, and Leipert (1998) stated that distance may not be a problem but said the concept exerts a strong influence in providing health care in rural areas. This view affirms Johnson, Ratner, and Bottorff's (1995) assertion that one's geographic location may influence or even determine the form of health-seeking behaviors rural residents demonstrate. In an article cited earlier, the older women described distance and geographical barriers with concern; yet, they seemed to take problems with accessibility "in stride" (Pierce, 2001, p. 52). However, the participants did express concern about the quality of nearby health services.

The remainder of the research all refuted the initial findings about distance and access to health care in Long and Weinert's (1989) theory-based article. Racher and Vollman (2002) stated that access to health care services is a major concern for residents across North America's rural and remote areas and the health professionals serving them. Fitzgerald, Pearson, and McCutcheon (2001) found that access to care is particularly a concern for Australian rural individuals with chronic illness; an expressed problem was finding the "best" doctor (p. 237). In a research-based computer intervention group of 142 women living in five sparsely populated western states, Winters and her colleagues identified that "distance was an overarching characteristic of the rural context that influenced the women's ability to self-manage their chronic health problems" (Winters, Cudney, Sullivan, & Thuesen, 2006a, p. 273). Buehler and Lee (1992) found the more rural the persons experiencing cancer, the more limited were formal health care resources available to assist them and their families.

"Distance and travel needs" were of prime concern for women seeking perinatal care in rural California (West, 2006, p. 105). Distance to emergency care was an expressed concern of service providers in rural areas (Lee & Winters, 2004) and of mothers of children living in frontier areas (Bales, 2006). In a survey of middle-aged women, Brown and colleagues (1999) concluded that experiencing difficulties with accessing health care results in greater reliance on self-treatment and self-care, thereby leading to development of "attitudes of independence and self-reliance" (p. 151).

Resources

In addition to distance, *availability of resources* is a concept that directly impacts access to health care services (Winters et al., 2006a, 2006b). Authors Gulzar (1999) and Racher and Vollman (2002) discuss the complexity of processes in accessing health services. The rurality or remoteness of a given place affects access to health services. Within the rural environment, such factors as geographical, political, and economical, as well as the acceptability and the education of health care providers, all influence the residents' access *to* and choice *of* health resources. Studying patterns of health care use and feedback loops among residents may add to the understanding of the complexity of accessing health care services in rural and remote areas (Racher & Vollman). Delivery of health services across sparsely populated areas presents unique challenges because of the vast distances involved and the scarcity of health professionals. For example, the greater the nurse-to-patient or physician-to-patient ratio and the more rural or remote the community is from large urban centers, the more limited the health resources are for rural and remote community members.

Health-Seeking Behaviors

Health-seeking behaviors were defined as "conscious behaviors designed to promote healthy relationships among physical, mental, social and spiritual aspects of one's life so that life balance in maintained" (Winters et al., 2006b, p. 34). The authors included three subthemes, SATL process, resources, and self-reliance, as part of health-seeking behaviors. The SATL process (Buehler et al., 1998) is used to describe the social process and identify symptoms of sickness, illness, or injury and then seek the appropriate level of requisite care. The level of care sought may be self, lay, or professional, depending upon the perceived seriousness and type of symptom. Accessing resources is a part of the SATL process. Self-reliance, defined as behaviors to promote or maintain health without seeking assistance from others, was prevalent in the data from Montana and the Canadian provinces of Alberta and Manitoba. Winters et al. considered self-reliance a subtheme of health-seeking behavior because of its paramount influence in seeking health care in sparsely populated rural areas.

Choice

Choice, the making of conscious decisions to live in a rural environment and access health care resources, was a new theme that emerged from the comparison study (Winters et al., 2006b). Explicitly evident in the Montana data and implicitly identified in the Canadian study through the participants' expressions of the benefits of living in rural environments, the theme is associated with the concept of "place." Although we think of place in a geographical context, it is a broader entity that shapes one's political, economic, spatial, geographic, and cultural views of the world (Kelly, 2003). De la Rue and Coulson (2003) found that rural participants' well-being and health were very influenced by the "geographical location of living on the land" (p. 5). "Place" provided these rural residents with a kind of emotional or spiritual connectedness that affected the outcomes of their health experiences.

Wathen and Harris (2007) thought that rural living affected the choice of resources the members of their Canadian study sample (n = 40) would consult about a chronic health concern or an acute medical problem. If they wanted to avoid "bothering" the doctor or their available rural doctor "might not be the best or too up to date" (p. 643), they chose to use their informal system (colleagues, friends, family), medical books, pharmacists, and/or the veterinarian.

Choice in making decisions related to accessing health care can be affected by several factors. Questions often asked to aid in determining a course of action are: Where is the closest facility that will provide the health care needed? What are the qualifications of the persons who staff that facility? What level of confidence is there in the local health care providers? Does familiarity with the professionals who staff the facility make a difference in making the choice of where to go? Is anonymity an important factor in this situation? Does the health care facility accept the insurance carried by the individual or family seeking care (Moran, 2005)? What hours does the facility stay open? What are the weather conditions? During stormy conditions (in winter, snow, freezing rain, and ice; in summer, rain, wind, and flooding), what roads are better maintained? In an acute emergency, can a fixed wing aircraft or helicopter land nearby? These represent only a fraction of the factors that may play into the decision-making for accessing health care.

Environmental Context

Appearing repeatedly throughout the literature reviewed were terms like *place* or *geographical location* or *rural context* or *environmental context*. According to Jones and Ross (2003), nursing practice is "shaped by its situatedness" (p. 16). Authors speak of the context of a place and the resources needed that are particular to a context or place (Andrews 2003a, 2003b; Andrews & Moon, 2005; MacLeod, Misener, Banks,

Morton, Vogt, & Bentham, 2008; Poland, Lehoux, Holmes, & Andrews, 2003; Thurston & Meadows, 2004; Winters et al., 2006a). According to Lauder, Reel, Farmer, and Griggs (2006), "'Context' is an important unit of analysis. . . . A rural health context is both physical and relational and aspects of rural environments . . . may enhance or impede health" (p. 75).

Health perceptions, needs, and actions of rural persons are also influenced by the environmental context. This was particularly evident in the research reported by de la Rue and Coulson (2003); Thomlinson et al. (2004); and Winters et al. (2006a). Winters and her colleagues found in their intervention study of rural women with chronic illnesses that four themes emerged through the "overarching characteristic of distance: (a) physical setting, (b) social/cultural/economic environment, (c) nature of rural women's work, and (d) accessibility/quality of health care" (p. 284–285).

Social Capital

Social capital is a concept that comes from sociology and has come into increasing importance over the last 20 years (Shookner, Scott, & Vollman, 2008). Rooker (2002, as cited in Lauder et al., 2006) defines the term as "forms of association that express trust and norms of reciprocity" (p. 75). The Policy Research Initiative (PRI) for the government of Canada (2005, as cited in Shookner et al., 2008) further clarifies social capital as the "networks of social relations that may provide individuals and groups with access to resources and supports" (p. 87). "Creating supportive environments is about building social capital" (p. 87) and is similar to the notion of building "rural capacity" (Hartley, 2005).

Nurses practicing in rural settings tend to be more actively engaged professionally and personally in the rural communities in which they live and work (Scharff, 1998; Bushy, 2000). However, the present role of nurses in creating supportive health care environments is not well understood; recognition, conceptualization, and measurement are needed "to more fully appreciate the impact nurses have on rural health access and services" (Lauder et al., 2006, p. 74).

Three qualitative studies about nurses spoke to the necessity of developing social capital within rural communities. Advanced practice registered nursing (APRN) graduates realized the importance of "rural connectedness" through development of support networks with other health care providers, relationships with urban health care centers, connections with local communities, and support through electronic means (Conger & Plager, 2008). Nurses providing maternity care realized that they needed to know "their community—who lives in their community, what their skills are, and whether they are available to address local health needs or respond to emergency situations" (MacKinnon, 2008, p. 6). Nurses in solo mental health practice recognized the necessity of assisting rural and remote clients "to achieve a level of social functioning to integrate the person back into their community network" (Gibb, 2003, p. 248). To do this they found that they needed to work more closely with the potential support structures identified within the clients' community. This was best achieved by fostering a caring home environment, trying to keep people with their families and in their place of employment (Gibb, Livesey & Zyla, 2003). By having such a support structure, rural mental practitioners can avoid sending the mental health client to a psychiatric institution when a crisis occurs.

SUMMARY

Theories are developed for the purposes of describing, explaining, and predicting phenomena (Fawcett, 2000). The intent of the early theory development work at Montana State University–Bozeman College of Nursing was to use the descriptive research data collected in sparsely populated rural areas to develop a middle-range theory, one that would provide a framework for nurses providing care to rural dwellers (Shannon, 1982). What evolved was a descriptive theory, the most basic type of middle-range theory (Fawcett, 1999). Middle-range theory focuses "on a limited dimension of the reality of nursing" and grows at the "intersection of practice and research to provide guidance for everyday practice and scholarly research rooted in the discipline of nursing" (Smith & Liehr, 2003, p. xi).

Although controversy exists about the placement and abstraction level of middle-range theories within the hierarchical structure of nursing theories (Peterson & Bredow, 2004), the basic theory structure, regardless of level, is similar—theoretical statements that describe or link key concepts (Fawcett, 1999). The interweaving of those concepts and statements provide a pattern of ideas that provide a new perspective of phenomena (Smith & Liehr, 2003). The pattern, once published and subjected to testing, should remain open to scrutiny, debate, change (if necessary), and the incorporation of new ideas.

By subjecting the middle-range rural nursing theory to testing in several studies (Bales, 2006; Bales et al., 2006; Lee & Winters, 2004; Moran, 2005; Thomlinson et al., 2004; Winters et al., 2006b) and the findings from several related studies, it has become evident that change has occurred over the past thirty years which has altered the applicability of the original published rural nursing theory base by Long and Weinert (1989). This change is demonstrated by revisions to the theoretical statements and in the newly emerging concepts reviewed above.

Vision for the Future

Because of the descriptive nature of the middle-range rural nursing theory, additional descriptive research is needed (Fawcett, 1999). Analysis methods can take several approaches, including the Wilson method (Walker & Avant, 1995), the evolutionary method (Rodgers, 1993), the empirical or inductive approach (Morse, 1995), or a combination thereof. Testing of the proposed changes to the rural nursing theory relational statements through qualitative studies (ethnography, grounded theory, phenomenology, narrative inquiry, historical inquiry, and photo voice) and participatory action research needs to take place in other sparsely populated areas. Development and testing of instruments to measure the concepts is also needed. Conducting surveys to measure attributes, attitudes, knowledge, and opinions using open-ended and semi-structured interviews and questionnaires is required (Fawcett). With a compilation of these focused research efforts can emerge a model, a schema, or a list of logically ordered statements that, when present, will provide guidance for the care of rural dwellers (Smith & Liehr, 2003).

Moving the Work Forward

A core group of nurse researchers from Montana and Alberta periodically meet to review and critique theoretical material and models. Members of this North American Study (NAS) group discuss and plan projects to further rural nursing theory development while offering research and educational opportunities to graduate students within their course work or independent studies. A rural nursing research and theory development listserv, developed at the Third International Congress of Rural Nurses in Binghamton, New York, provided a mechanism for online discussion for furthering rural nursing research and theory development. While this listserv is now dormant, two resources are potentially available for reestablishment of communication: (a) Nursing Theory Link Page, http://nursing.clayton.edu/eichelberger/nursing.htm, and (b) The International Council of Nurses (ICN) Rural and Remote Nursing Network, http://www.icn.ch/rrn_network.htm.

The NAS and listserv members did identify the following questions for exploration: (a) Are these health-seeking behaviors unique to rural residents? (b) Will health-seeking behavior activities of the SATL process fit under the same middle-range theory framework as those for health promotion? (c) How do illness variables affect rural persons' health-seeking behaviors? (d) How do illness variables affect rural people's choices of health care providers? (e) Are rural dwellers more accepting of "outsiders" if they are health care professionals working in partnerships with the rural community and local health professionals?

CONCLUSION

As we have argued in this chapter, the middle-range rural nursing theory as published by Long and Weinert (1989) is in need of revision. Advances in health service technologies and care along with the changes in the perception and behaviors of rural residents over the past 30 years may account for some of the emerging concepts that we have identified. Continued research and theoretical development efforts will increase the potential for a middle-range theory that can provide a structure for acceptable, adaptable, and appropriate nursing care to rural persons.

REFERENCES

Andrews, G. J. (2003a). Locating a geography of nursing: Space, place and the progress of geographical thought. *Nursing Philosophy, 4,* 231–248.

Andrews, G. J. (2003b). Nightingale's geography. *Nursing Inquiry, 10,* 270–274.

Andrews, G. J., & Moon, G. (2005). Space, place, and the evidence base: Part I—An introduction to health. *Worldviews Evidence-Based Nursing, 2,* 231–248.

Averill, J. B. (2002). Voices from the Gila: Health care issues for rural elders in southwestern New Mexico. *Journal of Advanced Nursing, 40,* 654–662.

Bales, R. L. (2006). Health perceptions, needs, and behaviors of remote rural women of childbearing and childrearing age. In H. J. Lee & C. A. Winters (Eds.), *Rural nursing: Concepts, theory and practice* (2nd ed., pp. 53–65). New York: Springer.

Bales, R. L., Winters, C. A., & Lee, H. J. (2006). Health needs and perceptions of rural persons. In H. J. Lee & C. A. Winters (Eds.), *Rural nursing: Concepts, theory and practice* (2nd ed., pp. 53–65). New York: Springer.

Blue, I., & Fitzgerald, M. (2002). Interprofessional relations: Case studies of working relationships between registered nurses and general practitioners in rural Australia. *Journal of Clinical Nursing, 11,* 314–321.

Brown, W. J., Young, A. F., & Byles, J. E. (1999). Tyranny of distance? The health of mid-age women living in five geographical areas of Australia. *Australian Journal of Rural Health, 7,* 148–154.

Buehler, J. A., & Lee, H. J. (1992). Exploration of home care resources for rural families with cancer. *Cancer Nursing, 15,* 299–308.

Buehler, J. A., Malone, M., & Majerus, J. M. (1998). Patterns of responses to symptoms in rural residents: The symptom-action-time-line process. In H. J. Lee (Ed.), *Conceptual basis for rural nursing* (pp. 318–328). New York: Springer.

Bushy, A. (2000). *Orientation to nursing in the rural community.* Thousand Oaks, CA: Sage.

Conger, M. M., & Plager, K. A. (2008). Advanced practice nursing practice in rural areas: Connectedness versus disconnectedness. *Online Journal of Rural Nursing and Health Care, 8*(1), 24–38. Retrieved January 24, 2009, from http://rno.org

Courtney, M., Tong, S., & Walsh, A. (2000). Older patients in the acute care setting: Rural and metropolitan nurses' knowledge, attitudes and practices. *Australian Journal of Rural Health, 8,* 94–102.

Davis, R., & Magilvy, J. K. (2000). Quiet pride: The experience of chronic illness by rural older adults. *Journal of Nursing Scholarship, 32,* 385–390.

de la Rue, M., & Coulson, I. (2003). The meaning of health and well-being: Voices from older rural women. *Rural and Remote Health, 3* (192), 1–10. Retrieved October 4, 2003, from http://rrh.deakin.edu.au

Fawcett, J. (1999). *The relationship of theory and research* (3rd ed.). Philadelphia: Davis.

Fawcett, J. (2000). *Analysis and evaluation of contemporary nursing knowledge: Nursing models and theories.* Philadelphia: Davis

Fitzgerald, M., Pearson, A., & McCutcheon, H. (2001). Impact of rural living on the experience of chronic illness. *Australian Journal of Rural Health, 9,* 235–240.

Gibb, H. (2003). Rural community mental health nursing: A grounded theory account of sole practice. *International Journal of Mental Health Nursing, 12,* 243–250.

Gibb, H., Livesey, L., & Zyla, W. (2003). At 3 am who the hell do you call? Case management issues in sole practice as a rural community mental health nurse. *Australasian Psychiatry, 11,* suppl., S127–130.

Gulzar, L. (1999). Access to health care. *Journal of Nursing Scholarship, 31,* 13–19.

Hanson, P. G. (2004). Canadian perspectives: Aboriginal perspectives in rural health promotion practice. In J. M. Wiegmann, Health promotion of families in rural settings (pp. 593–594). In P. J. Bomar (Ed.), *Promoting health in families,* chap. 20, pp. 581–604. Philadelphia: Elsevier.

Hartley, D. (2005). Rural health research: Building capacity and influencing policy in the United States and Canada. *Canadian Journal of Nursing Research, 37*(1), 7–13.

Hegney, D. (1997). Rural nursing practice. In L. Siegloff (Ed.), *Rural nursing in the Australian context* (pp. 25–43). Deacon Act, Australia: Royal College of Nursing.

Henson, D., Sadler, T., & Walton, S. (1998). Distance. In H. J. Lee (Ed.), *Conceptual basis for rural nursing* (pp. 51–60). New York: Springer.

Jirojwong, S., & MacLennan, R. (2002). Management of episodes of incapacity by families in rural and remote Queensland. *Australian Journal of Rural Health, 10,* 249–255.

Johnson, J. L., Ratner, P. A., & Bottorff, J. L. (1995). Urban-rural differences in the health-promoting behaviors of Albertans. *Canadian Journal of Public Health, 86,* 103–108.

Jones, S., & Ross, J. (2003). Describing your scope of practice: A resource for rural nurses. Christchurch, NZ: Centre for Rural Health. Retrieved February 6, 2008, from http://www.moh.govt.nz

Kelly, S. E. (2003). Bioethics and rural health: Theorizing place, space, and subjects. *Social Science & Medicine, 56,* 2277–2288.

Lau, T., Kumar, S., & Thomas, D. (2002). Practicing psychiatry in New Zealand's rural areas: Incentives, problems and solutions. *Australian Psychiatry, 10* (1), 33–38.

Lauder, W., Reel, S., Farmer, J., & Griggs, H. (2006). Social capital, rural nursing and rural nursing theory. *Nursing Inquiry, 13* (1), 73–79.

Lee, H. J., Hollis, B. R., & McClain, K. A. (1998). Isolation. In H. J. Lee (Ed.), *Conceptual basis for rural nursing* (pp. 61–75). New York: Springer.

Lee, H. J., & McDonagh, M. K. (2006). Further development of the rural nursing theory base. In H. J. Lee & C. A. Winters (Eds.), *Rural nursing: Concepts, theory, & practice* (2nd ed., pp. 313–321). New York: Springer.

Lee, H. J., & Winters, C. A. (2004). Testing rural nursing theory: Perceptions and needs of service providers. *Online Journal of Rural Nursing and Health Care, 4* (1). Retrieved September 16, 2004, from http://www.rno.org

Long, K. A. (1993). The concept of health: Rural perspectives. *Nursing Clinics of North America, 28,* 123–130.

Long, K. A., & Weinert, C. (1989). Rural nursing: Developing the theory base. *Scholarly Inquiry for Nursing Practice: An International Journal, 3,* 113–127.

MacKinnon, K. A. (2008). Labouring to Nurse: The work of rural nurses who provide maternity care. *Rural and Remove Health Care, 8,* 1–15. Retrieved January 20, 2008, from http://www.rrh.org.au

MacLeod, M. L. P., Browne, A. J., & Leipert, B. (1998). International perspective: Issues for nurses in rural and remote Canada. *Australian Journal of Rural Health, 6,* 72–78.

MacLeod, M. L. P., Misener, R., Banks, K., Morton, A. M., Vogt, C., & Bentham, D. (2008). 'I'm a different kind of nurse': Advice from nurses in rural and remote Canada. *Canadian Journal of Nursing Leadership, 21* (3), 40–53.

McConigley, R., Kristjanson, L., & Morgan, A. (2000). Palliative care nursing in rural Western Australia. *International Journal of Palliative Nursing, 6*(2), 80–90.

Niemoller, J. K., Ide, B. A., & Nichols, E. G. (2000). Issues in studying health-related hardiness and use of services among older rural adults. *Texas Journal of Rural Health, 18,* 35–43.

Moran, C. A. (2005). *Replication study of rural nursing theory: A Missouri perspective.* Unpublished thesis, Central Missouri State University.

Morse, M. J. (1995) Exploring the theoretical basis of nursing using advanced techniques of concept analysis. *Advances in Nursing Science, 17* (3), 31–46.

Peterson, S. J., & Bredow, T. S. (2004). *Middle range theories: Application to nursing research.* Philadelphia: Lippincott Williams & Wilkins.

Pierce, C. (2001). The impact of culture of rural women's descriptions of health. *The Journal of Multicultural Nursing and Health, 7,* 50–53, 56.

Poland, B., Lehoux, P., Holmes, D., & Andrews, G. (2005). How place matters: Unpacking technology and power in health and social care. *Health & Social Care in the Community, 13,* 170–180.

Racher, F. E., & Vollman, A. R. (2002). Exploring the dimensions of access to health services: Implications for nursing research and practice. *Research and Theory for Nursing Practice: An International Journal, 16,* 77–90.

Roberto, K. A., & Reynolds, S. G. (2001). The meaning of osteoporosis in the lives of rural women. *Health Care for Women International, 22,* 599–611.

Rodgers, B. L. (1993). Concept analysis: An evolutionary view. In B. L. Rodgers & K. A. Knafl (Eds.), *Concept development in nursing: Foundations, techniques and applications,* pp. 73–92. Philadelphia: Saunders.

Rosenthal, K. A. (1996). *Rural nursing: An exploratory narrative description.* Unpublished Dissertation, University of Colorado, Denver.

Shookner, M., Scott, C. M., & Vollman, A. R. (2008). Creating supportive environments for health: Social network analysis. In A. R. Vollman, E. T. Anderson, & J. McFarlane (Eds.), *Canadian community as partner: Theory & multidisciplinary practice* (2nd ed.). Philadelphia: Lippincott Williams & Wilkins.

Scharff, J. (1998). The distinctive nature and scope of rural nursing practice: Philosophical bases. In H. J. Lee (Ed.), *Conceptual basis for rural nursing,* pp. 19–38. New York: Springer.

Sellers, S. C., Poduska, M. D., Propp, L. H., & White, S. E. (1999). The health care meanings, values, and practices of Anglo-American males in the rural midwest. *Journal of Transcultural Nursing, 10,* 320–330.

Shannon, A. (1982). Introduction: Nursing in sparsely populated areas. In J. Taylor, Sparsely populated areas: Toward nursing theory. *Western Journal of Nursing Research, 4* (3) suppl., 70–71.

Smith, M. J., & Liehr, P. R. (Eds.) (2003). *Middle range theory for nursing.* New York: Springer.

Taylor, J. (1982). Sparsely populated areas: Toward nursing theory. *Western Journal of Nursing Research, 4*(3) suppl., 69–77.

Thomlinson, E., McDonagh, M. K., Reimer, M., Crooks, K., & Lees, M. (2004). Health beliefs of rural Canadians: Implications for practice. *Australian Journal of Rural Health, 12,* 258–263.

Thurston, W. E., & Meadows, L. M. (2003). Rurality and health: Perspectives of mid-life women. *Rural and Remote Health, 3* (219), 1–12. Retrieved November 6, 2003, from http://rrh.deakin.edu.au

Thurston, W. E., & Meadows, L. M. (2004). Embodied minds, restless spirits: Mid-life rural women speak of their health. *Women's Health, 34,* 97–112.

Walker, L., & Avant, K. (1995) *Strategies for theory construction in nursing* (3rd ed.). Norwalk, CT: Appleton-Century-Crofts.

Wathen, C. N., & Harris, R. M. (2006). An examination of the health information seeking experiences of women in rural Ontario, Canada. *Information Research, 11*(4). Retrieved October 26, 2008, from http://information.net/ir/11-4/paper267.html

Wathen, C. N., & Harris, R. M. (2007). 'I try to take care of it myself.' How rural women search for health information. *Qualitative Health Research, 17*(5), 639–651.

Winters, C. A., Cudney, S. A., Sullivan, T., & Thuesen, A. (2006a). The rural context and women's self-management of chronic health conditions. *Chronic Illness, 2,* 273–289.

Winters, C.A., Thomlinson, O'Lynn, C., Lee, H.J., McDonagh, M.K., Edge, D.S., et al. (2006b). Exploring rural nursing theory across borders. In H. J. Lee & C. A. Winters (Eds.), *Rural nursing: Concepts, theory and practice* (2nd ed., pp. 27–39). New York: Springer.

Exploring Rural Nursing Theory Across Borders

3

CHARLENE A. WINTERS, ELIZABETH H. THOMLINSON,
CHAD O'LYNN, HELEN J. LEE, MEG K. McDONAGH,
DANA S. EDGE, and MARLENE A. REIMER

The descriptive rural nursing theory first published by Long and Weinert in 1989, and republished in 1999, is widely accepted and frequently quoted in presentations and articles. However, little testing of the theory has taken place. Recently, the authors, nurse scientists from the United States and Canada, joined forces to validate the rural theory concepts. Lee and Winters (2004) conducted a qualitative study to explore rural persons' health perceptions and needs in the state of Montana, and Thomlinson, McDonagh, Reimer, Crooks, and Lees (2002) did the same in the Canadian provinces of Alberta and Manitoba. Then we compared the findings from these two studies. Our specific aims in the comparison were to (1) validate existing rural nursing theory concepts, (2) identify new emerging concepts, and (3) determine areas for further theoretical development and research.

BACKGROUND AND SIGNIFICANCE

Rural nursing is the provision of health care by professional nurses to persons living in sparsely populated areas (Long & Weinert, 1989). Rural nursing theory evolved because of a recognized need for a framework for practice that considers the special needs of this population. The

41

theory-building process began in the late 1970s with the collection of qualitative and quantitative data by Montana State University–Bozeman College of Nursing graduate students and faculty. A rich database resulted in the identification of several key concepts and the development of three theoretical statements related to understanding rural health needs and rural nursing practice. The first statement was that "rural dwellers define health primarily as the ability to work, to be productive, to do usual tasks" (Long & Weinert, 1989, p. 120). Two closely interrelated concepts associated with this statement pertain to work beliefs and health beliefs. Health is defined in relation to work, and health needs are secondary to work needs.

The second theoretical statement was that "rural dwellers are self-reliant and resist accepting help or services from those seen as 'outsiders' or from agencies seen as national or regional 'welfare' programs" (Long & Weinert, 1989, p. 120). Closely associated to this statement is the tendency of rural dwellers to rely on informal social networks for health care. Key concepts pertaining to this statement are self-reliance, outsider, insider, old-timer, and newcomer. Rural dwellers tend to engage in self-care and prefer the familiarity of the people and professionals who know them in contrast with the newcomer, or specialist, who is unfamiliar. Other concepts identified as important in understanding the health care-seeking behavior of rural residents are distance, isolation, and lack of anonymity, which are descriptive of the rural context in which these people live and work. The qualitative data from Montana, upon which the theoretical work was based, indicated that rural residents accepted distance as a normal part of living in a rural area. The degree of distance involved, whether actual or perceived, led some rural dwellers to experience a sense of isolation. Lastly, a lack of anonymity implies a limited ability for rural persons to have private areas in their lives, a phenomenon common to small towns and sparsely populated areas.

The third theoretical statement was that health care providers in rural areas "must deal with a lack of anonymity and much greater role diffusion than providers in urban or suburban settings" (Long & Weinert, 1989, p. 120). In a small community, everyone knows who the nurse is and this knowledge affects the nurse's effectiveness as a health care professional in that community. Furthermore, nurses are expected to function as expert generalists. For example, on a given day, a nurse working the day shift in a rural hospital may care for a laboring woman, recover an older man following surgery, triage in the emergency room, and prepare a pediatric trauma patient for transport to a regional medical center.

When the theory-building process began, literature and research related to rural health care were limited and focused primarily on rural health care delivery and access to service issues (Long & Weinert, 1989). A theoretical base for guiding rural health care did not exist. This prompted the faculty and students of Montana State University–Bozeman College of Nursing to begin the development of a theory base for rural nursing practice. Although rural nursing theory concepts are now widely accepted, a limited number of researchers have reported their efforts to test these initial findings. Our recent search of the literature resulted in only two citations for work that specifically focused on rural nursing theory (Nichols, 1989, 1999). Both were response articles to Long and Weinert's theory-based article. Much of the published rural literature and research continues to focus on issues related to health care delivery and access. Given the paucity of research, we designed a study to test the rural nursing concepts described nearly 30 years ago.

METHODS AND PROCEDURES

The Montana study and the Canadian study were similar in design and purpose but (Lee & Winters, 2004; Thomlinson, McDonagh, Reimer, Crooks, & Lees, 2002) planned and carried out separately. In both studies, we used an ethnographic approach (Miles & Huberman, 1994; Morse & Field, 1995; Rossman & Rallis, 2003). In an ethnographic study, researchers describe and interpret phenomenon of interest in a cultural or social group or system (Creswell, 1998). Consistent with this approach, we collected data through open-ended interviews of rural persons and observational field notes (Rossman & Rallis) that documented our insights, interactions with participants, and the physical and cultural context of the communities in which the participants lived. Through these activities, Lee and Winters and Thomlinson and her colleagues were able to identify the perceptions of the rural persons and learn what they understood about their health and how they managed their day-to-day health care situations. Using this open-ended approach, we found that themes emerged from the interview narratives (Miles & Huberman), allowing us to make comparisons with the concepts and statements contained in the rural nursing theory proposed by Long and Weinert (1989).

Montana Study

Montana is the fourth largest state in the United States covering 147,042 square miles and stretching 641 miles from east to west. The state is sparsely populated with a density of 6.2 persons per square mile *(Census 2000 Data for the State of Montana, n.d.)*. According to the 2000 Census, 90.6% of the state's residents are Caucasian; the principal minority population of 6.2% is Native American. Farming, fishing, and forestry occupations occupy 2.2% of the population, whereas 42.4% of the population is employed in service, sales, and office occupations *(Census 2000 Data for the State of Montana)*. The Rocky Mountains run north and south through the western part of the state, whereas eastern Montana is characterized by its rolling plains.

Lee and Winters (2004) conducted the Montana study according to the guidelines set forth by the Montana State University–Bozeman Human Subject Committee. They recruited participants through word of mouth (snowball sampling). Each participant signed a consent form that emphasized that only aggregate data would be reported. Lee and Winters maintained confidentiality of participants by removing names and identifiers. All participants were older than 18 years of age, employed in service occupations, and had lived in their respective communities for at least 5 years (see Table 3.1).

Table 3.1

DEMOGRAPHICS		
	MONTANA SAMPLE	**CANADIAN SAMPLE**
Men	14	13
Women	24	42
Ethnicity		
Caucasian	35	52
Native American	3	
Aboriginal		3
Age range, years	22–85 (m = 49)	18–84*
Education	7–18 (m = 13)	8–16*
Marital status		
Married	26	37
Divorced	5	5
Single	7	9
		(5 widow/widower)
Unknown		4

*Means not available.

Table 3.1

DEMOGRAPHICS (continued)		
	MONTANA SAMPLE	**CANADIAN SAMPLE**
Occupation		
Grocery store clerks	4	
Secretaries	3	
Hospital workers	3	
Restaurant workers	3	
Beauty shop workers	2	
Animal care workers	2	
Museum operators	2	
County employees	2	
Window treatment	2	
Post office workers	2	
Retirees		9
Ranchers		7
Education		19
Health care		3
Accountant		1
Bookkeeper		1
Other	13	15
Time in rural community, years	5–84 ($m = 34$)	3+*
Size of community, persons	70–1,728	50–5,000
County density, persons per square mile	0.8–29.8	Not calculated
Distance to nearest large town, miles	12–250 ($m = 60$)	Not asked
Distance to nearest emergency care, miles	0.1–110 ($m = 30$)	3–90*
Self-reported health status		
Excellent	5	Not asked
Very good	3	
Good	17	
Fair	8	
Poor	1	
Did not respond	4	
Health insurance		
Yes	29	All have health care insurance
No	8	
No response	1	

*Means not available.

Graduate nursing students enrolled in a rural nursing course conducted 38 interviews in the fall semesters of 2000 and 2001 with individuals living in rural towns with populations of 1,500 persons or less. Using open-ended questions, they asked participants about their perceptions of health and how they responded to illness and injury. Interviews lasted 30–60 minutes and were audio taped. Once transcribed, the students analyzed the interview narratives for themes. Students recorded observational field notes to document their activities, interactions, and insights. They wrote individual papers addressing the themes emerging from their interviews and field observations. Working separately, Lee and Winters (2004) coded the transcripts and field notes identifying common themes. They then met to compare their findings with those identified by the students. They continually compared data supporting the emerging themes until they arrived at a consensus on the findings. Four major themes emerged from the analysis: (a) definition of health, (b) distance and access to resources, (c) symptom–action–time-line process (SATL), and (d) choice (see Table 3.2).

Canadian Study

The provinces of Alberta and Manitoba are approximately equal in size, with each province covering 250,000 square miles or roughly one and three-quarters the size of the state of Montana. The geography of Alberta closely parallels Montana, with rolling prairie and the Rocky Mountains

Table 3.2

COMMON THEMES AND SUBTHEMES

THEME	SUBTHEME
Definitions of Health	a. Sickness b. Illness
Health-Seeking Behaviors	a. Symptom–Action–Time-Line (SATL) b. Resources c. Self-reliance
Choices	a. Residence b. Health care provider
Distance	a. Rural b. Northern

bordering the western edge of the province. The terrain in Manitoba varies from flat farmland in the south to the Cambrian Shield, an area of granite rock with thin soil, in the north. In the north are large tracts of land covered with muskeg and forest. A major geographic difference between the two provinces is that 17% of Manitoba is covered with water compared with 3% of Alberta *(Statistics Canada,* 2004). The geographic diversity was a major reason for selecting these two distinct sites for the study.

In Alberta the industries of farming, logging, ranching, and oil production employ 7% of the population, with sales, service, business, and finance employing 41% of Albertans. Similarly, in Manitoba farming, logging, mining, and fishing employ 7% of the population, whereas sales, service, business, and finance employ 41.6% of Manitobans (*Statistics Canada*, 2004).

Following ethical approval by the Conjoint Health Research Ethics Board at the University of Calgary, Thomlinson et al. (2002) sought participants through newspaper advertisements and through word of mouth from other participants. In the first stage of the study, they selected 29 participants from municipal districts and small towns within 300 kilometers of Calgary. In the second stage, they sought 26 participants living in central and northern Manitoba for interviews (see Table 3.1). As with the Montana study, all participants were over 18 years of age and signed consent forms that emphasized that only aggregate data would be reported. The confidentiality of participants was maintained through the removal of names and identifiers. Thomlinson and colleagues and nursing student research assistants conducted face-to-face, semistructured interviews lasting 45–60 minutes. Participants selected the locations for interviews, which were usually held in their homes.

Initially, four researchers (E. Thomlinson, M. McDonagh, K. Crooks, and M. Lees) coded five interview transcripts separately, then compared findings. Two of the researchers (E. Thomlinson and M. McDonagh) completed the analysis of the remainder of the transcripts. The major themes that emerged from the transcripts included definitions of health, health-seeking behaviors, resources that were accessed, and definitions of rural and northern.

DATA ANALYSIS

In June 2003, the authors met at the University of Calgary, Alberta. We developed agreements regarding steps in the process of data comparison, responsibilities of team membership, dissemination of findings, and authorship. Subsequent meetings were conducted via teleconference.

We began the process by viewing and comparing the demographic characteristics of the two samples. We compared the concepts, themes, salient characteristics, and relevant qualitative data excerpts from both studies and then displayed them using a concept-ordered matrix (Miles & Huberman, 1994). Concepts and themes having the same or very similar defining attributes were collapsed into a common theme. We further evaluated concepts and themes for differences in sample and methods and then added them to the matrix, resulting in a combined dataset. We then compared findings with rural nursing theory concepts and theoretical statements. In this manner, we maintained methodological rigor of consistency, neutrality, truth-value, and applicability (Morse & Field, 1995).

FINDINGS

After much analysis and discussion, we identified by consensus four common themes and nine subthemes (see Table 3.2 page 46) and summarized them below.

Common Themes

Definition of Health

We identified the theme *definition of health* in both studies. In the Montana study, health was described primarily as the absence of conditions that would interrupt work or play and included physical, mental, and emotional fitness. In the Canadian study, the definition of health was similar but included the importance of spiritual and environmental considerations. Participants from both studies spoke of health as a concept that was to some degree related to age and the absence of chronic illness with comments such as, "I'm healthy for my age." Following further examination of the transcripts and discussion, we agreed upon the common theme definition of health as a holistic perspective in which optimal ability to function at work or play and to pursue desired activities is maintained. Optimal ability is obtained through health-seeking and health-promoting behaviors to achieve holistic balance, resolution of short-term disruptions, and adaptation to long-term health challenges.

In addition, Canadian participants differentiated between *sickness* and *illness,* noting that sickness is short in duration and is curable; whereas illness is either chronic in nature or serious and life threatening. We then determined that sickness and illness were subthemes of definition of health.

Health-Seeking Behaviors

The theme *Symptom–Action–Time-Line* emerged from the Montana data and was used to describe the social process of identifying symptoms and seeking self, lay, or professional health care for illness and injuries (Buehler, Malone, & Majerus, 1998). SATL was similar to the theme health-seeking behaviors, which emerged from the Canadian data. We discussed the similarities and differences between these two themes noting that SATL focused on obtaining health resources once a health disruption is noted. Furthermore, the theme health-seeking behaviors incorporated SATL as well as behaviors designed to promote health and prevent health disruptions. We determined that health-seeking behaviors was a common theme and SATL was a subtheme of health-seeking behaviors. Health-seeking behaviors is defined as conscious behaviors designed to promote healthy relationships among physical, mental, social, and spiritual aspects of one's life so that life balance is maintained.

Resources

A theme identified in the Canadian data and defined as people and other sources of information and assistance one uses in health-seeking behaviors was named *resources.* Examples of resources that were provided by Canadian participants included community elders, trusted traditional healers, libraries, the Internet, and health care professionals who really listen. The Montana researchers also noted resources as a component of SATL. As a result, we determined resources to be an additional subtheme of health-seeking behaviors.

Self-Reliance

In reviewing the data, we noted a number of excerpts that described the self-reliance of rural dwellers. Participants engaged in self-care when managing illness and injury and when needed, chose to seek care first from friends and family members prior to seeing a health care professional. Participants commented that they kept their "medicine cabinets stocked," and when injured they would pull the edges of the wound together if only a "couple of inches long." They would see a health care provider for injuries they did not think they "could put a Band-Aid on" or handle themselves. Because of its prevalence in the data and the context in which the term appeared, we determined that *self-reliance* was a subtheme under health-seeking behaviors.

Choices

The conscious life choices one makes in terms of residence and accessing health services was a theme we identified as *choices*. The theme emerged from the Montana data based on participants' comments regarding their choice to live in rural areas and their decision-making processes regarding when and which health resources they access when ill or injured. Generally, participants expressed satisfaction with living in rural areas and commented on the benefits of rural living. The Canadian researchers did not initially identify choices as a theme. However, they did find that the participants exhibited a "taking charge" attitude, which we believed to be equated with making choices. And because the Canadian participants made comments similar to Montana participants regarding the benefits of rural living and how living in sparsely populated areas shaped their health care decision-making, we reached a consensus in identifying choices as a theme.

Distance

Thomlinson, McDonagh, Reimer, Crooks, and Lees (2002) classified participants in their study as either rural or northern, and asked the participants to describe what these terms meant to them. They noted that the Canadian government has six definitions of rural and defines northern as the region north of a north-and-south line determined by 16 combined social, biotic, economic, and climatic aspects of geography (McNiven, 1999). Distance was the factor that differentiated rural from northern for Canadian participants, in that northern residents are more isolated and distances to all services, not just health services, are much farther than those for rural residents. Distance was also described by the Montana participants, with comments focusing on distance to services, lack of service availability, and travel times to services. Thus, we determined that *distance* was a theme and *rural* and *northern* were subthemes of distance. Distance was defined as separation (space, time, and behavior) between the rural population and health care resources.

DISCUSSION

The definition of health we identified in this study, although more holistic than the original definition, continues to support the interrelatedness of work and health and provides partial support for the first theoretical statement identified by Long and Weinert (1989). Furthermore, the new definition of health adds to the original definition by including "ability to play," identifying the importance of mental and emotional fitness, and including the notion that health is qualified by age and the presence of illness. In addition, we determined health-seeking and health-promoting behaviors to be foundational to the maintenance of health.

Although variations existed within groups, health-seeking behaviors were demonstrated by participants from both countries. Therefore, we identified *health-seeking behaviors* as a common theme and described the processes participants used to promote healthy relationships among physical, mental, social, and spiritual aspects of their lives. Underlying the overall theme of health-seeking behavior were three subthemes: (a) SATL, (b) resources, and (c) self-reliance.

The acronym SATL described previously by Buehler, Malone, and Majerus-Wegerhoff (1998) is the social process of identifying symptoms and seeking self, lay, or professional health care for illness and injuries. With this process, participants choose the resources that they believe will be effective in promoting their health status or managing their health concern. We defined *resources* as people, other sources of information, and assistance one uses in health-seeking behaviors.

Self-reliance is described by Chafey, Sullivan, and Shannon (1998) as behaviors of accomplishing tasks without the help of others, stemming from values (such as autonomy) or contextual variables (such as barriers to resource access). Accordingly, we identified *self-reliance* in this collaborative study. Findings indicate that participants preferred to engage in self-care for illness and injuries and sought assistance from informal resources prior to seeking the services of health care professionals. The findings support the second theoretical statement (Long & Weinert, 1989), and the addition of three subthemes to *health-seeking behaviors* contributes to the expansion of the rural nursing theory base.

The theme *choices* refers to the participants' conscious decision-making processes regarding their places of residence and patterns of accessing health services. During data analysis, we realized that participants were constantly making choices, and these decisions affected their lifestyle, their personal health and health practices and that of their

families, and their livelihood. Examples of such choices include decisions regarding when, where, and from whom to seek care for an injury,
where they should reside (stay on the farm or move into town), and what
kind of foods they should be eating to maintain health and yet stay within
their allotted budget. Long and Weinert (1989) did not previously identify choices as part of rural nursing theory.

   Distance was an important concept that Long and Weinert (1989)
identified in their original descriptive theory, and we also found it important in the comparison study. We defined it as separation (space, time,
and behavior) between the rural population and health care resources,
and then further broke it down on the basis of the degree of remoteness recognizing that distances to *all* services, not just health services,
are much greater for isolated rural residents. Expanding the concept
of distance to include definitions of rural and northern is one way that
degrees of remoteness can be used to extend rural nursing theory. The
identification and explication of the themes *definition of health, health-
seeking behaviors, choices*, and *distance* have implications for furthering
health care providers' understanding of the health care-seeking behaviors, practices, and preferred resources of rural dwellers.

Implications for Rural Nursing Theory and Practice

The findings of this comparison study validate and expand upon existing rural nursing theory concepts and provide partial support for the
first and second theoretical statements identified by Long and Weinert
(1989). As the focus of this study was on the health perceptions and
needs of rural persons, it is beyond the scope of this project to address
the rural nursing theory concepts germane to the third theoretical statement regarding the role of rural health care providers.

   Through the expansion of the previous understanding of health, educators and practitioners are provided the opportunity to view their specific rural population's health needs in a broader context. The data also
reveal that a variety of health-seeking and health-promoting behaviors is
important to rural dwellers. The information gained from this study about
SATL, choices, and distance has significant implications for further rural
nursing theory development and practice. By increasing the amount of
information gathered and the breadth of the rural population sampled,
the theory base solidifies its applicability to rural nurses and thus has the
potential to positively affect the health care delivery to rural dwellers
in North America. Understanding the health care decision-making pro-

cesses used by rural dwellers will assist nurses to provide care appropriate to their clients' needs and rural lifestyle.

Although distance is not a new concept in the rural nursing theory base, our understanding of distance and what it means to specific rural groups has been expanded in this study. The data support the notion that distance is not constant; it is variable among specific populations and their contexts. This has implications for how the context of rural dwellers is understood by rural nurses and has the potential to affect future programs for health education and health-program delivery.

Although each of the four themes and nine subthemes require further examination, the aforementioned findings suggest that major tenets of rural nursing theory can be applied across the western United States–Canadian border. This finding provides contextual information important to the further development of rural nursing theory. Additional research that compares and contrasts the health perceptions and needs of persons living in differing rural environments is necessary to further build upon the theory base. In addition, replication of this study is needed internationally as well as in other North American rural and remote areas to provide the necessary rigor and applicability of rural nursing theory. Finally, studies are needed that address the third theoretical statement, which focuses on the issues facing nurses practicing in rural and remote areas. A more solid base for rural nursing theory is required to guide the delivery of nursing care to rural and remote populations.

ACKNOWLEDGMENTS

This research was funded by Montana State University–Bozeman College of Nursing Block Grant; Sigma Theta Tau International, Zeta Upsilon Chapter; and Visiting Scholar, University of Calgary, Alberta, Canada.

REFERENCES

Buehler, J., Malone, M., & Majerus, J. (1998). Patterns of response to symptoms in rural residents: The symptom-action-time-line process. In H. J. Lee (Ed.), *Conceptual basis for rural nursing* (pp. 318–328). New York: Springer.

Census 2000 data for the state of Montana. (n.d.). Retrieved December 15, 2002, from http://www.census.gov/census2000/states/mt.html

Chafey, K., Sullivan, T., & Shannon, A. (1998). Self-reliance: Characterization of their own autonomy by elderly rural women. In H. J. Lee (Ed.), *Conceptual basis for rural nursing* (pp. 156–177). New York: Springer.

Creswell, J. (1998). *Qualitative inquiry and research design: Choosing among five traditions*. Thousand Oaks, CA: Sage.

Lee, H. J., & Winters, C.A. (2004). Testing rural nursing theory: Perceptions and needs of service providers. *Online Journal of Rural Nursing and Health Care, 4*. Retrieved July 5, 2004, from http://www.rno.org/journal/issues/Vol-4/issue-1/Lee_article.htm

Long, K. A., & Weinert, C. (1989). Rural nursing: Developing the theory base. *Scholarly Inquiry for Nursing Practice, 3* (2), 113–127.

Long, K. A., & Weinert, C. (1999). Rural nursing: Developing the theory base. 1989. *Scholarly Inquiry for Nursing Practice, 13* (3), 257–269.

McNiven, C. (1999). North is that direction. Canadian Social Trends, pp. 8–11. *Statistics Canada—Catalogue No. 11–008*. Retrieved July 23, 2004, from http://estat.statcan.ca/content/english/articles/pop-a.shtml

Miles, M. B., & Huberman, A. M. (1994). *Qualitative data analysis* (2nd ed.).Thousand Oaks, CA: Sage.

Morse, J. M., & Field, P. A. (1995). *Qualitative research methods for health professions* (2nd ed.). Thousand Oaks, CA: Sage.

Nichols, E. (1989). Response to 'Rural nursing: Developing the theory base.' *Scholarly Inquiry for Nursing Practice, 3,* 129–132.

Nichols, E. (1999). Response to 'Rural nursing: Developing the theory base.' 1989. *Scholarly Inquiry for Nursing Practice, 13,* 271–274.

Rossman, G. B., & Rallis, S. F. (2003). *Learning in the field* (2nd ed.). Thousand Oaks, CA: Sage.

Statistics Canada. (2004). Retrieved May 27, 2004, from http://www.statcan.ca/start.html

Thomlinson, E., McDonagh, M. K., Reimer, M., Crooks, K., & Lees, M. (2002). Health beliefs of rural Canadians: Implications for practice [Abstract]. *Charting the course for rural health in the 21st century, 18*.

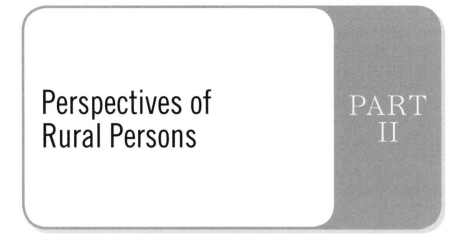

Perspectives of Rural Persons

PART II

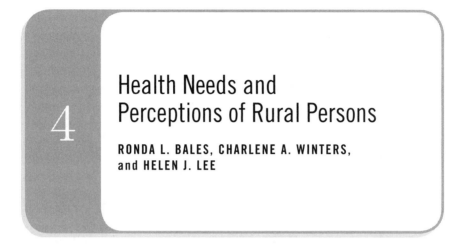

4

Health Needs and Perceptions of Rural Persons

**RONDA L. BALES, CHARLENE A. WINTERS,
and HELEN J. LEE**

Health practices of rural dwellers are known to be influenced by their perceptions of health and illness. Long and Weinert (1998) remarked on the individuality of health perceptions among rural dwellers and noted that those assumptions regarding concepts of health cannot be generalized among rural populations. Understanding the health perceptions, needs, and behaviors of an individual, family, or community can be instrumental in health promotion planning. This chapter addresses the health needs, perceptions, and behaviors of six individuals living in one community in rural Montana.

INTRODUCTION TO THE COMMUNITY

With an elevation of 7,651 feet above sea level, the echoed phrase "closer to heaven than I may ever get" is a vivid reference to the vast and beautiful wilderness known as Montana City.[1] The community is nestled in the midst of mountain peaks and lies just east of the northeast entrance to a national park (Glidden, 1982). The location of Montana City is one of its unique attributes with access to and from the community varying from summer to winter. Although travel in and out of Montana City during the summer may be slow because of the winding mountain roads, it is not limited. The winter months, however, bring additional challenges beyond distance to the members of this community that other rural Montanans may not face. When the snow begins to fly in October, residents are faced with isolation in terms of travel outside their community. From October to May, when the snow typically melts, the only passable route by automobile is 55 miles on a narrow, winding highway through a national park with an additional 55 miles to expanded health care services (*National Geographic Road Atlas*, 2000). Passage via this route is dependent on snowplows to keep the roads passable. An alternative route out of Montana City is available. This route allows for travel to towns and cities in Montana and a neighboring state, about 100 and 120 miles, respectively (Glidden; *National Geographic Road Atlas*). There is a catch, however; this route includes a stretch of road over a pass approximately 10 miles long that is left unplowed during the winter (Fahlberg, 1983). Therefore, access to and from Montana City via this route during the winter months is limited to those with snowmobiles. Thus, one can visualize that winter brings challenges to these rural dwellers that affect access not only to health care but also to all dimensions of life outside the community.

METHODS

Ronda L. Bales: My purpose in this study was to explore the health needs and perceptions of rural persons living in Montana City, Montana. I chose descriptive qualitative research methods for this research project because they provide an opportunity "to try to understand how people make sense of their worlds" (Rossman & Rallis, 1998, p. 8). In this case, it allowed me an opportunity to understand how, when, where, and why the residents of Montana City seek health care and the factors that influence health care behaviors, access, and usage.

After obtaining informed consent, I conducted semistructured interviews with members of the community. Initially, I identified participants through a key informant who owned a cabin located within the community. I approached the remaining participants directly and asked about their interest in participation in the study.

Sample

The convenience sample consisted of five women and one man, aged 37–76 years. The participants had lived in the community 3–30 years.

Montana City met the definition of remote rural described by Koehler (1998): "a community with a population of 2,500 or less located forty miles or further from a city with a population of 50,000 or greater. Remote rural communities do not have a hospital or medical assistance facility" (pp. 238–239).

Data Collection and Analysis

I collected data by using a semi-structured interview guide. Questions were open-ended and intended to elicit information regarding the individuals' health perceptions and needs. Interviews were audio taped and transcribed. Field notes were kept to document observations and impressions about the community and persons interviewed. I analyzed the transcribed interviews and field notes for emergent themes.

FINDINGS

Montana City

The population of this community varies drastically in accordance with the change of seasons. The participants of the study estimated the year-round population to be 70–100 persons and stated that it tripled during the summer. All participants identified themselves as "year-round" residents of the community.

I identified two main groups within the sample: (a) those who had lived in the community for a number of years, and (b) those who had recently moved there. A comparison was provided by one participant who gave a description of the long-time members of the community.

> If you live here long enough, you can tell who lives here by how they dress, the snowmobiles they drive, the clothes they wear are patched up with duck tape. They have the old style stuff, but then maybe that's a sign of the culture too. I just think that some of that goes with it, that you choose to live that way because you want to. It is not important, material things are not important here. I am really speaking generally cause there are people moving in who have a lot more money to spend and they have the nicer homes. So you see, we are seeing a change in our culture here.

Health Care

Health care resources within the community of Montana City were limited. There was no clinic, hospital, or other formal health care. However, Emergency Medical Services (EMS) was available. The EMS network was composed of volunteers from the community who were mainly trained at the First Responder level and one member who was prepared to practice at the Emergency Medical Technician (EMT) level at the time I conducted the interviews. There was a dedicated ambulance for the national park located at the entrance and the park ranger stationed there was an EMT. The EMS process was explained by a participant.

> If someone calls 911, they call me or someone on the roster. Then I go and appraise the situation and call for the ambulance if it is needed. See, we do have an ambulance available, but it is at the gate [to the national park]. But the park administration doesn't think the community should rely solely on the Park for its EMS services. So that is why they call someone on the list first, and then if we need it, we call for the ambulance.

The park ambulance is equipped for advanced life support and can travel to a clinic located in Maryville, approximately 55 miles through the national park. If transport to a hospital was necessary, a second ambulance from Littlewood had to meet the park ambulance and transport the patient. Medical flight services are typically not available to the community because the location presents a dangerous situation for helicopters.

All participants interviewed identified a retired doctor who lived in the community as a health care resource. Participants indicated they had accessed him at one time or another and that he helped them make judgments about whether or not it was necessary to obtain further or immediate care for a health-related issue. The identified retired physician had lived in Montana City for 5 years at the time I conducted the study. I contacted and interviewed this individual, not as a participant of the study, but rather to gain insight into the health care needs of the community in general. The retired physician indicated that he was available for emergencies and did what he could "on the spot," but that he did not encourage members of the community to use him as their regular health care provider. He also stated that he made the decisions about what he would treat and how far he would go in treating patients before sending them to a medical facility because he had very limited resources and equipment available to him in Montana City. He commented that he had very little besides his "five senses" with which to provide care.

Health Status

Two participants described themselves as having major medical illnesses. Several other participants made reference to the fact that there were a number of people in the community who had suffered major illnesses. According to the retired physician, the illnesses suffered by members of the community included heart failure, stroke, cancer, leukemia, pulmonary hypertension, and pheochromocytoma. Furthermore, he had the impression that the incidence of serious illness in the community was higher in comparison with other communities of similar size. Several interviewed participants also indicated that there appeared to be a high rate of smoking and alcohol consumption within the community. As one participant stated,

> There is a high rate of alcohol consumption and drugs too here, even for a small community. And that is a big factor in health issues here. And smoking, that is another issue, everybody smokes. I am sure for the percentage of smokers in a community we are way off the top end.

Data such as average income, poverty rates, and unemployment percentages were not available for Montana City. Therefore, I could not draw any conclusions about these data for the community.

Themes

Six major themes emerged from the analysis of the data. They included *self-reliance, hardiness, conscientious consumer, informed risk, community support,* and *inadequate insurance.* Two themes (*self-reliance* and *hardiness*) were reported previously in rural nursing literature (Chafey, Sullivan, & Shannon, 1998; Wirtz, Lee, & Running, 1998). Four themes (conscientious consumer, informed risk, community support, and inadequate insurance) were new.

Self-Reliance

Self-reliance has been defined as "the capacity to provide for one's own need" (Agich, 1993, as cited in Chafey et al., 1998). Each participant expressed that they take care of themselves first. However, varying degrees of self-reliance were described. Two participants, a married couple who moved into the community to retire, expressed self-reliance but also stated they probably accessed formal health care more quickly than long-time residents of the community. Factors that may have influenced their self-reliance included good health insurance, easy access to health care prior to moving to Montana City, and one participant's diagnosis of pulmonary hypertension. They explained,

> We are a little different because we retired here from a very different background and there are several other couples like that. So you are seeing some different things in the rural areas than maybe before because our experience is to take advantage of good medical care where we were and so we sort of expect or do the same thing here, although it is a bit harder, but I think we would be much more apt to take advantage of it than people who have lived here for 50 years. They have had to do things on their own and are very resourceful and they take care of things on their own. But we are spoiled the other way and so it is a little [different].

Another participant who also moved into the community to retire stated, "It has to be pretty bad [to seek health care]. I usually wait it out or take care of it myself." Then he described a contrast between himself and long-time residents of the community.

> I think that a lot of people here, because they have lived here all their life and haven't had access to immediate care, wait it out. The locals definitely try to treat themselves first and do wait it out when they probably should leave right away and get there before it is too bad. So, in a way, I guess we are probably different from some of the people who have lived here a long time.

Another example of self-reliance was reported by a participant when she described how she and her husband planned for surgery.

> We chose May because we knew we wanted to come home after his surgery so he could recuperate up here. Since we live on Montana Pass and there was still snow that meant we still had to get him to the house, and that had to be by snowmobile. The doctor said not to sit on the snowmobile, but that he could stand on our pull sled. So, I drove the snowmobile and he stood up on the pull sled and I took him home.

Hardiness

The participants demonstrated several characteristics of *hardiness* identified by Wirtz, Lee, and Running (1998). Those included adaptability, positive attitude, and endurance. The following excerpt from the interview with the participant who was suffering from pulmonary hypertension demonstrates adaptability and a positive attitude.

> I suppose I am concerned [about my health], but I happen to know this is a progressive disease and it's just going to progress and so we will just deal with it as it comes. I think by nature I am an up person and so you just do it.

Another participant who suffered from a major medical condition causing her severe pain demonstrated adaptability and endurance. She commented, "I just worked . . . I just go until I drop." "Our thing is we go until I scream [because of pain] and if I scream, I go in."

An older participant recovering from surgery also demonstrated endurance while caring for her terminally ill husband.

> I was in the hospital with my new shoulder when they called me at the hospital and told me that I had to either have him out of the hospital by the tenth of June or come up with $118 a day. I can't afford $118 a day. They said I couldn't take him home with [my] shoulder and I said, 'well, I am going to. I don't have $118 a day.' My grandson came and stayed with me for four days and that really helped until I learned how to handle him, getting him in and out of bed and I had to lift. I felt more comfortable when I had him [my husband] at home, though I didn't sleep much, but I knew he was taken care of and that is where he wanted to be.

Conscientious Consumer

The theme of *conscientious consumer* was a new theme identified in this study. Many participants made reference to making decisions about where to seek care depending on the type of illness or injury involved and the time of year. "In the summer you can go to Conway or Robertson or Littlewood, or Bowman or Lackwood. We have those options depending on how important it is." Another participant, a little over 8 months pregnant at the time of the interview, made a statement about selecting a health care provider and making arrangements for the birth of her child.

I chose the Littlewood clinic but Conway would actually be a little closer but they have sometimes a little bit more weather concerns, whereas the road to Littlewood is always open. I chose it [Littlewood] after comparing it with Lackwood and other places.

Another participant demonstrated the concept of *conscientious consumer* by his explanation of his decisions about emergency care.

That [miles to emergency care] depends on what type of emergency. If right now I cut my finger off working with the saw over there, I would head for Conway. If I was having chest pains, if I was able to make a conscious decision, I would be heading to Lackwood. Now they do have the clinic in Maryville and they are very good there. They have a really good doctor, but he is in the process of leaving. And it depends on who comes in there. If I like the doctor, I would go there for some things. If I don't like him, I wouldn't go back for anything. And in a few months if I cut my finger, I would be heading to the clinic in Maryville and then on to Lackwood because the road to Conway will be closing. And it really does depend on what is going on. I would base my decision on where to go on the situation and the problem.

Informed Risk

Informed risk was a second new theme that emerged from the analysis. Informed risk was evidenced by the two participants with major health problems. One participant, who had pulmonary hypertension, explained that she was aware of the health risks associated with where she lived, but chose to remain in Montana City because of other benefits it provided that she valued. In other words, the risk was worth it to her because she was where she wanted to be.

There are times when I wonder if I will be here in the morning and sometime I probably won't, but there is no future in worrying about it. I probably shouldn't be at this altitude, but what we have up here, what we enjoy [is here], and so we loath to give that up.

She further explained that she was aware of the implications of living in Montana City.

I am aware [of the risks and concerns] because the doctors keep telling me that I probably shouldn't be at this altitude, but obviously I'm still here so that must tell you something about my attitude. It would probably be more convenient closer to the hospital and yet I don't really want to live having to be close to the hospital when friends and activities are all up here. It's more fun to be up here and have to deal with whatever happens because I shouldn't be here.

The husband of the above participant was also involved in the research project and stated,

Well, there were a lot of concerns when this [diagnosis of pulmonary hypertension] first happened. The doctors in Denver were very concerned about us coming back here without what they considered any back up. All the patients they have treated have been with[in] twenty minutes of the hospital and a backup. See, with primary pulmonary hypertension, the literature has showed that within 20 minutes of the prostacyclin infusion being stopped, there are severe, rebound reactions, including death in some cases. The infusion must be continuous, and if something happens, say the pump is dropped and it pulls on the catheter, or if she falls and it somehow stops, or even if the catheter gets clogged, but if the infusion is stopped for any reason, you must start another IV. . . . We are aware of what the doctors think and we know what it might mean to live here because of the altitude or problems with the catheter.

He further explained and defined *informed risk* in the following statement:

The altitude here is a problem and the doctors really think we should move. This altitude is not good for [my wife] and the pulmonary hypertension can be worse because of it, but we know that and like I said, maybe one day we will have to move to Lackwood or whatever, but right now this where we want to be.

Another participant who also suffered from a major disease process stated,

As far as being this far away, we have talked about it, my surgeon and I talked about it. I mean jeepers, if it is time to go in [to the hospital], it is time to go in. And if it is too late, it is too late. I don't have a concern about that at all, at all.

She further explained by stating:

I would never move just for medical care, just simply because I love it here. I mean how can you not go out here [outside her home] and think, 'oh cool.'

It is a heart song and it is a peace of heart for me to be here and that is a lot of help. It really is. I can go out there and look at the mountains and get something out of that and that makes the difference.

Another participant stated, "those of us who have been here for years, we just try to take care of ourselves without having to get any medical attention. Sometimes that is ok. We realize the risk we are taking."

Community Support

Another theme that emerged was *community support*. Each of the individuals made statements that the community pulls together when someone needs help. The hardy individual described previously who cared for her husband stated,

There is a lot of people here I could have called. That is one thing about Montana City. If you ever need help, even if you are a stranger to them, you get help. That is one thing about up here. It is a great community.

Another participant shared her perception of support.

The people in the community are great. Every time I am having a bad day all we have to do is make a phone call or stand out on the street and they are here, taking care of my boys and my business. It is incredible. It really is. They had a benefit auction for us one time when I was in the hospital. And those times too, the boys get spoiled rotten by the whole community.

Inadequate Insurance

All participants had insurance. Five stated that insurance was a concern for them. Four commented it was expensive, had high deductibles, or was inadequate. One participant stated,

Yes, we have health insurance. It is very expensive and we pay it all ourselves. That has been a real burden. And a lot of people up here do not have health insurance, at all. I don't know if any business has health insurance and benefits, or even provides part of it. So that is a very difficult thing here. When you don't make a lot of money and the health insurance keeps going up all the time. A major part of our income goes to health insurance. That is a real burden.

Another long time resident of the community stated she had health insurance, "but it doesn't leave me much to live on. I live on about $250 a month after that." Two retired participants brought medical insurance with them from their jobs. One stated, "we are different than a lot of people here in the community in that we brought our insurance here with us. A lot of people here do not have insurance, or do not have adequate insurance."

All participants stated their health insurance coverage did not affect how they accessed care. When I asked a long-time member of the community if her health insurance affected how she sought care, she stated,

> No, I don't think so. I know it does for a lot of people here, if they don't have health insurance which a lot of them don't, I think it affects them as a choice of going to the doctor, or the hospital, or not seeking care.

Participants estimated that one-half to three-quarters of the members of the Montana City community did not have insurance.

DISCUSSION

The themes that emerged provided valuable information for comparison to previously identified concepts in the rural nursing literature. The primary characteristics of *self-reliance* included "self-reliance as learned, decisional choice, and independence" (Chafey et al., 1998, p. 162). Self-reliance as learned was demonstrated by several participants and was clearly more evident in those who had lived in the community for a long period of time. The individuals who had more recently moved into the community considered themselves self-reliant, stating that they try to take care of things themselves first. They also acknowledged that those who had grown up in the community or had lived there a long time did more for themselves than they did.

Self-reliance as a decisional choice was not as clear in the data from the Montana City participants. Participants inferred they made many choices on a daily basis, but never indicated that was of great importance to them. They all mentioned a sense of security provided by knowing a retired doctor lived in the community who was willing to provide information as they engaged in the decision-making process.

Hardiness is another theme that emerged. As previously discussed, the data from Montana City participants showed evidence of adaptability, positive attitude, and endurance, characteristics of hardiness (Wirtz et al., 1998). All participants expressed in some manner that one must adjust to what life had to offer" (p. 262). Two long-time residents demonstrated learned experience, an additional characteristic of hardiness, by making statements such as "the way it had always been" or "that's all we have ever known." Overall, the Montana City residents demonstrated hardiness congruent with hardiness previously described in the rural nursing literature.

Four of the themes I identified were new themes or variations of existing themes. *Conscientious consumer* was a theme that I identified in the Montana City data and it appeared to be similar to concepts previously discussed in the nursing literature. Distance played a role in where the Montana City participants accessed care for a particular injury or illness. Mileage, time, and perception are attributes of distance (Henson, Sadler, & Walton, 1998). Mileage and time are congruent with the attributes of *conscientious consumer* as the participants weighed these two factors when determining where to seek care for a particular health problem. For the Montana City participants, weather was a key factor that the conscientious consumer had to consider in their decision-making process.

The theme of *conscientious consumer* also paralleled health resources concepts (Ballantyne, 1998). Ballantyne stated, "if the client is motivated to seek health care beyond the immediate boundaries of the community, factors such as transportation, distance, inclement weather, and finances become important issues" (p. 182).

Informed risk was a new theme or perhaps a variation of an existing theme. Informed risk was not specifically found in the nursing literature. Informed risk means that individuals are aware of the risks or consequences of their decisions, but desire for quality of life outweighs the risks presented. The participants acknowledged that there may be some risks in living where they did, but they also were weighing their options when making these decisions.

Community support has been discussed in the nursing literature in a variety of ways. The concept of *community support* may be related to previously presented concepts (e.g., informal networks [Grossman & McNerney, 1998] and familiarity [McNeely & Shreffler, 1998]). Community support was clearly demonstrated by "rallying," "benefit auctions," and "helping take care of my business and my kids."

Inadequate insurance had an impact on a number of participants. *Inadequate insurance* was not a concept in itself, but I identified it as a potential modifying factor for health care usage in the community. Although I did not identify a concept that paralleled *inadequate insurance* in the nursing literature, it is an issue related to resource accessibility and health care access that warrants further investigation.

IMPLICATIONS FOR NURSING PRACTICE

Informed risk affects the way health care practitioners relate to their clients. It is important that the practitioner confirm that it is truly informed risk and individuals are able to make informed decisions. For example, it was important for the individual with pulmonary hypertension to understand the risk of being further than 20 minutes away from an appropriate medical facility and the risk she was taking with the prostacyclin infusion. It was also important for her to understand physiologically the impact altitude may have on the progression of her disease. Once practitioners are clear that their client is truly informed, then it is important to respect their decisions. Furthermore, once the decision has been made by the individual to remain in a particular environment or situation, the practitioner should provide the appropriate information and education, teach the client and family necessary skills, and assist them in identifying available resources. Even if a practitioner disagrees with a client's informed decision, the individual's choice should be respected.

Health care practitioners should be aware of modifying factors such as time and distance that affect access to care and the health care decision-making process of *conscientious consumers*. The participant who was 8 months pregnant at the time of the interview provides an example.

> When they [practitioners in general] tell you 'well leave your house when your contractions are five minutes part,' well that could make for a child born in Gateway. They [rural doctors in Littlewood] do realize that even if you are racing it is a good two-hour drive and at night you cannot go that fast.

In this example, inaccurate perceptions on the part of providers caring for pregnant clients may result in babies being born in the back seat of an automobile in the middle of nowhere. Therefore, it is imperative for providers to understand conscientious consumers when making decisions relative to health care. Discussing what-if scenarios with rural clients, particularly in relation to distance, time, and weather, will help them be the best and wisest conscientious consumers.

Self-reliance and *hardiness* both have an impact on when, why, and how rural individuals will seek care. As with informed risk, health care providers should work with individuals in an attempt to provide the necessary information, skills, and available resources although allowing persons to be self-reliant.

Understanding the presence or lack of *community support* for clients in rural communities gives the practitioner insight into the availability of resources. For example, individuals who have been hospitalized and want to return home rather than stay on a transitional care unit may be able to do so with strong community support.

Inadequate insurance affected participants' use of health care. High deductible, out-of-pocket expenses, distance, and availability of services also influenced health care decision-making for these isolated rural residents. The combination of these issues warrants thorough investigation to fully understand health care access.

As indicated by Long and Weinert (1989), "continued research can provide a more solid base for the nursing theory that is required to guide practice and the delivery of health care to rural populations" (p. 126). Thus, previously identified concepts as well as newly emerging concepts or themes warrant further investigation to help health care practitioners provide the highest quality care to rural individuals.

NOTE

1. The names of the all communities in this chapter were changed to maintain anonymity of participants.

REFERENCES

Ballantyne, J. (1998). Health resources and the rural client. In H. J. Lee (Ed.), *Conceptual basis for rural nursing* (pp. 178–188). New York: Springer.

Chafey, K., Sullivan, T., & Shannon, A. (1998). Self-reliance: Characterization of their own autonomy by elderly rural women. In H. J. Lee (Ed.), *Conceptual basis for rural nursing* (pp. 156–177). New York: Springer.

Fahlberg, L. (1983). *Nine months of winter.* Montana City: Pilot Peak.

Glidden, R. (1982). *Exploring the Montana high country: History of the Montana City area* (2nd ed.). Montana City: Ralph Glidden.

Grossman, L. L., & McNerney, S. (1998). Informal networks. In H. J. Lee (Ed.), *Conceptual basis for rural nursing* (pp. 200–208). New York: Springer.

Henson, D., Sadler, T., & Walton, S. (1998). Distance. In H. J. Lee (Ed.), *Conceptual basis for rural nursing* (pp. 51–60). New York: Springer.

Koehler, V. (1998). The substantive theory of protecting independence. In H. J. Lee (Ed.), *Conceptual basis for rural nursing* (pp. 236–256). New York: Springer.

Long, K. A., & Weinert, C. (1989). Rural nursing: Developing the theory base. *Scholarly Inquiry for Nursing Practice: An International Journal 3*, 113–127.

McNeely, A. G., & Shreffler, M. J. (1998). Familiarity. In H. J. Lee (Ed.), *Conceptual basis for rural nursing* (pp. 89–101). New York: Springer.

National Geographic Road Atlas. (2000). Canada: MapQuest.com, Inc.

Rossman, G. B., & Rallis, S. F. (1998). *Learning in the field: An introduction to qualitative research.* Thousand Oaks, CA: Sage.

Wirtz, E. F., Lee, H. J., & Running, A. (1998). The lived experience of hardiness in rural men and women. In H. J. Lee (Ed.), *Conceptual basis for rural nursing* (pp. 257–274). New York: Springer.

Strategizing Safety: Perinatal Experiences of Rural Women

5

KATHARINE S. WEST

The health of mothers and infants is of critical importance to a community. Health statistics related to maternal and infant morbidity and mortality reflect the current health status of women and serves as a predictor of health of the next generation (U.S. Department of Health and Human Services, 2000). Maternal/child statistics closely mirror the general health of the community and its prevailing socioeconomic conditions. To support maternal/child health, and thereby the health of the community, health care programs must respond not only to the biological needs of and risks to mothers, but also to their beliefs and customs and to the social fabric of their lives (Hoffmaster, 1986).

Maternity care must not only be available, but also accessible and acceptable to clients. *Availability* refers to the existence of a particular service, including the necessary personnel to provide that service. *Accessibility* refers to whether a person has logistical access to services, including the resources to pay for them. *Acceptability* refers to whether the service offered is a good fit with the values and beliefs of the client (Bushy, 1994). Women living in rural areas have limited access to receiving available prenatal services that are acceptable to them (Conrad, Hollenbach, Fullerton, & Feigelson, 1998; Gertler, Rahman, Feifer, & Ashley, 1993; McManus & Newacheck, 1989). A lack of appropriate care can contribute to poor perinatal outcomes (Hoffmaster, 1986). Thus, it is likely that the experiences of rural women differ from urban or suburban women.

The nursing community may benefit from a better understanding of what it is like for mothers to have a baby when living in a rural area, identifying what internal and external factors influence their experiences, and what strategies the mothers use to optimize birth outcomes. At a time when disparities in service delivery between metro and nonmetro areas are increasing, both federal and state governments acknowledge the importance of providing standardized services (California Department of Health Services [CDHS], 2000a, 2000b; California Department of Public Health, 2007; Centers for Disease Control and Prevention [CDC], 2007). One way to accomplish this is to provide client-specific information to the local public health nursing service. Assessing what mothers know, and specifically what rural mothers know, is important information for improving the acceptability of health care services. Incorporating women's knowledge and values into community plans to meet state and federal health goals is critical for developing plans that will be successful, and ultimately improve birth outcomes. Mothers may have different definitions and concerns than the government has regarding birth services, and it would be prudent to investigate this. It is also desirable to tap into the creative solutions that mothers may have developed for themselves and further develop these ideas for the rural community.

The study described in this chapter contributes information from the woman's perspective related to access, support systems, perceptions, and expectations related to perinatal care. Furthermore, the results of this study promote public health nursing through the increased knowledge and assessment of the community of rural pregnant women. Kuehnert (1991) stated that nursing interventions enable and empower communities to change public policy affecting accessibility, availability, and affordability of health services, and other social conditions underlying many health problems. The public health nurse who provides maternal/child health care addresses the particular needs of mothers and children, may improve patient outcomes by influencing policy development, and may provide policy advocacy in partnership with the community, thus improving pregnancy outcomes for rural women.

PURPOSE

I designed this qualitative descriptive study to discover how pregnant women living in a rural area seek and experience perinatal health care. My second purpose was to give a voice to rural women and their ways of knowing and functioning during the perinatal period.

In this study, I focused specifically on experiences of women having babies while they were living in Mariposa County, California, to understand and identify internal and external factors that influenced their experiences and pregnancy outcomes. The findings show how mothers viewed their interactions with the health care team and their experience of having a baby in a rural area, behaviors and emotions that typified a mother's response to managing her pregnancy, and factors that influenced these interactions and experiences.

METHODS

Symbolic interactionism is a conceptual framework that provides a way to focus on human behavior, how people define the events in their lives (their beliefs), and how they act in relation to their beliefs (Chenitz & Swanson, 1986). Humans ascribe definitions and meaning to events in their lives through an understanding of self and through shared social interaction. Interaction with the health care system is only one factor in a rural client's engagement with the health care system. When there are many factors present, the symbolic interactionist approach allows the researcher to conceptualize behavior in complex situations in a new and different way. By using this approach, I gained insight into the strategies employed by rural women seeking perinatal care and the importance they ascribed to their experiences. I used the discovery mode of grounded theory (Glaser, 1978) with this study to focus on women's concerns, as no prior descriptive research was found on this specific topic. Research findings from this study provide a description of the core variables or the basic social process underlying the experience of the subjects. Grounded theory is especially suited to studying rural women and their pregnancies because it provides a means to discover a theory of experience since there are few theories to explain or predict the behaviors of this special population.

Setting

Mariposa County is a mountainous county located in the western Sierra Nevada range near the center of the state of California. At the time of the study, the county encompassed an area of 1,455 square miles with an estimated population of 15,950. There were no incorporated cities. Half of the county was classified as nonmetro-rural and the other half as nonmetro-frontier. Two-thirds of Yosemite National Park is located within the county.

The setting for the study was the area south of the Merced River. The western portions of this region encompassed rolling foothills dotted with oaks and pines and ranch land with some of the richest grazing areas in the state. The majority of county health care services were located in Mariposa, the county seat and largest town, with an estimated population of 1,900. Transportation had been a point of concern relating to health care services in all of Mariposa County, as there had been limited public transportation through the years. Because of the large geographic area and the minimum driving distance of 40 miles to the next major metropolitan area, it has been a significant challenge to deliver comprehensive perinatal health care to the residents of the county (Mariposa County Health Department [MCHD], 1999).

With a steady birth rate of approximately 130 babies per year and no physicians providing delivery services within Mariposa County, the majority of Mariposan mothers delivered in one of three neighboring counties. Regular local obstetrical services were discontinued in 1982 when the town's general practitioner retired. A local clinic provided childbirth classes and offered prenatal care every other week by a visiting family practice physician from the next county. High-risk obstetrical care was only available by traveling to one of four neighboring counties. Most women drove a minimum of 1–2 hours one-way to prenatal appointments and to reach the hospital of delivery (MCHD, 1999).

Data Collection

The inclusion criteria for the study were women who (a) had current residence in Mariposa County, (b) were currently pregnant at the time of the interview or delivered within the county since 1982 when obstetrical deliveries ceased, and (c) provided written consent to participate in the research study. I obtained a convenience sample from referrals by family ministries at churches in the county. Demographic data were collected at the time of consent. Individual study participants were interviewed using semistructured, open-ended questions until no new information was forthcoming (data saturation).

Collectively, at the time of the interviews, the nine study participants had been pregnant 32 times, with 22 pregnancies completed and one in progress. Eighteen of the 32 pregnancies qualified for inclusion in this study because those pregnancies occurred in Mariposa County after in-county deliveries had ceased. Prenatal care was begun at an average of 8 weeks with a range of 4 to 16 weeks gestation. Four women were delivered by an obstetrician-gynecologist (OB-GYN), one by a perinatologist, two by a midwife in a hospital setting, and one by a midwife at home. Five women delivered babies in Fresno County, two in Merced County, and one at home in Mariposa County. The newborns weighed an average of 2,679 grams (range: 816–4,196 grams). One preterm infant born less than 27 weeks gestation received care in a regional neonatal intensive care unit. Each woman had 1 to 8 living children aged 8 months to 32 years, including one set of twins and one term infant who died in the postneonatal period from complications of a congenital birth defect.

Using an interview guide and carefully worded broad questions allowed me to explore the women's experiences and to better understand what it is like to be pregnant in a rural county. I encouraged the women to freely share their experiences and to identify factors that influenced their pregnancies. Because attitudes are difficult to measure, overt questions about attitudes were not asked. Rather, attitudes were allowed to emerge from answers regarding social interactions. In a similar manner, standard health care concerns were not directly addressed but allowed to emerge from the data.

Data Analysis

I audio taped the interviews and transcribed them. QSR N-Vivo™ (2000) was used to manage the data and facilitated the recognition and understanding of information presented in the interviews. The constant comparative method of analysis required that, initially, I coded interviews to reflect the substance of what was said and then compared each interview with subsequent interviews for similarities and differences. I then compared and clustered codes, labeling clusters as categories emerged (Chenitz & Swanson, 1986). I examined all variables in the study data until the categories that emerged were united by a core category.

FINDINGS

Pregnant women in Mariposa County were confronted with the same decisions as pregnant women everywhere: They had to (a) select a caregiver, (b) choose behaviors that support a healthy pregnancy, (c) prepare for labor, and (d) experience a successful delivery. However, women in

Mariposa County have one significant difference: they must also come to terms with at least one hour of travel across rural countryside during active labor so they and their health care provider can meet for the birth. The women all voiced concerns about an unattended precipitous delivery.

The mothers' main concern was having an unattended delivery on the highway with its potential complications and problems, which they resolved by engaging in the basic social process of *strategizing safety*. Strategizing safety best tied together all the variable categories that emerged from the data. In one way or another, every person volunteered concern about the distance and the plans she made to cope with this concern. One mother explained, "It's just the travel distance and having to make alternate plans that most people wouldn't have to make. We had kind of a mock OB [obstetrical] kit in the car just in case."

The Basic Social Process: Strategizing Safety

The basic social process of *strategizing safety* has four phases (see Figure 5.1): (a) seeking information, (b) choosing, (c) following through, and (d) fine-tuning.

For the Mariposa women in this study, strategizing safety in pregnancy commenced upon confirmation of the pregnancy and concluded

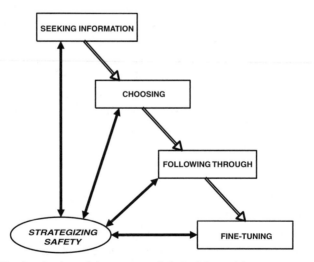

Figure 5.1. The four basic social processes of strategizing safety.

with the birth. The first phase, *seeking information,* involved fact-finding about the various types of obstetrical care that were available, locally or at a distance. Interpretation of the facts was filtered through personal beliefs and previous experience. The second phase, *choosing,* included deciding on a caregiver for the pregnancy—either a physician or a midwife or a combination of the two. In making her choice for caregiver, a woman committed herself to a location for delivery. The third phase, *following through,* began with the initiation and continuation of prenatal care. As pregnancy progressed, changes in circumstances or development of complications sometimes required an alteration in decisions. Coping with the pregnancy was managed with the help of the woman's social support network and her own inherent abilities. The fourth phase, *fine-tuning,* included preparation for labor and the experience of delivery. The labor experience included getting to the right place for delivery at the right time and was the core of the basic social process. Stressors and circumstances unique to the peripartum dictated changes in plans at this phase. Medical interventions were sometimes guided by the need to resolve what one mother termed "the one hour of worry" because of the distance involved.

Seeking Information

[My last baby] was kind of a surprise. My first thought was, oh dear. Moved up to this place where I don't know anybody. There are no OB-GYNs listed in the phone book. How am I going to find a doctor?

The first phase of strategizing safety is *seeking information.* Initially, a woman had " . . . a suspicion about being pregnant. And then I went looking for a doctor to confirm it." Sometimes they found the physician or midwife through friends, relatives, or current health care providers. "I got my referral through my sister and her midwife." "And then I just went with that group because everybody, you know, [the midwife] just delivered all the babies, so I just went with them." One woman pregnant for the first time sought additional information about types of health care providers and possible delivery options. Being a primipara and the newcomer in town, she did not have a relationship with an obstetrical caregiver and required information before she could make her choices.

To some degree, personal history influenced the kind of information participants wanted. For example, one participant gathered information about home delivery because she was born at home.

> My grandma had [her] children here; most of them at home. . . . I think I liked the idea [of a home delivery] because, well, my mom had . . . her children at home, and I thought if she can do it, surely I could do it.

In this first phase, the women were seeking information based on what they learned from people they knew, or where they believed they might find obstetrical services. From the very beginning, they were already considering the one hour of worry. This became more evident in the next phase as they made their choice.

Choosing

The second phase of strategizing safety is *choosing*. Choosing is accomplished as a direct result of the information obtained in the first phase. Elements and facts surrounding the circumstance influenced individual choices. The meaning and importance of the decision to the person making the choice also influenced choice.

In the case of the experience in Mariposa County, women chose between a physician and a midwife, and both types of providers were available to attend hospital deliveries in neighboring counties. However, few midwives were available to attend home births in Mariposa County.

> My sister-in-law had a baby at home. . . . I asked her if her midwife would come over here, but she doesn't travel that far. But then I asked for a referral. That's how I found out about the midwife here. The reason I wanted to do that, I was a little, I mean part of you is a little nervous because you don't know if something could go wrong. I did have a doctor for back-up if there were problems.

Other women made their choices by first deciding on the location for delivery and then finding a caregiver on staff at that location. This was sometimes influenced by the report from other women.

> I called around. I asked people for names and I called around and asked the offices questions. I had made the decision that I didn't want to go to [a particular town]. I didn't want to deliver [there] . . . because I heard a lot of bad stories, that they didn't like it. They didn't like the doctors there. They didn't feel comfortable in the hospital. They didn't like the nurses. They didn't like either one of the hospitals [there]. I don't think I've ever heard a success story. . . . So, I knew that I wanted to deliver in [another] area.

Prenatal visits were available at the midwifery clinic in a nearby town where "[a]t least that's a compromise. You still have to travel in labor, but you can have your visits closer." Finally, there were visits offered at physicians' offices outside of Mariposa County: "And that's exactly what we do when we came down for my prenatal visits. We'd usually plan them for early in the morning, get that done first, and then we'd go shopping and go eat lunch, you know."

Ultimately, choosing hinged on several factors, but time and distance were always the major influences of the final decision. Mariposa women weighed all these options in their minds, balancing the pros and cons of travel considerations for prenatal care with considerations for delivery. Travel concern was the constant factor, with the main point being to resolve fear and worries. The one hour of worry was the compelling factor that guided their choosing.

Following Through

Following through, the third phase of strategizing safety occurs after information has been obtained and a choice has been made. Following through is evidenced by the woman's behaviors as related to the specific circumstance for which safety must be strategized. Coping and adaptation behaviors that enable one to follow through during this phase are derived from a combination of personal experience, self-care, and social support from friends and family.

During the perinatal experience of the Mariposa women, following through was contingent on the distance the women must travel to reach their caregiver or the distance the caregiver must travel to reach the patient. For instance, the resolve to keep her appointments was reflected by the mother, who admitted,

> I had to go. What choice did I have really? Some days I was just plain tired. But I think that was the hardest part, and being so far away. The one time that I was spotting, I was thinking, "What am I going to do?" I could have gone to [a nearby hospital] but I don't know any of those doctors, and I want my own doctor.

The health care provider sometimes shared the travel burden with the mother. "Actually [for] my exams, the doctor would come up to a clinic up here. But [for my other pregnancies], I'd just go to her office in town."

Women frequently combined their prenatal visits with other activities. "I would usually go after . . . work in the morning, and then I would go in the afternoon to the midwife. So it worked out okay that way." Sometimes, alternative plans were developed in conjunction with the women's support networks and health care providers. One woman was offered an option when ". . . people from church came up and told me that they work in [town], and that they'd be more than happy to take me in."

Fine-Tuning

Fine-tuning begins with final preparation for the event that indicated a need for safety in the first place. Fine-tuning may come about from actions of the woman who is strategizing safety or may result from the actions of others. Fine-tuning may also be imposed on the situation by the environment. Stressors may develop leading to further fine-tuning. Similar coping skills that were useful in the following-through phase may become significant in this phase as well. Social support from family and friends continue to help the woman achieve a conclusion to the event.

For pregnant women in Mariposa County, fine-tuning was synonymous with labor and delivery. At the onset of labor, the one hour of worry was most acutely experienced and fine-tuning was implemented. As one woman noted,

> Our plan was that if I had a long labor, we were going to get a hotel room down the street from the hospital and labor in a hotel. They had suites just down the road from the hospital. And so the plan was to labor at the hotel, and then when [contractions] got closer, to go to the hospital.

Distance and travel needs were foremost in the women's minds. Mariposa's families constantly weighed the odds for a successful delivery during the phase of fine-tuning: "The only hard thing is the emergency. [Mariposa County emergency services are] not really worth much at all . . . it's kind of just a helipad and a band-aid dispenser." The experience of labor proved whether their particular strategy for safety was adequate. Labor in the right place attended by the right people and a successful birth was the outcome the women sought. The details of their labor guided their choice of caregiver and influenced the steps they followed throughout pregnancy.

Once labor began for the rural woman, "getting there" was the observable critical behavior during the one hour of worry. Getting there sometimes involved more than transportation; sometimes getting there required fine-tuning by coming up with an alternative travel route:

> We were a little concerned with the road conditions and you have to go up this one grade called Briceberg. We were a little concerned what the weather was going to be like. Sometimes they just close the roads and they won't let you go through.

Because some of the roads could be covered with snow, the winter season demanded a different sort of fine-tuning. One family who lived between Mariposa and Yosemite had to plan for a winter due date. The mother reflected that had the road to town been snowed over, "We could go up to Yosemite, although they don't really have those kind of services, they do have a clinic there. They have a hospital, and probably the doctor could have helped us there."

The original plan sometimes included an alternative labor support person in the event that the woman could not contact her preferred labor support.

> We had my mom who lives next door, so if I was here, and [my husband] wasn't here, then my mom was to drive. If [my husband] were here, then of course he would drive me. And we had back-up plans with neighbors.

However, if the woman found herself in early labor, and already at or near to the planned location of delivery, the one hour of worry sometimes resulted in fine-tuning the labor plan. One woman was in early labor at the hospital when she fine-tuned her plans:

> [We all] talked about that openly. [My doctor], the nurses, myself and my husband said, 'If you had someplace to go here, I would just send you home. But since you live so far away,' and he just had to think about us going to a hotel. He just didn't agree with that. That was an issue. So . . . had we been up here, I think that it would have been a different ending.

The birth itself sometimes demanded immediate fine-tuning as described by the mother who delivered in an ambulance along the highway on the way to the hospital.

> Well, you've got your gurney, which is not wide. Actually, I just got on all fours and really, that's not a bad way to have a baby. Because there was

nothing to hold on to or anything. Actually, I . . . just kind of squatted down and held on because there was nothing. There was no way to really get comfortable. . . . And I was pretty upset to think [an emergency medical technician was going to do the delivery] because I wasn't sure what his skills were. So they didn't have to do anything really. Just catch the baby, but they did fine.

Fine-tuning concluded with the birth of the infant. With the arrival of the newborn, strategizing safety was completed with all the corresponding fears of an unattended delivery; the one hour of worry had ended.

Summary of Strategizing Safety

The identified social process in this study, *strategizing safety* under the circumstance of rural perinatal care, was completed with the infant's birth. For Mariposa women, the safe arrival of the newborn was the result of nine months of their strategizing to optimize the situation surrounding the one hour of worry. Although the same is certainly true that urban women seek safe delivery for their infants, urban women's concern for safety during travel in labor does not usually manifest, if it manifests at all, until the final weeks of pregnancy. On the other hand, women in Mariposa County strategized safety from the beginning of pregnancy, throughout pregnancy, occasionally during that significant hour of travel, and sometimes even after arriving at the planned location for delivery. One mother summed up the situation:

> I would love to have my babies where I wouldn't have to travel fifty-five or sixty miles. Maybe because I have healthy pregnancies and deliveries, I don't have that worry so much, but I just think a clinic or someplace to go to have my babies. I don't like traveling in labor. . . . Like I said, I do have healthy pregnancies, but I think it would be wonderful to have a place up here to have my babies.

DISCUSSION AND IMPLICATIONS

Research about the inner world of the pregnant woman has been published in the nursing and psychological literature since the middle of the twentieth century. Much of the field of maternal/child nursing is based on the seminal work of Rubin (1961, 1967a, 1967b, 1975). According to Rubin's long-accepted research (1975), there is a sequence to the psychological tasks of pregnancy and a different focus during each phase. According to Rubin, the mother's focus is inwardly aligned and the fetus is interpreted as being a part of her physical self. Nesting behaviors and thoughts of delivery help her prepare for birth, including solving logistical issues such as transportation at the time of labor. Only in the final weeks of a full-term pregnancy does she change to an outwardly aligned focus with thoughts toward alternative plans or contingencies as she prepares for the trip to the hospital. Rubin called this set of behaviors *safe passage.*

Corbin (1981) also identified how women manage safety during pregnancy-related illness through the task of *protective governing.* Corbin found that women actively managed "their problems . . . to guard the fetus and herself against morbidity and mortality" (p. iv), noting the importance of the social setting in which this occurred.

Patterson, Freese, and Goldenberg (1990) conducted research to explore how women utilized health care during pregnancy. The major concern of women was identified as *seeking safe passage* throughout pregnancy and childbirth by means of several processes that were described as largely psychological, or internal, in nature. Patterson et al. also stated that seeking safe passage might consist of a single approach with the ultimate outcome being the enrollment in prenatal care.

Similar processes were also identified in this study of rural women with one notable difference. Women in Mariposa County were specifically concerned with the external environment and the attendant implications for safe passage throughout pregnancy and ending with delivery. Mothers in Mariposa began to prepare for the trip to the hospital, at least mentally, immediately upon confirmation of pregnancy. These thoughts pervaded their entire pregnancy. Specifically, it was the one hour of worry—the concern with delivering en route to the hospital—that influenced all of their decisions and choices. Seeking safe passage for them was far more than an internal exercise at the beginning of pregnancy. *Strategizing safety* was the process by which the women attempted to manage risk and bring control to their external environment throughout their pregnancy in anticipation of the birth of their newborn.

The women in Mariposa identified a yearning for local obstetrical services. One mother noted, "It would be wonderful if we had someplace close to go for prenatal and postpartum care here at our hospital." Having access to both outpatient and inpatient obstetrical care becomes especially important for residents in rural areas with the chronic shortage of physicians. In both urban and rural settings, obstetrics accounts for a similar number (17%) of inpatient procedures (Hall, Owings, &

Shinogle, 2006). Yet research into the challenges of providing health care in a rural setting tends to focus on the recruitment and retention of primary care physicians or, less explored, how to make specialty physician services accessible to rural residents (Drew, Cashman, & Savageau, 2006). Numerous suggestions have been made, but only a few have included the addition of a visiting physician specialist who maintains a rural ancillary practice. Hospital administrators view visiting specialists as a growing trend and are actively recruiting them to fill specialty needs. Interestingly, in light of the Mariposan mothers' concerns about the one hour of worry of travel, Drew et al. noted that very few visiting specialists (11%) indicated that they were willing to travel more than one hour to their rural clinic.

In addition, local county health departments could supplement health care teams by deploying rural public health nurses to work in partnership with urban perinatal programs. The rural nurse with additional training in expanded roles, such as registered nurse (RN) obstetrical ultrasound certification, could further increase access using such technologies via telemedicine.

The advent of telemedicine increases options for access to specialty care. Using telemedicine in rural obstetrics with fetal ultrasonography, including three-dimensional ultrasound and fetoscope images, shows promise for alleviating the shortage of specialists with enhanced access to quality obstetrical care (Reddy, Bartlett, Harnett, McManamon, & Snelgrove, 2000).

An area of recent focus in rural care has been on how specialists manage high-risk pregnancies from a distance. Some of the observations were that urban health care providers seemed unaware of the special challenges rural women faced with access. Several nurse researchers suggested there would be value in helping nurses and other health professionals become sensitized to the special needs of rural pregnant women and not simply focus on the complicating factor of pregnancy. For instance, when the complication was crack cocaine use, Pursley-Crotteau (2001) noted that there was a particular lack of awareness on the part of staff to focus on the developmental and special physical needs of these women.

Notably absent in these studies are rural nurses, yet there is a role for both rural nurses and advanced practice nurses (APNs) in meeting access to care needs. One approach for improving rural access to obstetrical services was "First Steps," a public health nursing care pathway for maternity-support services managed through the rural health department in the state of Washington. "First Steps" was a legislated program to first implement a maternal health care pathway (Olds, 1997). The results were well received by both health care team and family members when the maternity care pathway brought prenatal care services directly into the community.

Increasing utilization of the APN in rural areas is another possibility for increasing access to the health care team. Nearly 30 years ago, there were discussions with rural communities in California to use certified nurse midwives (CNMs) to meet their basic maternity care needs (Nesbitt, Connell, Hart, & Rosenblatt, 1990). Unfortunately, this remains an underutilized approach. California passed the first Midwife Practice Act in 1974, with the Midwifery Practice Act of 1993 further authorizing "licensed midwives and certified nurse midwives to attend cases of normal childbirth and to provide prenatal, intrapartum, and postpartum care, including family-planning care, for the mother, and immediate care for the newborn" (California Business and Professions Code, 1993) According to the California Nurse Midwives Association (CNMA; n.d.), "CNMs have been practicing in California since 1960 and practice in all settings including private hospitals, public health departments, HMOs [health maintenance organizations] family planning clinics, homebirth practices, and universities" (para. 2). California has the highest number of practicing CNMs in the country (CDC, National Vital Statistics System [NVSS], 2006), with 1,186 actively licensed CNMs in 2009 (California Board of Registered Nursing [CA BRN], 2009). According to the CDC, California midwives delivered nearly 44,000 babies, or 7.8% of births in the state in 2006, but 96.5% of those deliveries took place in a hospital (CDC NVSS, 2006). Legislation was passed in 1996 that allowed APNs—certified clinical nurse specialists (CNSs), nurse practitioners (NPs), and CNMs—to directly bill Medicare for services in both rural and urban areas (Minarik, 1997). Although this was meant to be a positive measure to encourage reimbursement for services in a rural area, an impediment may be the lack of affordable liability insurance for APNs providing perinatal care. Like obstetricians across the country, CNMs/APNs are experiencing a professional liability crisis that is having a negative impact on providing accessible rural obstetric care.

COMMENTARY

Community-driven solutions must be developed locally, in the public health model of partnership with local public health agencies taking the lead with local community businesses. The partners should identify outcome measures appropriate for their own community, and then devise the most appropriate strategies to address the unmet needs, both internal and external, of rural mothers. Ultimately, it is the family's choice to live in a rural area with its advantages and disadvantages. However, because of this choice, women believe they are solely responsible to strategize their own safety and that of their babies. Health care teams must become attuned to the special concerns of mothers.

Even though their one hour of worry influences their decisions for 9 months, the women in this study believed the trade-off was worth it. "It's like having your own path to heaven" to live in a rural area, according to one mother. Another described the reasons she chose to have her children in a rural area when she said:

> It's just a joy to see a child go outside and entertain himself all day long with the grass, the rocks, the trees, and the animals rather than something artificial, and not to have to be entertained by something artificial all the time. Although we own all of those things. I mean we have the Nintendo's and the Game Boys and whatever else, but just the opportunity to experience God-given entertainment. It's worth it to me. It doesn't mean it's wrong or right for anybody else, but to me that makes it all worth it.

Finally, to sum it up, another mother affirmed:

> But I think I just love being up here so much better then, looking back, it's still worth it. The drive is still worth it. I wouldn't move down there just to get closer to medical care because I think all the benefits are worth it. But it would be nice if we had someplace close to go for prenatal and postpartum care here at our hospital.

ACKNOWLEDGMENT

The author acknowledges the collaboration of Barbara Artinian, PhD, Professor of Nursing, Azusa Pacific University, for her invaluable guidance with this study.

REFERENCES

Bushy, A. (1994). When your client lives in a rural area, Part I: Rural health care delivery issues. *Issues in Mental Health Nursing, 15*, 253–266.

California Board of Registered Nursing (CA BRN). (2009). *Monthly Statistics.* Retrieved March 2, 2009, from http://www.rn.ca.gov/about_us/stats.shtml, California Business and Professions Code, § 2507(a) (1993).

California Department of Health Services (CDHS). (2000a). *Comprehensive perinatal services program (CPSP)*. Retrieved December 24, 2000, from http://www.dhs .ca.gov/prp/mchb/Comprehensive_Perinatal.htm

California Department of Health Services (CDHS). (2000b). *Federal performance measures*. Retrieved December 24, 2000, from http://www.dhs.ca.gov/prp/mchb/ Federal_Performance_Measures.htm

California Department of Public Health (CDPH), Maternal, Child, and Adolescent Health Division (MCAH). (2007). *Maternal Child Health Services Title V Block Grant, State Narrative for California*. Retrieved June 23, 2009, from http://www. cdph.ca.gov/programs/mcah/Documents/MO-CA-Narratives-09-19-08.pdf

California Nurse Midwives Association (CNMA). (n.d.). *FAQ—Nurse midwifery in California*. Retrieved February 28, 2009, from http://www.cnma.net/

Centers for Disease Control and Prevention (CDC). (2007). Preconception and Interconception Health Status of Women Who Recently Gave Birth to a Live-Born Infant—Pregnancy Risk Assessment Monitoring System (PRAMS), United States, 26 Reporting Areas, 2004. *MMWR 56(SS10);1–35*.

Centers for Disease Control and Prevention (CDC): National Vital Statistics System (NVSS). (2006). 2006 Birth data, State detail: MRSTATE by ATTEND by BFACIL3 (n06-state). Table produced on 3/3/2009 2:22 from n06-state.ivx

Chenitz, W. C., & Swanson, J. M. (1986). *From practice to grounded theory: Qualitative research in nursing*. Menlo Park, CA: Addison Wesley.

Conrad, J., Hollenbach, K. A., Fullerton, J. T., & Feigelson, H. S. (1998). Use of perinatal services by Hispanic women in San Diego County: A comparison of urban and rural settings. *Journal of Nurse Midwifery, 43*, 90–96.

Corbin, J. C. (1981). Protective governing: Strategies for managing a pregnancy-illness. (Doctor of Nursing Science, dissertation, University of California, San Francisco, 1980). Retrieved March 3, 2009, from *Dissertations & Theses: Full Text Database*. DAI-B 43/02, p. 382, Aug 1982 (Publication No. AAT 8214917).

Drew, J., Cashman, S. B., & Savageau, J. A. (2006). The visiting specialist model of rural health care delivery: A survey in Massachusetts. *The Journal of Rural Health, 22* (4), 294–299.

Gertler, P., Rahman, O., Feifer, C., & Ashley, D. (1993). Determinants of pregnancy outcomes and targeting of maternal health services in Jamaica. *Social Science Medicine, 37*, 199–211.

Glaser, B. G. (1978). *Theoretical sensitivity*. Mill Valley, CA: Sociology Press.

Hall, M. J., Owings, M. F., & Shinogle, J. A. (2006). Inpatient care in rural hospitals at the beginning of the 21st century. *Journal of Rural Health, 22* (4), 331–338.

Hoffmaster, J. E. (1986). Rural maternity services: Community health nurse providers. *Journal of Community Health Nursing, 3*, 25–33.

Kuehnert, P. L. (1991). The public health policy advocate: Fostering the health of communities. *Clinical Nurse Specialist, 5* (1), 5–10.

Mariposa County Health Department (MCHD). (1999). *Family Health Outcomes Project (FHOP) Report*. Mariposa, CA: Author.

McManus, M. A., & Newacheck, P. W. (1989). Rural maternal, child, and adolescent health. *Health Services Research, 23*, 807–848.

Minarik, P. (1997). Medicare reimbursement for nurse practitioners and clinical nurse specialists passes; States' Legislative and Regulatory Forum II. *Clinical Nurse Specialist, 11*, 274–275.

Nesbitt, T. S., Connell, F. A., Hart, L. G., & Rosenblatt, R. A. (1990). Access to obstetric care in rural areas: Effect on birth outcomes. *American Journal of Public Health, 80,* 814–818.

Olds, S. (1997). Designing a care pathway for a maternity support service program in a rural health department. *Public Health Nursing, 14,* 332–338.

Patterson, E. T., Freese, M. P., & Goldenberg, R. L. (1990). Seeking safe passage: Utilizing health care during pregnancy. *Image—Journal of Nursing Scholarship, 22,* 27–31.

Pursley-Crotteau, S. (2001). Perinatal crack users: Becoming temperant: The social psychological processes. *Health Care for Women International, 22,* 49–66.

QSR N-Vivo™. (2000). Qualitative data analysis software program (Version 1.2) [Computer software]. Melbourne, Australia: QSR International Pty Ltd.

Reddy, E. R., Bartlett, P. J., Harnett, J. D. M., McManamon, P. J. & Snelgrove, C. (2000). Telemedicine and fetal ultrasonography in a remote Newfoundland community. *Canadian Medical Association Journal, 162*(2), 206.

Rubin, R. (1961). Basic maternal behavior. *Nursing Outlook, 9,* 683–686.

Rubin, R. (1967a). Attainment of the maternal role: Part I. Processes. *Nursing Research, 16,* 237–245.

Rubin, R. (1967b). Attainment of the maternal role: Part II. Models and referents. *Nursing Research, 16,* 342–346.

Rubin, R. (1975). Maternal tasks of pregnancy. *Maternal-Child Nursing Journal, 4,* 143–153.

U.S. Department of Health and Human Services. (2000). With Understanding and Improving Health and Objectives for Improving Health. Objective 16: Maternal, infant, and child health, in *Healthy People 2010* (2nd ed.). Washington, DC: U.S. Government Printing Office, November 2000. 2(B), 16-3.

Health Perceptions, Needs, and Behaviors of Remote Rural Women of Childbearing and Childrearing Age

6

RONDA L. BALES

Montana is a rural state characterized by vast open spaces, a sparse population, and large geographical distances between cities and towns. An estimated 70% of the state's population live in towns with fewer than 15,000 inhabitants, and 80% of Montana communities have a population of fewer than 3,000 people (Montana Office of Rural Health, 1999). In 2002, the Health Resources and Services Administration (HRSA) designated 35 of Montana's 56 counties as Health Professional Shortage Areas (HPSA) (HRSA, 2002). In 2009, the number of counties designated as HPSAs increased to 39 (HRSA, 2009); 9 counties have no physician in active practice (Montana Office of Rural Health, 2008). More than 25% of Montanans live in a primary care health professional shortage area (HRSA, 2004).

Rural health research identified common health perceptions among rural individuals. Aspects common to rural dwellers included their definition of health as the ability to work, reliance on self and informal systems of care, and decreased willingness to use health care services provided by outsiders (Weinert & Long, 1990). The unique characteristics of rural dwellers may affect how and when they seek health care. Internal factors, such as self-reliance and reliance on informal support systems of family, friends, and neighbors, may lead to a delay in seeking formal health care services (Long, 1993). These factors, as well as external factors including long distances and lack of adequate health care resources, may put the rural individual at increased risk for illness, disability, and premature death (Long; Veitch, 1995).

Few researchers have explored the impact of rurality on the health of midlife women or those of childbearing and childrearing age (Hemard, Monroe, Atkinson, & Blalock, 1998). Women of childbearing and childrearing age, regardless of geographic location, have common health care needs. Early detection and treatment of diseases common in women, such as breast and cervical cancers, can reduce death and disability associated with these diseases. However, access to care has been a factor that influenced whether or not women participate in the screening processes for breast and cervical cancers (Wilcox & Mosher, 1993; Nuovo, Melnikow, & Howell, 2001). Although the gap is narrowing, rural women continue to have more children than their urban counterparts, as well as experience their first pregnancy at an earlier age (Bescher-Donnelly & Smith, 1981). Therefore, in addition to screening for cervical and breast cancers and general health maintenance, women in this stage of life have needs for adequate birth control, family planning, prenatal care, and childbirth education.

Women of childbearing and childrearing age may experience stress because of multiple demands placed on them by family relationships and home and work responsibilities (Kenney, 2000; Bigbee, 1984). The number of women working outside the home has steadily risen and rural women account for a significant portion of this growth (Walters & McKenry, 1985). Rural women have less educational opportunities and less occupational choices and therefore often work at low-wage jobs (Bescher-Donnelly & Smith, 1981). Rural women working outside the home also have fewer provisions for quality childcare (Bigbee). These factors, added to the primary responsibilities for home and family management, intensify the multiplicity of roles experienced by rural women. Research has indicated that stress and illness may be closely related and multiple stressors can compromise the immune system, therefore putting the individual at increased risk for acute and chronic illnesses (Kenney).

Women oversee their own health care as well as the health care of their family members. Rural women often act as health officers or gatekeepers of health care for the entire family (Bushy, 1993a; Hemard et al., 1998; Tevis, 1994; Ross, 1982). Therefore, the manner in which women conceptualize health is integral to the health and health practices of the family. However, women's perceptions of health have rarely been solicited (Bushy, 1993b, 1994; Ross, 1982).

Long (1993) has emphasized the importance of providing care consistent with the way rural individuals conceptualize health. Little has been written about the health perspectives of women of childbearing and childrearing age in remote rural areas. The purpose of the study described in this chapter was to explore the health perceptions, needs, and behaviors of remote rural women of childbearing and childrearing age living in Montana for greater than 5 years. *Remote rural* was defined as:

> . . . a community with a population of 2,500 or less located 40 miles or further from a city with a population of 50,000 or greater. Remote rural communities do not have a hospital or medical assistance facility. A practicing physician does not reside in a remote rural community. (Koehler, 1998, pp. 238–239)

METHODS

I used grounded theory approach for this study (Byrne, 2001; Chenitz & Swanson, 1986; Strauss & Corbin, 1990). Following approval by the Montana State University–Bozeman Institutional Review Board and after obtaining informed consent, I conducted semistructured interviews with women of childbearing and childrearing age living in remote rural areas in Montana. I knew the initial participants personally and identified other participants through personal contacts. I obtained subsequent participants by using the snowball technique.

Sample

The convenience sample consisted of 11 women aged 28–49 years (M = 37.7 years) who had lived in remote rural communities in Montana for greater than 5 years. An attempt was made to vary the sample as much as possible by contacting potential participants who comprised the full age range appropriate for this study, 18–49 years, as well as by contacting potential participants from different geographical locations within the state.

The communities in which the participants lived had a population of 850 or less. The women had lived in their respective communities 5–40 years with an average length of time in the rural community of 17.9 years.

Educational preparation ranged from 12–18 years (M = 14.7 years) making the participants more educated than the general population of Montanans. Six of the 11 women (54%) held a bachelor's degree and one had a master's degree, whereas an estimated 11.7% of the general Montana population have baccalaureate degrees (U.S. Bureau of the Census, 2000).

All participants were married and had children. Two women worked full-time, five worked part-time, and four were not employed outside the home. All but one woman had children living at home at the time of the study. For the women with children at home, the number of children in the household ranged from one to five. The age of the children who lived at home ranged from 2 months to 17 years (M = 7.7 years).

Nine of the women had health insurance and two did not have any insurance. The participants stated cost as the major factor for lack of insurance. For the nine women with health insurance, seven were part of a family involved in farming, ranching, or small business and all seven women reported that their insurance had a high deductible and premium.

Distance to emergency medical care ranged from 10–114 miles (M = 44.8 miles) with travel time ranging from 12 minutes to 2.5 hours one way. The participants cited the hospital or medical assistance facility located in the nearest large town and ambulance service to the nearest town as their source of emergency care. In addition, the participants identified local individuals with medical training as a source of assistance in an emergency. Rural road conditions, weather conditions, geography, and road construction were some of the variables influencing travel time to emergency care.

Data Collection and Analysis

I conducted four in-person and seven telephone interviews. The questions were open-ended and intended to elicit information regarding the women's health perceptions, needs, and behaviors and how their perceptions and conceptualizations of health affected their health behaviors. I audio taped interviews and later transcribed them. I analyzed the qualitative data for common themes using the methodological technique of grounded theory known as constant comparison (Strauss & Corbin, 1990).

EMERGENT THEMES

Seven themes emerged from the data: (a) distance as a way of life, (b) distance as a disadvantage in an emergency, (c) episodic evaluation, (d) children first, (e) prevention for life, (f) access within reason, and (g) holistic health.

Distance as a Way of Life

The participants identified that distance, although an inconvenience at times, was not a disadvantage. They accepted as part of everyday life that they lived some distance from health care as well as from a variety of other general services. At times it was noted to be inconvenient, but "just the way it is." The women reported "enjoying the lifestyle" that a rural environment provided and the small inconvenience that distance presented in some circumstances was worth the experience of living in a rural setting.

The women reported that distance did not deter them from seeking health care or cause a delay in seeking health care. One participant made the following comments about distance to health care:

If we are sick, if one of the kids is sick, we are going to go to the doctor if we need to. You just get used to living out here so it doesn't make a difference. I mean you think 30 miles, you know you are going to drive there if you are sick and need the health care services or whatever. Just like you do to go out to pizza, you drive to health care.

The distance, it doesn't seem very long [70 miles]. Usually we pick up grandma who is halfway and we always have something else to do besides go to the doctor, like get groceries or something, so it doesn't seem bad.

The women did not find distance to be a significant concern in regard to their past pregnancies and impending deliveries. Although they took some precautions and thought about what the distance might mean, none of the women had specific concerns about their delivery in light of the distance that needed to be traveled to get to the hospital.

I guess growing up 30 miles from town, you know what that is like. So living 60 miles from town now, you don't think about it. It is just the way it is. You know that you have miles to travel and you can get there in around an hour and that is just the way it is. You can't worry about it. My husband wasn't concerned about having to deliver the baby if we didn't make it in time. Our big joke was that he was going to bring the calf pullers in. That is just a typical rancher. We deal with animals all the time. Calving and foaling and little animals and birthing and the whole reproductive situation. I guess it is just a natural thing. It is not something that you dwell on. You think about it, what if something happens, but like I said, you just deal with it if something happens.

When considering distance during pregnancy, the women recalled factors that could cause a delay in their travel, such as weather and road construction. "It was in the back of our minds, what if a storm comes or whatever. You think about it a little bit, but you know also realizing that comes with this lifestyle."

Another issue the women consistently identified about planning for their labor and delivery was the importance of their health care providers being "in tune" to the fact that they lived some distance from the hospital and that their provider helped them plan for their delivery. The women reported that their doctors gave them advice, such as "come in when things start" or "head to town, don't just wait." The women seemed more comfortable with the distance because of their relationship with their health care providers and the fact that their providers appreciated their situation.

Two women had experienced breast cancer in recent years. Although both women had access to health care providers and a hospital within 15 miles, they were forced to travel longer distances to a larger medical center to receive specialized care for cancer. Both women traveled a distance of 60–80 miles, one way, 5 days a week for 6 weeks for radiation treatment. One of the women had to travel for chemotherapy as well. Their perspective on traveling for health care for treatment of a disease was somewhat different from the rest of the sample who only traveled for routine health care, and on a much less frequent basis. For the two women with breast cancer, traveling the longer distance was seen as even more of an inconvenience and somewhat of a disadvantage when considering access to health care. Both women discussed that although the daily travel was an inconvenience, the support of friends and neighbors in the community was an advantage that balanced out the situation for them.

> One problem is that we are kind of far away from certain medical facilities that we might need, but in my case at least making the 80 mile trip for radiation did work out really well because I had the advantage of friends and neighbors who were really helpful. I think that is one advantage of the rural situation. The more specialized things you need to go farther away for. They can handle most things locally, but if you have cancer or heart problems or something that requires more specialized care, then you have to go farther away. You are at a disadvantage in some ways because you are farther from care, but you have got good friends and neighbors to help you out too. I think that is the advantage that maybe people in a larger area wouldn't have.

Although distance was occasionally viewed as an inconvenience, all of the women were accustomed to traveling some distance for general services, routine health care services, and the delivery of their children. If health care was needed, it was obtained. Distance to health care services did not result in a delay in seeking care, if the care was deemed necessary.

Distance as a Disadvantage in an Emergency

All the women verbalized that distance was a distinct disadvantage in the case of an emergency. They were aware that in an emergency distance presented the risk of serious consequences to their health, the health of their family, or even death. They noted, "It would take you awhile to get somewhere," and "It takes time for them to get to you." One woman stated, "You know the distance is there if something really happens." One woman recounted her concern and thought processes during an acute illness experienced by one of her children:

> We were working in the yard and I took my eyes off my son for 2 seconds. The next thing I knew he was throwing up. We took him inside and changed his clothes, but he couldn't stop throwing up and then he was finally throwing up bile and he had a horrible color, pasty white. All the color was out of his lips. I wasn't sure what he had gotten into. We called Ask a Nurse because now he has fallen asleep and we can't really keep him awake between throwing up. They told me to give it 4 hours for whatever it is to work out of his system. His breathing was rapid and shallow and he was unable to stay awake. I was taking his pulse the whole time, for 4 hours that is what I did. Then four hours went by and he woke and said, thirsty, and he was crying. But that was a long 4 hours and then I thought to myself, if he is not okay in 4 hours and they told me to bring him in, and it takes an hour and half to get there, should I leave in 2 hours to be part of that four. I really remember not liking the distance at that moment.

The issue of distance, travel time, and how an emergency would be handled was considered by one woman.

> With us, we live 30 miles out so it would take at least 20 minutes. I am sure they go fast and stuff, but you still can't go that fast. I would never sit with my kid in an emergency and wait for an ambulance. That is at least 45 minutes. It would be an hour by the time they came, put somebody on the

stretcher, put them in the ambulance and got back to town. I couldn't sit there and calmly wait. I would get in the car and just tell them I would meet them. I think I would get them that much closer and sooner to getting help. I would call the ambulance and then I would take off.

The women had also identified individuals in their local communities with medical training who could assist should an emergency arise. They felt these people might be of great assistance in an emergency, especially while waiting for an ambulance to arrive.

Although they consistently identified distance as a disadvantage in emergent situations, they were well aware of the risks involved and accepted this as the one disadvantage to rural life.

I learned early in life that things are going to happen. You are going to have accidents. You just have to deal with it when it happens, whatever the severity of it. If you have an accident, you know you are going to have to wait for the ambulance. If you have to pack somebody up in the pickup and bring them to town, you do it. When you grow up with that and make the decision to live out here, you just take those things into consideration and that is just the way it is.

It is something you live with when you are this far out. You just know that there is always that chance that something real major, a bad emergency, could happen and your chances are a lot slimmer than if you are living right in Billings, Montana.

Episodic Evaluation

A third theme to emerge was episodic evaluation. The women used their experiences and best judgment to consider each injury or illness episode to make a decision about how to manage it. Episodic evaluation was something they did for themselves as well as their children.

For each illness episode, symptoms present, length of the illness, severity of the symptoms, and the progression or resolution of symptoms were considered. The impact of the illness on daily life and whether or not the illness affected their ability to go to work or their children's ability to go to school were factors influencing their decision to seek formal health care. All the women began with informal care or self-care behaviors, such as home remedies and over-the-counter medicines, and illnesses were allowed to "run their course" unless the symptoms progressed, continued for a long period of time, or significantly affected the individual's daily activities.

If someone gets where they are absolutely miserable for a few days and I can see they are not going to shake whatever they have, then we will go. If it is something that is affecting their everyday life or if they are missing school, then I will go see a doctor.

You just kind of see how they are doing. If after a couple of days they don't get better, you take them in. You think we are this far out, what if it gets worse. You would rather have it taken care of than have it get worse and then that is more of an emergent state. Then you think, gosh, we are 30 miles out or whatever. Then 30 miles makes a huge difference.

Most women elicited advice from their mothers, sisters, friends, or neighbors during some illness episodes. The women inquired how others had handled similar situations and the types of treatments that helped resolve the problem. "I talk to my mom. I trust her judgment." "I ask around, see what others have tried." Others sought advice from their health care provider over the telephone.

The women used the same type of episodic evaluation when considering whether an injury could be handled at home or if accessing professional health care was necessary. The type of injury, the quantity of blood involved, and the pain level were factors influencing their decision to handle the injury on their own or see a health care provider.

I have handled kids getting bucked off horses, cuts, and scrapes. You look at how deep it is and try to decide, do we need stitches, or is there a concussion or what. I guess you just assess the situation and it just depends on how bad it is.

If they had initially decided to handle an injury at home, the mothers reevaluated the injury as time went on. They sought formal health care if bleeding continued, the pain worsened, the injury did not seem to be healing, or infection seemed to be present. The women indicated they did not delay seeking care for themselves or their children if the care was deemed necessary.

Children First

The women consistently indicated that they sought health care sooner for their children than they did for themselves. They used the episodic evaluation process with their children just as they did for themselves, but reported that they took their children to a formal health care provider more readily. The women indicated they took their child to the doctor sooner than they would go themselves because it was difficult to judge how someone else was feeling and how the illness was affecting them. This was especially true for younger children and infants who could not verbalize how they were feeling. As children got older, mothers were more inclined to "let things run their course" and to evaluate whether to take them in based on what the child was telling them.

> I definitely take the kids in sooner. I guess because I don't want it to go on too long with them. I don't want them to get sick. You know how you feel yourself, but you don't really know how your child feels. You only know what they tell you and what you observe. I don't like to let it get out of hand.

The women also indicated that they were the one in the family who determined whether a child was ill and if they needed to see a formal health care provider. Mothers were also consistently responsible for taking their children to the doctor. "Mom takes them to the doctor and mom sits in the waiting room." "You deal with it because you are the mom, you are the woman, and you take care of everything. They are your children." These responsibilities were predicated on the fact that mothers spent more time at home with the children than their spouses. "I am more tuned into it because I am with them more during the day. My husband might say, her nose is running or whatever, but I am usually a step ahead of him because I am around more."

Women stated that gauging someone else's illness or pain is difficult to do, particularly when the other person is a very small child. Although they handled many illnesses at home without the help of a formal health care provider, they were quick to seek care if they were unsure about how their child felt or uncertain of the severity of the illness or injury.

Prevention for Life

The women indicated that routine health care and illness prevention strategies were important activities in life. They reported that it was important to detect illness or disease early so that they could be treated properly and have a better chance at a long healthy life. Ten women participated in yearly health screening activities citing prevention as the main reason for choosing to participate in health maintenance activities. Prevention for life was important for "catching things early" and "staying healthy." The women who had experienced breast cancer realized the importance of health maintenance and yearly exams and credited these activities for saving their lives.

The women verbalized they were more aware of the importance of health maintenance activities after becoming mothers because their children relied on them to be healthy and to be there to take care of them. They educated themselves on health issues through a variety of sources and actively sought information, especially on issues of specific importance in their lives. The mothers were primarily responsible for providing health education for their children. Prevention for life was a strategy practiced by the women to keep themselves and their families as healthy as possible.

Access within Reason

All the women believed health care was accessible within reason for the area in which they lived. Most were unable to identify any type of health care service that they wished they had available to them in their local community that was not currently available. Even when considering the disadvantage of distance in an emergency, one participant stated, "We have access. We just have to get there. It just takes time. That is the way it is out here."

Access was also seen as having the ability to obtain advice from someone over the phone, to have questions answered, "flexible hours," and "getting hold of someone if I need to." One woman who did not have health insurance defined access to care as "money and insurance." However, cost was an issue for all women. Seven women who had health insurance reported high premiums and high deductibles and had to pay out-of-pocket for routine health care and office visits. Most stated that their insurance was for "major medical." However, high deductibles did not result in a delay in seeking care for these women. They obtained health care if they believed it to be necessary.

> Having to pay out-of-pocket doesn't keep us from going to the doctor. I want to keep everybody healthy and we will pay for it one way or another, so you might as well go in and get it taken care of early. It doesn't have an effect on whether I go or not just because I know I have to pay for it.

Holistic Health

Health was defined holistically. Good health included (a) a lack of major health problems, (b) minimal or no use of routine medications, (c) being mentally and physically active, and (d) having the ability to perform necessary tasks without limitations or undue stress. Good health also included being (a) physically fit, (b) eating well, and (c) having an overall sense of well-being. Poor health affected day-to-day activities, but most of the women, unless they were experiencing an acute illness episode, did not feel their health had a negative effect on their daily life.

IMPLICATIONS FOR NURSING PRACTICE AND RESEARCH

I identified several implications for nursing practice. First, although distance was perceived as a "way of rural life," health care providers should remain cognizant of the distance and time traveled for routine health care and plan follow-up care accordingly. In addition, nurses and other health care providers should educate expectant mothers on the appropriate precautions to take when traveling to a community where they will deliver their babies.

Second, concerns were raised about the time it took to access care in an emergency. Nurses should explore this issue with rural dwellers. The availability of emergency resources (persons, services) in their local communities should be discussed. Education regarding planning for and handling various emergencies can be addressed during routine health care visits.

Third, the women were clearly interested in maintaining their health and participating in screening activities to identify illness early in the course of a disease process. Therefore, when seen in the office women should be counseled regarding age-appropriate screening activities. Written information regarding preventive health and health maintenance activities for their children should also be offered at each encounter. Other strategies that may be implements to deliver health education include local seminars on women and children's health issues. Providing addresses for Internet-based health information should be included with each educational intervention.

I also identified several implications for nursing research. Distance continues to be an interesting concept in the rural literature. Much controversy remains as to the impact of distance on health care utilization and whether individuals who live at increasing distances from health care engage in more self-care behaviors and delay seeking formal health care. Further research is warranted concerning this concept; comparison between rural women and their urban counterparts may provide important information about similarities and differences in self-care behaviors and utilization of formal health care.

Other areas to explore include the experience of illness and the effect of stress on the lives of childbearing and childrearing remote rural women. The women in this study who suffered from breast cancer and traveled for treatment viewed distance as more inconvenient than the women who traveled less frequently for routine health care. They also verbalized significant community support that counterbalanced the inconvenience of daily travel of 60 miles or more, one way. Furthermore, the women were not specifically questioned regarding their stress level. The health perceptions of women of childbearing and childrearing age who have suffered from a life-threatening illness or have experienced stress have rarely been solicited and may add valuable data to the rural health literature.

Finally, research is needed that addresses the health perceptions, needs, and behaviors of rural childbearing and childrearing women who live in different geographical areas and at varying distances from health care services. The health needs of women in their early childbearing years may differ from those who are raising older children. Therefore, more research is needed to understand further the health perceptions, needs, and behaviors of women in this stage of life.

REFERENCES

Bescher-Donnelly, L., & Smith, L. W. (1981). The changing roles and status of rural women. In R. T. Coward & W. Smith, Jr., *The family in rural society* (pp. 167–186). Boulder, CO: Westview Press.

Bigbee, J. L. (1984). The changing role of rural women: Nursing and health implications. *Health Care for Women International, 5,* 307–322.

Bushy, A. (1993a). Defining rural before tackling access issues. *The American Nurse, 25* (8), 20.

Bushy, A. (1993b). Rural women: Lifestyle and health status. *The Nursing Clinics of North America, 28* (1), 187–197.

Bushy, A. (1994). Women in rural environments: Considerations for holistic nurses. *Holistic Nursing Practice, 8* (4), 67–73.

Byrne, M. (2001). Grounded theory as a qualitative research methodology. *Association of Operating Room Nurses, 73* (6), 1155. Retrieved October 22, 2001, from Expanded Academic ASAP@http://www.galegroup.com

Chenitz, W. C., & Swanson, J. M. (1986). *From practice to grounded theory: Qualitative research in nursing.* Menlo Park, CA: Addison-Wesley.

Health Resources and Services Administration (HRSA). (2002). *Health Professional Shortage Areas (HPSAs).* Retrieved April 10, 2002, from http: //belize.hrsa.gov/newhpsa/newhpsa.cfm#

Health Resources and Services Administration (HRSA). (2004). *The Health Care Workforce in Eight States: Education, Practice and Policy Project Description.*

Health Resources and Services Administration (HRSA). (2009). *Health Professionals Shortage Areas (HPSAs).* Retrieved February 27, 2009, from http://hpsafind.hrsa.gov/HPSASearch.aspx

Hemard, J. B., Monroe, P. A., Atkinson, E. S., & Blalock, L. B. (1998). Rural women's satisfaction and stress as family health care gatekeepers. *Women and Health, 28,* 55–73.

Kenney, J. W. (2000). Women's 'inner balance': A comparison of stressors, personality traits and health problems by age groups. *Journal of Advanced Nursing, 31,* 639–650.

Koehler, V. (1998). The substantive theory of protecting independence. In H. J. Lee (Ed.), *Conceptual basis for rural nursing* (pp. 236–256). New York: Springer.

Long, K. A. (1993). The concept of health: Rural perspectives. *The Nursing Clinics of North America, 28* (1), 123–131.

Montana Office of Rural Health. (1999). *Montana Statistics.* Retrieved October 21, 2001, from http://healthinfo.montana.edu/ruralhealth/default.html

Montana Office of Rural Health. (2008). *Montana Physicians.* Retrieved February 27, 2009, from http://healthinfo.montana.edu/Montana%20Physicians.html

Nuovo, J., Melnikow, J., & Howell, L. P. (2001). New tests for cervical cancer screening. *American Family Physician, 64,* 780–786.

Ross, H. M. (1982). *Women and wellness: Defining, attaining, and maintaining health in eastern Canada.* Unpublished doctoral dissertation, University of Washington, Seattle.

Strauss, A., & Corbin, J. (1990). *Basics of qualitative research: Grounded theory procedures and techniques.* Newbury Park, CA: Sage.

Tevis, C. (1994). Partners for health and safety. *Successful Farming, 92* (8), 1–2, 57–58. Retrieved October 22, 2001, from Expanded Academic ASAP@http://www.galegroup.com

U.S. Bureau of the Census. (2000). *Census 2000 data for the state of Montana.* Retrieved October 21, 2001, from http://www.census.gov/census2000/states/mt.html

Veitch, P. C. (1995). Anticipated response to three common injuries by rural and remote area residents. *Social Science and Medicine, 41,* 739–745.

Walters, C. M., & McKenry, P. C. (1985). Predictors of life satisfaction among rural and urban employed mothers: A research note. *Journal of Marriage and Family, 47,* 1067–1071.

Weinert, C., & Long, K. A. (1990). Rural families and health care: Refining the knowledge base. *Marriage and Family Review, 15,* 57–75.

Wilcox, L. S., & Mosher, W. D. (1993). Factors associated with obtaining health screening among women of reproductive age. *Public Health Reports, 108,* 1–10, 76–86. Retrieved October 21, 2001, from Expanded Academic ASAP@http://www.galegroup.com

Rural and Remote Women and Resilience: Grounded Theory and Photovoice Variations on a Theme

7

BEVERLY D. LEIPERT

Canada is the second largest country in the world, and approximately 22% of its population resides in rural and remote areas (Canadian Institute for Health Information [CIHI], 2006). In this vast country, health status declines as one moves farther from urban centers (Romanow, 2002). Rural people have shorter life expectancies, lower incomes, fewer years of education, more social isolation, and higher rates of crime, death, infant mortality, unemployment, smoking, alcohol consumption, and obesity compared to the national average (CIHI; Health Canada, 2003; Northern Secretariat of the BC Centre of Excellence for Women's Health, 2000).

Rural women must address these issues in various ways in order to maintain and promote their health. In this chapter, I explore the resilience of women in rural and remote Canada as perceived and depicted in two research studies conducted with rural women in northern British Columbia (NBC study) and southwest Ontario (SWO study).

PURPOSES OF THE STUDIES

The purpose of the NBC study was to examine how women perceive and maintain their health within geographical, social, economic, and other contexts within northern British Columbia (BC), Canada. The purpose of the SWO study was to explore the nature of pictorial and descriptive data about social and health promotion needs and resources provided by older rural women in southwest Ontario using the photovoice method. The resilience of rural women emerged as a theme in both studies.

METHODS

Both studies were guided by a feminist theoretical approach. Feminist inquiry considers not only women's individual voices and experiences, but also larger sociopolitical, economic, and cultural structures that influence women's lives (MacDonald, 2001). The NBC study also used a grounded theory method to identify and describe complex and hidden processes (Morse, 2001) related to rural and northern women's health. The SWO study used a unique method called photovoice which was developed specifically for research with rural women (Wang, Burris, & Ping, 1996). Using this method, cameras were provided to participants so that they could take pictures of social and health promotion needs and resources in their rural communities (Leipert, Landry, McWilliam, et al., under review). The women also recorded perspectives in log books and participated in two focus groups to discuss the pictorial and narrative data and their perspectives.

Setting

The NBC study included both urban and rural settings in northern BC. Northern rural settings are characterized as rural, rural remote, and rural isolated. Rural communities have a population of less than 1,000 people with less than 400 people per square kilometer (Statistics Canada, 1993). Rural remote communities are 80–400 kilometers or 1–4 hours travel in good weather to a major regional hospital (Canadian Association of Emergency Physicians, Rural Committee, 1997). Rural isolated communities are more than 400 kilometers or 4 hours travel in good weather to a major regional hospital (Rennie, Baird-Crooks, Remus, & Engel, 2000). In the north, both urban and rural settings are considered remote and isolated because of their distant location from health care and other resources.

The SWO study was conducted in four counties in southwest Ontario. These counties are considered rural because they are "outside of urban centres with 10,000 or more population" (du Plessis, Beshiri, & Bollman, 2002, p.1). Although distances are less and the number of people are greater in southwest Ontario compared to northern BC, southwest Ontario is still considered rural because farmland covers 75% of the land area (Turner & Gutmanis, 2005) and major amounts of agricultural products are grown there (Caldwell, Brown, Thomson, & Auld, 2006).

Sample

In the NBC study, the sample was constructed using theoretical sampling (Glaser, 1978) and consisted of 25 women who had lived in northern settings for a minimum of 2 years. The women were aged 21–86 years (the majority within 41–60 years), had less than Grade 9 to university education, and had incomes of less than \$10,000 ($n = 2$) to over \$60,000 ($n = 5$). The women reported Aboriginal, Métis, South Asian, British, Swiss, and Canadian cultural backgrounds. The majority of the women were married or living common law, employed full-time or part-time, and in good health. Two-thirds ($n = 17$) of the study participants resided in rural and remote settings (farms, ranches) as well as in villages of less than 100 residents and in small towns, whereas the remaining one-third ($n = 8$) of the participants resided in Prince George, population 75,000, the only city in the north.

In the SWO study, purposeful snowball sampling (Patton, 2002) was used to create a sample of 31 women who ranged in age from 55 to 89 years, had less than Grade 9 to a university degree, and had incomes of less than \$10,000 ($n = 1$) to over \$50,000 ($n = 3$) (not all participants answered all of the sociodemographic questions). The women claimed Aboriginal, Mennonite, Dutch, Belgian, and Canadian cultural backgrounds. The majority of the women were widowed ($n = 18$), lived in towns of 250 to 7,500 residents ($n = 14$) or on farms ($n = 4$), and reported good ($n = 11$) or excellent ($n = 8$) health.

Data Collection

Prior to data collection in the NBC study, ethical approval was obtained from the University of Alberta Health Research Ethics Board and University of Northern British Columbia Ethics Review Board. Narrative data were then collected through semistructured interviews using open-ended questions; observational data were also collected during travels to interviews on farms and ranches and in northern communities as well as from written documents, such as maps, tourist guides, community histories, and newspapers (Leipert, 2006). Each participant was interviewed three times; the first interview was in person and the second and third interviews were predominantly by telephone. The first and second interviews were taped and transcribed, then imported into the NVivo

(Version 1) computer program for analysis. Pseudonyms selected by each woman were used in transcribing to protect participants' identities. Notes taken during third interviews and memos containing researcher reflections subsequent to interviews were also collected.

Prior to data collection in the SWO study, ethical approval was obtained from the University of Western Ontario Health Research Ethics Board. The 31 participants consisted of five groups in four rural communities. Each group participated in two group interview sessions; both group sessions were audio taped. In the first group session, the research was explained and cameras were demonstrated and provided to the women, along with log books for recording perspectives (Leipert et al., under review). Participants were invited to photograph images and record reflections in log books about social and health promotion needs and resources for older rural women in rural settings. After two weeks, the cameras and log books were retrieved and the films were developed. At the second group session, the photos were returned to the women, and they were invited to select two images: one that best represented a social and health promotion need and one that best represented a social and health promotion resource. Participants were asked for titles for each of these pictures and discussion ensued as to the meaning of the pictures and their importance regarding social and health promotion needs and resources of rural older women. The second interview session concluded with participants completing a brief sociodemographic questionnaire.

Data Analysis

In the NBC study, analysis was conducted concurrently with data collection and followed the grounded theory constant comparative method (Glaser, 1978, 1992). With the assistance of the NVivo (1999) computer program, I reviewed interview transcripts line by line and coded them for categories and themes. Participants clarified, elaborated upon, and verified emerging categories, subcategories, and relationships in second and third interviews. A fourth interview was conducted with three participants for verification of the theory that emerged in the study (Leipert, 2006). Analysis and data collection ceased when no new information or insight was forthcoming about the categories and their relationships and when the theory seemed to be elaborate in complexity and clear in its articulation of the central problem and the process used to address it (Glaser, 1978).

In the SWO study, data were analyzed using a rigorous three-phase process. In the first phase, the second group interview participants: (1) identified key data by selecting their photos, (2) contextualized data by explaining the meaning of their photos, and (3) codified data by identifying issues, concepts, themes, and theories (Wang & Burris, 1997). These audio taped data were transcribed and, in the second phase, were analyzed by a minimum of two researchers using NVivo to determine themes related to rural social and health promotion needs and resources (Leipert et al., under review). As a result of this analysis, themes related to rural women and resilience also emerged. In the third phase, a three-stage analysis process (Oliffe, Bottorff, Kelly & Halpin, 2008) was used. In the first stage, *preview,* the researchers viewed participants' photographs alongside the narratives about each picture in order to understand intended representations and to situate the participants within the context of their photographs. In the second stage, *cross-photo comparison,* the researchers developed themes that were reflected in the entire photograph collection. We reviewed the total data set of 575 usable pictures taken by the participants. The final stage, *theorizing,* allowed the researchers to develop abstract understandings by linking the themes to the feminist theoretical approach of the study. As resilience began to emerge as an important theme in the original analysis, the photos were reanalyzed using this rigorous three-stage process to determine more consistently and accurately findings regarding rural women and resilience.

Limitations

A limitation of the NBC study is the exclusion of non-English speaking women; for both the NBC and SWO studies representation of various groups of women, such as very remote women, lesbian women, and women who live in extreme poverty, were limited. In addition, the grounded theory and photovoice methods used in the two research studies differed to some degree. Nonetheless, data analysis in both studies revealed rich information regarding the resilience of rural women in two diverse locations in Canada.

FINDINGS

The NBC Study

The findings and theory that emerged regarding resilience in the NBC study have been elaborated elsewhere (Leipert, 2006). Only some elements of the theory will be summarized here; the main focus in this section of the chapter will be on the findings regarding the nature of the resilience revealed by the women in the NBC study.

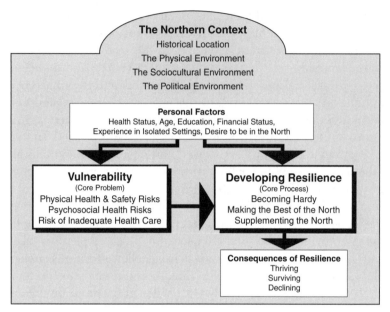

Figure 7.1. Northern Canadian women's health: Developing resilience to manage vulnerability.

The intent of grounded theory is to generate a theory that explains a process of how individuals respond to a main concern or problem (Glaser, 1978). The main problem for the women in this study was vulnerability to health risks, in particular, physical health and safety risks, psychosocial health risks, and risks of inadequate health care. Women responded to these health risks by developing a process of resilience which included strategies of becoming hardy, making the best of the north, and supplementing the north (Leipert, 2006) (see Figure 7.1).

Developing Resilience

In response to vulnerability to health risks, women in the study engaged in a core process of developing resilience. This process involved strategies of becoming hardy, making the best of the north, and supplementing the north.

Becoming Hardy

Becoming hardy for northern women involved taking a positive attitude, following spiritual beliefs, developing fortitude, and establishing self-reliance. Taking a positive attitude helped women put northern challenges into perspective and deal with them, thereby enhancing their commitment to northern life. Spiritual beliefs provided personal comfort, meaning and balance, opportunities for cultural and social connections, and a sense of peace, control, care, and belonging. Spirituality included religious and cultural beliefs, as well as friendships, personal reflection, and communing with nature. Establishing self-reliance increased women's confidence, courage, and skills to tackle new and difficult challenges. Examples of self-reliant strategies included learning to drive, using various strategies to defend oneself against wildlife and threatening humans in isolated settings, and learning to suture wounds if women lived in remote locations.

Women were better able to develop hardiness if they were healthy and motivated to be in the north, could address isolation and other northern context issues, were able to learn about and purchase resources, and had a social support network. Women who were ill, in low income or remote situations, worked outdoors, or traveled on isolated or winter roads were especially challenged in becoming hardy. Adequate personal and social resources were essential in becoming hardy. Carmen noted, "You have to have an upbeat attitude. What makes you hardy is the fact that you don't dwell on the fact that you're living where it's cold and remote"; Lilac recommended "having things to amuse you at home in winter"; and Gert valued "the company of women."

Making the Best of the North
Making the best of the north meant that women used and developed available resources and opportunities. These included participating in northern activities, making decisions about health care services, seeking education and information, seeking and providing social support, and working on financial and employment issues.

Women participated in northern activities by (a) enjoying the ready access to outdoor activities, such as camping and hiking; (b) developing indoor interests, such as quilting, painting, and computer use; and (c) volunteering for community groups. Sometimes making the best of the north through participation required a conscious effort. Carmen explained, "When you live in more remote areas, you have to make yourself be positive. It's not something that just happens." For example, Carmen planned trips to Prince George for entertainment and "to do something different."

Study participants made a variety of decisions about health care. They tried to circumvent inadequate care by seeking a second opinion from another physician or by changing their physician. These circumventions were not always possible because of a scarcity of physicians and physician refusals in small communities to provide advice to patients of colleagues. Women also sought the more accessible and sometimes more appropriate services of public health nurses. Public health nurses were valued because they were "approachable" and took a "holistic approach to health" (Rosie), and because they accorded time, education, and respect to women. Other times, women sought health care in another northern community or outside the north. However, women with low incomes and women who were older, ill, or disabled often had to settle for inadequate care provided locally. To supplement the limited health care in the north, and because alternative therapies were believed to be legitimate in their own right, women also made decisions to use alternative health care such as massage and naturopathic options. Health needs, age, cultural and educational backgrounds, economic circumstances, available time, and their knowledge about care accessibility and quality influenced women's decisions about health care.

Women also developed resilience by seeking education and information from nurses, physicians, universities, community colleges, and distance education programs. Education and information helped to change attitudes, enhanced job and career opportunities, increased knowledge and abilities regarding health and health care, and enriched quality of life. Factors that affected women's ability to access educational resources included women's geographic location; their access to finances for tuition and travel; time for study and travel; and access to technology, such as electricity, telephones, computers, roads, and automobiles.

Social support provided women with instrumental (practical), emotional, affirmational, and informational resources (House & Kahn, 1985). Marie explained, "When people in the north go out of town shopping, they always ask their friends, 'Is there anything you want me to pick up for you?'" Signe noted that it was important "to find somebody to talk to, to ease the loneliness of the long dreary winters." Frequently, northern residents had left extended family to seek employment in the north. Thus, friends often took the place of family. In addition, social support, especially by women, helped women who were new to a community become an insider and thus better able to secure friends, information, support, employment, and other resources.

Financial and work issues included limited employment options for women, lack of child care, male attitudes about what women can and should do, inadequate remuneration, lack of respect, sexual harassment at work, and reluctance of communities to employ women who were new to the community. The boom and bust nature of northern resource-based economies compromised job prospects for men, with resultant financial implications for their female partners. Study participants addressed these limitations by engaging in diverse full-time and part-time employment in both the public and private sector. Part-time work decreased risks by decreasing travel in dangerous climates and terrains and helped women maintain control and make the most of their talents, interests, and opportunities. However, part-time employment also decreased women's incomes.

Nevertheless, women in the study illustrated that through resourcefulness, assertiveness, and effective decision making, part-time and full-time work sometimes improved their financial and employment situations. For example, Casey capitalized on her computer and ranching resources and developed part-time employment "helping a friend do a seed catalogue, babysitting, baking, I [have] eggs and we have hay. . . ." Ruhi developed assertiveness skills to deal with harassment at her restaurant job, and other women made decisions to work part-time, change jobs, or do volunteer work to address employment situations. With adequate incomes, women were better able to access health resources both near and far.

Supplementing the North

Supplementing the north involved being political (personally and for the community) and leaving the north, temporarily or permanently. Supplementing the north included adding to, as well as changing, what presently existed in the north, thereby enriching northern resources and minimizing vulnerability.

The main mode of political action used was that of advocacy, speaking out for themselves and others. Leah advised, "It's important to learn to advocate for yourself with your doctor," and Casey believed that "being your own advocate will take you far." Women engaged in community advocacy to increase awareness about and access to resources. Community advocacy activities included participating in Take Back the Night walks, subscribing to and writing for a regional publication that focused on northern women's interests, and serving as a member of a community committee that met with the Premier of the province about local health matters. Participation in this research was also seen as a political act. Eileen explained, "Women up here feel disempowered, under, and invisible . . . this research will help women become more visible to themselves and that's part of becoming more empowered." Women needed time and finances, as well as commitment, courage, assertiveness, and tact to be successful as political activists in and for northern communities.

Leaving the north temporarily was a strategy that every participant used to decrease exposure to vulnerabilities and to supplement resources. Obtaining health care in southern locations increased the quality, timeliness, and appropriateness of care, and for women who required special or more diverse care, their ability to obtain any care at all. Goods and services obtained from southern locations increased women's quality of life by increasing choices and decreasing costs of living in the north. Women who were able to travel to vacations and events outside the north brought back expertise and experiences that enriched their lives and the lives of other northerners. Women who were poor, ill, or very geographically isolated often had greater need to leave the north; however, their ability to leave was also compromised by their needs and circumstances.

Leaving the north permanently was a resilient strategy because it required courage and self-assertion to leave friends and family and an established life in the north. Leaving permanently was a strategy that was considered especially salient for single women and for women who wanted enriched education, employment, and sociocultural options. Eileen, a single mother, was considering leaving because she felt that people in her community "look at single moms as having made mistakes, not quite fitting in, as being peripheral." Marie, a single retired woman, was looking forward to leaving the "redneck rough crude" north to lead "the quality of life I want to lead." Leah, a young single woman, was moving south where "all my friends are" and where she could access desired education. Although leaving permanently may increase women's resources and quality of life, their leaving would mean that the north would lose vital resources—women with an informed vision of how northern women's health could and should be advanced.

Women's location within the northern context, the degree of vulnerability they experienced, and personal factors (age, health and financial status, and cultural background) affected the degree to which women could develop and use resilient strategies. Although older women and women who were isolated, ill, or poor experienced greater vulnerability to health risks and a greater need for resilience, their ability to be resilient was compromised by their situations. Thus, those with the greatest needs were often the least able to address their needs.

The SWO Study

Similar to the NBC study, rural older women in the SWO study also experienced vulnerability risks. Physical health and safety risks were associated with poor climate, especially in winter; broken sidewalks and limited rails along walking trails, which contributed to unsafe sites for physical exercise; and spraying and other farming practices. For Aboriginal women, the increased use of alcohol and other drugs on their reserve contributed to physical health risks not only for the users but also for women who lived close by. Although most of the women were retired, and thus not employed, one woman in her 80s still actively farmed and, although she did not comment on employment risks to her health, working around farm machinery could pose a risk to her physical health.

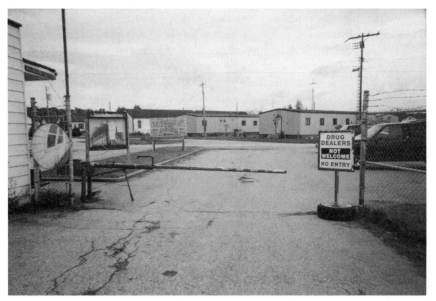

Figure 7.2. Drug dealers not welcome.

Psychosocial health risks were perhaps a larger concern for women in the SWO study. Although they were not as geographically isolated from each other compared to the NBC participants, nonetheless for this group of older rural women isolation was an issue. Isolation from friends and family due to limited transportation or the inability to no longer drive, lack of access to family members such as spouses who were deceased or in distant long-term care facilities, limited abilities to travel in winter, and not having access to exercise resources in winter, such as an indoor pool, contributed to feelings of loneliness and depression. Histories of abuse and neglect experienced by Mennonite and Aboriginal women and the frequent closure of rural churches contributed to mental health and spiritual concerns. The following quotes illustrate these issues:

> All our children . . . were raised there. . . . We went . . . across the road to the church all the time. I don't know what I'll do when they close [the church]. . . . We bought [our home here] because we figured the church would be there . . . you could walk [across the road] to church in your old age but you can't do that I guess. . . .
>
> I got married . . . had eight children. . . . This was not [a] very good . . . marriage . . . my husband left . . . I was always scared of him, all the time. . . . Until we finally came across the border [from Mexico] into the States . . . I finally felt better . . . I didn't have to watch all the time.
>
> Residential schools . . . caused a significant loss in native cultural/identity. This can be seen in areas such as language, parenting skills, family and community values and roles, loss of living in ancestral land base, day to day living values and belief systems. [The] inflict[ion]of physical, psychological, emotional and sexual abuse . . . resulted in . . . generations of mental health issues . . . post traumatic stress disorders . . . all of these factors have affected me during my childhood, youth, adult life and as a senior.

The older rural women in this study also experienced risks of inadequate health care. Closure of pharmacies in rural communities, lack of access to hospitals that were close by, and poor or distant long-term care facilities were major areas of concern. The following quote illustrates this latter issue:

> This is the nursing home where my husband lived. The reason we chose [it] is because it was close to where we lived. . . . [When it closed] we had to take the first one that came up . . . 23 km away [from home].

Developing Resilience

Becoming Hardy

The older rural women in this study also developed hardiness as they took a positive attitude and followed spiritual beliefs, as exhibited in the numerous comments ("I go to church every Sunday . . . I feel it helps me when I pray. I feel if there's any problems in your family, you know, it's like a support to you . . . that's my opinion.") and pictures of rural churches, and bibles (especially in the pictures taken by the Mennonite women); developed fortitude; and established self-reliance.

One woman spoke about the importance that taking a nursing aide course had been for her in her younger years and the challenges she endured in order to take this course, "Well I had always wanted to be a nurse from the time I was twelve years old. . . . [Being an RNA] changed my life. . . . It gives me more incentive of living now [in my senior years]." The fortitude and self-reliance that this woman exhibited resulted in a sense of accomplishment and pride in her ability to care for others and to complete an education program especially when almost overwhelmed with childbearing, child care, and farming responsibilities.

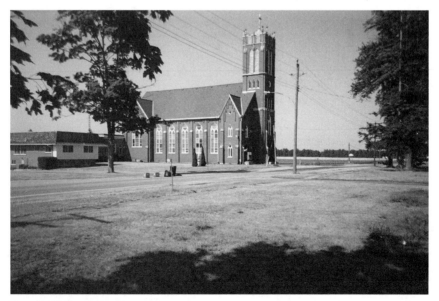

Figure 7.3. Rural church.

Another woman, aged 83, revealed elements of fortitude and self-reliance in her narratives of active farming and tractor driving activities, "I used to work nights all the time. . . . I loved to come home . . . jump on the tractor . . . go out to the fields . . . think . . . I can watch the birds . . . the trees . . . the sand blow, how relaxing to get away from the stressful night's work."

The hardiness of one of the Aboriginal women was revealed in the poetry she wrote in which she addressed past injustices and hopes for the future:

> *Our hopes and dreams*
> *became a war zone . . .*
> *May our Nation*
> *give us peace in heart*
> *As we come together*
> *from a broken promise*
> *We speak with one voice*
> *through the wisdom*
> *Given to us by our ancestors*
> *many moons back.*
> *Arise, and come together*
> *our First nation*
> *Together we'll heal from*
> *a broken promise*
> *Let our drums beat*
> *coming together lock*
> *Step of the way: stamping*
> *our feet, good spirits coming together.*

These activities helped the women contribute to their families and communities in the past and in the present, and gave them a sense of accomplishment, pride, independence, and agency.

Of all the above attributes of hardiness, perhaps the most important attributes for participants in this study were their attitudes toward themselves and their past and present lives. The women in this study frequently spoke about the importance of accepting some of life's situations, not engaging in self-pity, and enjoying what one has without constantly striving to have more and better, as these quotes exemplify:

I am happy. I have a good life. We are going through hard times but, hey, that's life. But I am not unhappy because of circumstance. I'm glad we came to Canada.

I think everyone here has been a role model in some way to family or friends and yet there may be a reluctance to claim that, to say that you've done that, even though you have been a role model . . . none of us really see ourselves as a leader . . . [but] as a mother or a daughter or anything you are a leader no matter how you look at it.

These attitudes provided peace of mind as well as the ability to be inspired and objective when considering issues and ways to address them. The many challenging situations with which the participants in this study engaged throughout the course of their lives, and the many ways they needed to develop resilience in the past to address difficult circumstances no doubt provided rich experience that formed the basis for these hardy attitudes. For example, participants had experienced extreme poverty, societal discrimination, oppression and abuse by spouses, issues related to adapting to a new country, having to learn a new language (English), raising a (often large) family in challenging circumstances, and making new friends in a new land. Thus, life experiences and fortitude developed over the years in stressful and

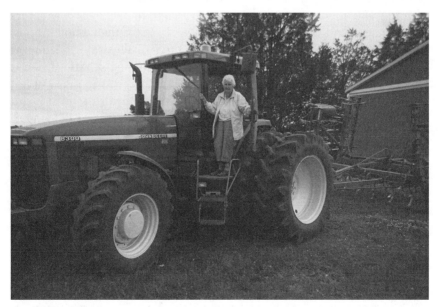

Figure 7.4. The love of John Deere.

challenging circumstances may assist in the development of resilience for a satisfying older age in rural contexts.

Making the Best of the Rural Context

Several women in the study were proud of their ability to drive, even if this was only during the good weather and road conditions in the summer. For women who were older, who lived alone, and who lived in an area where resources were decreasing or nonexistent, being able to drive afforded them access to resources in other communities and social support from friends and families. A participant summarized the perspectives of most of the women in the study when she stated, "Without wheels, we're stuck. We can't go anywhere . . . there's no bus stopping where I live. . . . When stores are closing . . . and no new stores come in . . . makes you feel like there's something missing. . . . Like you can't get what you would get, say, in a larger community."

Examples of titles that participants gave to pictures related to their vehicle included "My Best Companion" and "Freedom." Women with sufficient funds were able to purchase electric carts that helped them get around in town situations, although these were of limited use in more rural and unpaved contexts.

Participants enjoyed the outdoors, especially in the summer. The planting and tending of gardens was a major theme in the women's development and enactment of resilience. Titles of their photographs, such as "Peace/Happiness" and "My Sanctuary," illustrate the importance of gardens to these women, as do their comments: "My garden is like my haven . . . my peace of mind. . . . It's the best way to relax, sit out there and read. . . . Look at the flowers in the morning. . . . It's just beautiful"; and "My little garden creates a feeling of peace and enjoyment which of course, makes me happy and healthy."

In addition, participants enjoyed physical activities such as swimming in the neighborhood or their own outdoor pools, lawn bowling, biking, and walking. These activities helped them stay physically healthy, facilitated mental health as they interacted with grandchildren, neighbors, and friends, and helped participants support future generations, as this participant remarked:

> I believe in setting a good example [for my grandchildren] for their physical health. . . . The other day my daughters were talking to me and they said, 'Our parents have taught us to be physical [and] they're still in their 70's . . .

and we have all followed suit'. . . I do feel good that they have all . . . said to me that I have been a good example.

Participants also believed that it was important for one's mental health to keep busy in the winter months, when it was more difficult and risky for older people to be physically active outdoors. Some of the resilient activities in winter included meeting with friends for card and board games, quilting, baking gatherings, and indoor exercise classes.

In addition, pets, such as birds, dogs, and cats, provided companionship and meaning to their lives, and helped participants be resilient in the face of isolation and loneliness brought about through the loss of a spouse or the enforced isolation of being housebound in winter. Titles of pictures of pets revealed how important they were to participants, for example "Joy," "Happiness," and "The Loves of My Life."

Participants were also able to be resilient in the face of adversity and health challenges because of their contributions from and to their communities. For women who lived alone, helpful neighbors who could be relied on to do chores, such as check smoke detectors and pick up groceries in winter, were essential and very much appreciated: "My

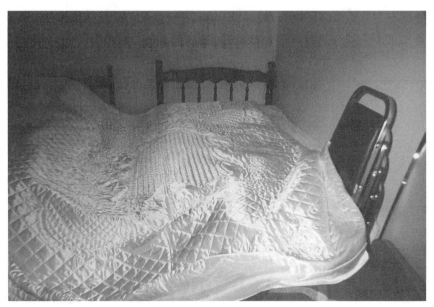

Figure 7.5. Made out of love.

neighbor . . . [helped] change the battery on the smoke alarm. . . . Women that live alone need to have good friends and neighbors . . . we get so we depend on them."

Home delivery of prescription drugs by pharmacies and access to local or home visiting health care resources such as nurses, massage therapists, and housekeeping services were also very welcome. Because participants were assisted in these and other ways to be resilient and independent, and because they could see the need for and the value of their contributions, participants were able and eager to give back to their rural communities. Thus, they contributed in many and several ways, including assisting at church and other community events, volunteering at community agencies such as the Mennonite Central Committee which provides clothing and other resources to the Mennonite community, and providing services such as transportation to others in the community.

Supplementing the Rural Context

Participants supplemented the resources in their rural communities by traveling to other towns and cities for goods and services. They also

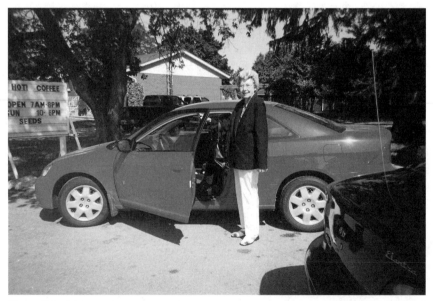

Figure 7.6. Driving to keep an appointment.

provided transportation to others and often carpooled so that they could access distant resources.

Women with sufficient funds valued traveling to warmer climates in winter so as to avoid dealing with winter challenges ("I'm very fortunate that I am in Florida in the wintertime, but not everybody's that fortunate"). Participants who did not have access to funds for travel supplemented their resilience, especially during the isolating winter months, by cultivating enjoyment of local available resources such as seniors centers and in their creation of activities that could be experienced individually or with others, such as quilting, cooking, watching TV, reading, and enjoying pets. In addition, some women who still actively farmed enhanced their safety and peace of mind by learning to use technology as this 83-year-old participant noted:

> What's helping more is the younger farmers all have cell phones in their tractors. If you get alarmed, you can phone 'em . . . or they can phone you. . . . They've got me educated on how to use one 'cause I'm out driving the tractor. . . . He [her son] can phone me and say 'Are you alright mother?'

Whether and how participants wanted to, needed to, or could supplement the rural context with resilient approaches depended on several factors. Women who were healthy could physically manage to access distant resources such as health care and shopping. Women who needed health care resources were often compromised in their ability to be resilient and travel, especially in winter, to health care resources which were at a distance. Women with financial and social resources could purchase what they needed, rather than do without or with limited or delayed resources available more locally; occasionally, friends, spouses, and children assisted with funds and support. Several women in the study, especially those who were older and more isolated and the First Nations and Mennonite women, depended on their spiritual beliefs and each other to help them be resilient so that they could meet needs or develop acceptance of limitations, as these comments indicate: "My church is the most important part of my physical, mental, social and general well being. . . . I travel quite a long distance to attend services. . . ." And, "When [I] go to church, I feel him [my husband] in the seat with me . . . he's not there but . . . he is in spirit. . . ." Another said,

> I believe that to have a healthy sense of well being, it has to be holistic including social/emotional, physical, cognitive and spiritual. Native people . . .

embrace their spirituality in a strong and meaningful sense . . . usually in a belief system that can be Native Traditional, or Christian belief. In our community most people chose one of these belief systems [for] a sense of identity, belonging, and self worth.

DISCUSSION AND IMPLICATIONS FOR NURSING

Findings from both of these studies revealed that rural women in the NBC study and the SWO study develop resilience in response to a number of factors, such as life experiences, stages in life, resources and needs, and the nature of rural contexts. Although the nature and degree of resilience may have varied according to participant circumstance, geographical location, and other factors, the elements of resilience of *becoming hardy, making the best of the context,* and *supplementing the context* remained relevant for women in both rural settings.

The findings also reveal some interesting differences in resilience between the two research groups. Participants in the north tended to develop and experience resilience in more geographically challenging environments that included vast distances, difficult terrain, extreme weather, presence of wild animals, and sparse populations and resources. Although participants in the south also experienced some of these challenges, such as those related to weather and limited resources, the challenges were less extreme. For example, the weather in southwest Ontario is not as cold in winter and the cold does not last as long as in northern BC. Accordingly, and perhaps because of the increased age of the participants in the SWO study compared to those in the NBC study, the resilience developed and enacted by the participants in the SWO study tended to be more affected by age and mobility issues. In addition, the challenges faced by Aboriginal and Mennonite women in the SWO study illustrate the need to understand cultural experiences, needs, and resources, and how these might affect the nature of the resilience developed by women in various cultures. These differences, to name only three, influence how, when, and if rural women need to and can develop resilience, and obviously have implications for the nature of rural nursing practice within these contexts. Clearly, more research is needed to understand effects of the rural geographical location on the resilience of rural women of various ages, cultures, abilities, and needs. In addition, future research should explore how rural nurses can and do facilitate the development of rural women's resilience.

It must be noted that the diverse research methods used in these two studies provide differing types of data which can both enrich and limit understanding. For example, the in-depth repeated one-on-one interviews conducted in the NBC study facilitated participants' expressions of intimate and complex perspectives and experiences, whereas the focus group method used in the SWO study facilitated an overview perspective (Morgan & Krueger, 1998) (although several women did share intimate details of their lives in the group interviews and log books). The use of the photovoice method in the SWO study provided rich pictorial data that enhanced data collection, analysis and understanding, and dissemination and impact of findings. Thus, the diverse methods used revealed important data regarding rural women and resilience and serve to recommend the notion that combining two research approaches (such as grounded theory individual interviews and photovoice focus group interviews in combination with participants' pictures and log book recordings) in subsequent studies could provide enhanced understanding of the nature and context of rural women's resilience.

The SWO study revealed that the photovoice method includes some value added features. Throughout the study, photovoice contributed to the development of enhanced knowledge, social support, confidence, agency, and resilience. Participants often remarked upon the value of participating in the photovoice study, how they had learned and grown, and how participation in the study enhanced their lives, "I had a chance to do something with other women . . . it gives me a chance to think for myself"; and "[It was] very interesting. . . . Educational. . . . You're not alone in your thoughts . . . [you] get other points of view [of different people]."

To facilitate ongoing development of SWO participants' resilience and community change, a Booklet of Findings will be provided to each participant. This booklet, which will include a summary of the study findings and examples of quotes and photos, can be used by participants to illustrate to health care practitioners, policy-makers, and local officials, such as mayors, some of the health promotion challenges that need to be addressed in their communities. In addition, the booklet will illustrate the resilient resources of participants, suggesting strengths upon which health care practitioners and others can build to promote the health of rural older women. Successful aging and rural women's health have been characterized as including the ability to plan ahead, be intellectually curious and in touch with creative abilities, physical activity, serenity and spirituality, caring for friendships and other social connections, and volunteering and civic responsibilities (Coward, Davis, Gold, et al., 2006; Glicken, 2006; McPherson & Wister, 2008). Clearly, the photovoice method acted not only as a research approach, but, as importantly, it assisted women in the SWO study to successfully age. As such, photovoice is obviously a method to consider in rural research with rural women in other locations and age groups to assist them to develop abilities and perspectives that may help them to advance their resilience and age successfully.

Implications of the research for health care practice and health-related policy indicate that services must be expanded in rural and northern communities to include more diverse and enriched health care providers and services that address health promotion and illness prevention as well as diagnostic and treatment needs of rural and northern women. This is particularly so for older rural residents who comprise a significant and growing population in rural communities and who also may require enhanced health care support (Clark & Leipert, 2007; Keating, 2008). Indeed, in some rural communities in Canada seniors presently comprise up to 40% of the population (Statistics Canada, 2001), and it is anticipated that by 2021 one in four seniors will reside in a rural setting (Health Canada, 2002). As women tend to live longer than men and often experience greater chronic conditions and isolation (Ministry of Industry, 2006; Keating, 2008; McPherson & Wister, 2008), attention to the health of older women is an especially important aspect of rural health care.

Women form the backbone of rural communities and provide significant family and community support (Keating, 2008; Leipert & Smith, 2008; Sutherns, McPhedran, & Haworth-Brockman, 2004). Clearly, enhancing the resilience of rural women will support not only the women themselves but also their families and communities. Although findings in both the SWO and NBC studies revealed that rural and northern women were indeed resilient, their resilience does not absolve governments of their responsibilities to strengthen system deficiencies and enrich rural health care resources. As health care planning moves forward, these studies clearly indicate that rural women should be included as equal partners in health care planning, policy, and practice that address rural health and health care and rural women's resilience.

Increased efforts must be made to recruit and retain health care professionals who can provide respectful and appropriate care to women in northern and other rural settings. Northern and rural health care professionals must be comfortable living and working in small communities that are under-resourced and culturally diverse, where lack of anonymity and traditional gender roles and expectations prevail, where isolation and distance are facts of life, and where newcomers may be regarded as outsiders (Lee & Winters, 2006; Leipert, 1999; Leipert, Kloseck, McWilliam, et al., 2007; Rennie, Baird-Crooks, Remus, & Engel, 2000). In addition, health care practitioners must include respect, empowerment, advocacy, community development, and coalition-building approaches in their practices with rural women (Coward et al., 2006; Leipert & Reutter, 1998). These approaches are particularly important to help make the most of resources in sparsely populated communities and to increase support, resilience, and power for and with rural and remote women.

This study and others (Coward et al., 2006; Leipert & George, 2008; Leipert & Smith, 2008; Sutherns, McPhedran, & Haworth-Brockman, 2004) indicate that more feminist qualitative research is needed in isolated settings, particularly regarding the health issues and resilience of women who may be more vulnerable to health risks, and women who were not well represented in this study, such as those in very remote settings and disabled women. Additional qualitative and quantitative research could expand and test components of the theory revealed in the NBC study with women in other rural and remote settings. Additional research that explores aspects of resilience, such as factors that facilitate and hinder rural women's resilience, would provide important information for rural health care practice and policy.

REFERENCES

Caldwell, W., Brown, C., Thomson, S., & Auld, G. (2006). *The urbanite's guide to the countryside.* Guelph, ON: University of Guelph.

Canadian Association of Emergency Physicians, Rural Committee. (1997). *Recommendations for the management of rural, remote, and isolated emergency health care facilities in Canada.* Ottawa, ON: Author.

Canadian Institute for Health Information [CIHI]. (2006). *How healthy are rural Canadians? An assessment of their health status and health determinants.* Ottawa, ON: CIHI.

Clark, K., & Leipert, B. (2007). Strengthening and sustaining social supports for rural elders. *Online Journal of Rural Nursing and Health Care, 7* (1), 13–26.

Coward, R., Davis, L., Gold, C., Smiciklas-Wright, H., Thorndyke, L, & Vondracek, F. (Eds.). (2006). *Rural women's health: Mental, behavioral, and physical issues.* New York: Springer.

du Plessis, V., Beshiri, R., & Bollman, R. (2002). Definitions of rural. *Rural and Small Town Canada Analysis Bulletin, 3* (3), 1–16. Statistics Canada, Catalogue 21-006-XIE.

Glaser, B. (1978). *Theoretical sensitivity.* Mill Valley, CA: Sociology Press.

Glaser, B. (1992). *Basics of grounded theory analysis: Emergence vs. forcing.* Mill Valley, CA: Sociology Press.

Glicken, M. (2006). *Learning from resilient people: Lessons we can apply to counseling and psychotherapy.* London: Sage.

Health Canada. (2002). *Canada's aging population.* Ottawa, ON: Minister of Public Works and Government Services Canada.

Health Canada. (2003). Rural health in rural hands. Retrieved July 23, 2003, from http://www.hc.sc.gc.ca/english/ruralhealth/rural_hands.html

House, J., & Kahn, R. (1985). Measure and concepts of social support. In S. Cohen & S. Syme (Eds.), *Social support and health* (pp. 83–108). Orlando, FL: Academic Press.

Keating, N. (2008). *Rural ageing: A good place to grow old?* Bristol, UK: The Policy Press.

Lee, H.J., & Winters, C.A. (2006). *Rural nursing: Concepts, theory, and practice* (2nd ed.). New York: Springer.

Leipert, B. (1999). Women's health and the practice of public health nurses in northern British Columbia. *Public Health Nursing, 16,* 280–289.

Leipert, B. (2006). Rural and remote women developing resilience to manage vulnerability. In H.J. Lee and C.A. Winters (Eds.), *Rural nursing: Concepts, theory, and practice* (pp. 79–95). New York: Springer.

Leipert, B., & George, J. (2008). Determinants of rural women's health: A qualitative study in southwest Ontario. *The Journal of Rural Health, 24* (2), 210–218.

Leipert, B., Kloseck, M., McWilliam C., Forbes, D., Kothari, A., & Oudshoorn, A. (2007). Fitting a round peg into a square hole: Exploring issues, challenges, and strategies for solutions in rural home care settings. *Online Journal of Rural Nursing and Health Care, 7* (2), 5–20.

Leipert, B., Landry, T., McWilliam, C., Kelley, M., Forbes, D., Wakewich, P., & George, J. (under review). Rural women's health promotion needs and resources: A photovoice perspective. In J. Kulig and A. Williams (Eds.), *Rural health: A Canadian perspective.*

Leipert, B., & Reutter, L. (1998). Women's health and community health nursing practice in geographically isolated settings: A Canadian perspective. *Health Care for Women International, 19,* 575–588.

Leipert, B., & Smith, J. (2008). Using photovoice to explore older rural women's health promotion needs and resources. In P. Armstrong (Ed.), *Women's health: Intersections of policy, research, and practice* (pp. 135–150). Toronto: Women's Press.

MacDonald, M. (2001). Finding a critical perspective in grounded theory. In R. Schreiber & P. Stern (Eds.), *Using grounded theory in nursing* (pp. 113–157). New York: Springer.

McPherson, B., & Wister, A. (2008). *Aging as a social process: Canadian Perspectives.* Don Mills, ON: Oxford University Press.

Ministry of Industry. (2006). *Women in Canada: A gender-based statistical report.* Ottawa, ON: Statistics Canada.

Morgan, D., & Krueger, R. (1998). *The focus group kit.* London, UK: Sage.

Morse, J. (2001). Situating grounded theory within qualitative inquiry. In R. Schreiber & P. Stern (Eds.), *Using grounded theory in nursing* (pp. 159–175). New York: Springer.

Northern Secretariat of the BC Centre of Excellence for Women's Health. (2000). *The determinants of women's health in northern rural and remote regions.* Prince George: University of Northern British Columbia.

NVIVO. (1999). Version 2.0. QRS NUD*IST Vivo. Melbourne, Australia: Qualitative Solutions and Research Pty, Ltd.

Oliffe, J., Bottorff, J., Kelly, M., & Halpin, M. (2008). Analyzing participant produced photographs from an ethnographic study of fatherhood and smoking. *Research in Nursing & Health.* Retrieved June 18, 2008, at www.interscience.wiley.com

Patton, M. (2002). *Qualitative research and evaluation methods* (3rd ed.). London, UK: Sage.

Rennie, D., Baird-Crooks, K., Remus, G., & Engel, J. (2000). Rural nursing in Canada. In A. Bushy (Ed.), *Orientation to nursing in the rural community* (pp. 217–231). London, ON: Sage.

Romanow, R. (2002). *Building on values: The future of health care in Canada.* Ottawa, ON: Commission of the Future of Health Care in Canada.

Statistics Canada. (1993). *Census of agriculture: Selected data for Saskatchewan rural municipalities.* Ottawa, ON: Government of Canada.

Statistics Canada. (2001). *Urban and rural population counts for Provinces and Territories.* Ottawa, ON: Minister of Industry.

Sutherns, R., McPhedran, M., & Haworth-Brockman, M. (2004). *Rural, remote, and northern women's health: Policy and research directions.* Winnipeg, Manitoba: Centres of Excellence for Women's Health.

Turner, L., & Gutmanis, I. (2005). *Rural health matters: A look at farming in southwest Ontario: Part 2.* London, ON: Southwest Region Health Information Partnership.

Wang, C., & Burris, M. (1997). Photovoice: Concept, methodology, and use for participatory needs assessment. *Health Education and Behavior, 24,* 369–387.

Wang, C., Burris, M., & Ping, X. (1996). Chinese village women as visual anthropologists: A participatory approach to reaching policy makers. *Social Science and Medicine, 42,* 1391–1400.

Rural Family Health: Enduring Acts of Balancing

SONJA J. MEIERS, SANDRA K. EGGENBERGER,
NORMA K. KRUMWIEDE, MARY M. BLIESMER,
and PATRICIA A. EARLE

Rural families are unique as they respond to health experiences and the expectation of the modern health care system that families be actively involved in the care of their members. The rural family, as a unique interrelated system, has health beliefs and utilizes health care in ways that are distinctly different from urban dwellers (Armer & Radina, 2006; Bushy, 2000). Theory building identifies commonalities and differences in nursing practice across all rural settings so that relevant nursing care approaches can be proposed (Blake & Bisogni, 2003; Long & Weinert, 1989). The focus of this study was to understand the health experience of families in a rural midwestern setting. Specific aims of the study were to: (1) define rural family health, and (2) describe the process that families in a particular rural setting employ in creating health.

BACKGROUND AND SIGNIFICANCE

Nursing practice has historically acknowledged the relationship of family to health (Nightingale, 1855, 1858; Whall, 1986; Whall & Fawcett, 1991; Harmon Hanson, Gedaly-Duff, & Kaakinen, 2005). However, nursing science with a focus on caring for the family as a whole has received little attention until the last decade (Wright & Leahey, 2005; Eggenberger & Nelms, 2007). Family scholars call for a commitment to family care in the nursing discipline (Wright & Leahey) since research findings (Paavilainen, Seppanen, & Astedt-Kurki, 2001; O'Brien, 2007; Ray & Street, 2007) highlight the significance of the family to the health and well-being of individual members, as well as the influence of a family member's illness on the family. Family members are often concerned for each other, resulting in watchful attention and other actions aimed to support members' development, health, and illness needs (Denham, 2003, p. 127; Hebert & Schulz, 2006). Yet, family nursing literature describes deficiencies in the state of family nursing science and emphasizes the need for family research to advance nursing knowledge and family nursing theory that can guide family nursing practice (Hauenstein, 2008; Feetham & Meister, 1999; Gilliss & Knafl, 1999; Denham).

Family-focused research in psychology, psychiatry, counseling, medicine, family science, and nursing has predominantly resulted in overview texts and periodicals regarding the family system, the family life cycle, family interaction, and family coping (Duvall, 1977; Hill, 1949, 1958; Kitrungrote & Cohen, 2006; Rosenblatt, 1994; Olson, Russell & Sprenkle, 1989; Walsh, 1993; Wright & Leahey, 2005). Therefore, knowledge development in the emerging field of family nursing, with a focus on caring for and with the entire family, is in its infancy (Baumann, 2000). Current family nursing scholars (Wright & Leahey; Denham, 2003; Chesla, 2005) identify a need for nursing research focused on understanding family processes that enhance family health experiences. A key emphasis in this knowledge development must be to identify and describe the foundational concept of family health.

Clarity regarding the meaning of family health nursing is necessary as a central concern to the development of theory and practice, a worthy focus since the need for family care is increasing in all settings (Baumann, 2000; Hebert & Schulz, 2006). Individuals in rural areas define health, access health care, and engage in treatment for illness in unique ways (Lee, 1998; Armer & Radina, 2006). Rural families tend to define health as being able to do work and, as a result, symptoms that do not decrease the ability to be active and work may be ignored until absolutely necessary. Rural individuals and families tend to be more self-reliant than their metropolitan counterparts and not as easily accepting of others, especially those with positions of power and status such as health care providers (Bigbee, 1991).

Research regarding how the rural family unit manages its health is minimal and investigations using a theoretical framework created deliberately for use in a rural nursing context are extremely rare (Cody, 2000; Denham, 1999a; Winstead-Fry, 1992). In a study of rural Appalachian families, health was described by Denham as a "dynamic and complex construct consisting of multiple member interactions within and across the boundaries of households nested within social contexts" (p. 133). Denham's family research (2003) highlights the need for nursing practice that addresses processes supporting family health. To enhance the understanding of rural family health, the research question focus for this study was "How do rural families create family health?"

METHODS

We used a qualitative design with grounded theory methodology to guide this study. This research explored the family social process of creating health and described the dimensions of this interactive process, thereby contributing to theory development (Glaser & Strauss, 1967).

Setting and Participants

In this study, we used the definition of *rural* from the Office of Management and Budget (2005). Families who lived in an economically and socially integrated area of a less than 50,000-person population in south central Minnesota were eligible for the study. We recruited families who were not dealing with an active health problem to establish a baseline understanding of the nature of family health. We used this study as preparation for future studies with families dealing with acute or chronic illness. Family membership for this study was self-defined.

We obtained approval for the study from the Institutional Review Board of Minnesota State University–Mankato, prior to recruitment of participants. Prior to interviews, adult participants signed consent forms and children, 9 years and older, signed assent forms. We assured all participants confidentiality and anonymity.

Theoretical Sampling

We used a theoretical sampling technique simultaneously with the process of data collection. We identified the initial family as an eligible family from the professional network of one of the researchers. This family had been articulate regarding health issues in community conversations where the researcher was involved. We identified additional families through a snowball sampling technique. As the analysis proceeded, we enrolled families who could further illuminate the family process of creating health. For instance, as the category of transitions evolved, we made a strategic decision to enroll a family that could be assumed to be experiencing transitions. This sampling technique resulted in data being obtained from 12 families identified as A–L over a 24-month period of sampling and analysis (see Table 8.1). The families included 53 individuals ranging in age from 1 year to 78 years with a median family income between $50,000 and $59,999.

Table 8.1

FAMILY DESCRIPTIONS

FAMILY	AGE OF FEMALE ADULT	OCCUPATION OF FEMALE ADULT	AGE OF MALE ADULT	OCCUPATION OF SECOND ADULT	AGES (YEARS) & GENDER OF CHILDREN
A	39	RN	40	County Worker	19m, 18m, 15m, 9m
B	44	Bookkeeper	45	Mechanic	18m
C	37	Cosmetologist	—	—	12m, 9f
D	44	Medical Secretary	45	Farmer	21f, 18m, 15f, 11m
E	68	RN	70	Skilled Laborer	34m, 33m, 16m
F	41	Education Paraprofessional	42	Agribusiness	15f, 13m
G	30	RN	32	Sales	3f, 1m
H	37	Homemaker	38	Health Care Administrator	9f, 7f, 5f
I	66	Retired Sales	78	Retired Mechanic	—
J	45	RN	46	Business Consultant	24f, 2f
K	46	Farmer	47	Farmer	19f, 18f, 15f, 11m, 10f, 8m
L	53, 42	Counselor	—	Professor	21m

Note: f = female and m = male.

Data Collection

We invited all family members to participate. All research members conducted interviews at one time or another. Two members of the research team conducted each interview with the family as a family group in the family home. In all instances, we interviewed minor children in the presence of their parents; all members were present at the interview with the exception of one family in which we interviewed the college-aged son separately because of scheduling conflicts.

Each of the two researchers present interacted with the family to enhance comfort and conversational style. We used a semistructured format with audio taped interviews lasting 1–2 hours. We used the following probes to enhance interaction: (a) "Describe your family for us," (b) "What is your definition of family health?" and (c) "Describe good times and bad times for your family."

Prior to transcription, we completed preparation of data, including subject identification, and instructions to the transcriptionist regarding how to notate pauses or laughter. The interviewers recorded facial expressions and body movement as audio field notes. The transcriptionist transcribed these notes and included them as an addendum with each interview to provide the interview context for analysis (Sandelowski, 1995). The interviewers verified the accuracy of the interview transcription by listening to the original audiotapes while simultaneously reading the transcripts.

The Process of Data Analysis

We analyzed interview data following the process described by Strauss and Corbin (1990). Each of us open coded the verbatim transcripts to determine phenomena that comprised the family health experience as a social process. We worked in pairs to review the conceptual labels and validate interpretations. We then reviewed these interpretations as a team and began to assemble the labels into categories of processes. We identified properties and dimensions of the category. We subsequently reviewed all transcripts according to this process until we analyzed 375 pages of data text.

We then subjected the data to the process of axial coding, a set of procedures whereby data are put back together in new ways to make connections between categories (Strauss & Corbin, 1990). As the analysis proceeded, we identified similarities and differences of categories were identified. Finally, we identified a core category, the central phe-nomena around which all other categories were integrated.

Trustworthiness

We directed our attention toward establishing rigor in this qualitative study through the measures of transferability, credibility, dependabil-ity, and confirmability as detailed by Lincoln and Guba (1985). Our use of exemplars in reporting findings enhances the possibility that other researchers can judge the appropriateness of transferring the study find-ings to another setting. We achieved credibility by reviewing data text in dyads followed by team analysis to clarify and confirm categories. In addition, conducting family interviews in the naturalistic setting of the home enhanced the credibility of the data. We achieved dependability by the use of audio taped, transcribed verbatim interviews. We all dis-cussed the core category and reached consensus on a hypothesis state-ment regarding relationships between categories. Empirical grounding of the study is evident in the findings as the categories and labels are directly linked to the data. Such empirical grounding is necessary so that the discipline of nursing can determine usability of the resultant theory (Strauss & Corbin, 1990). We established confirmabilty by recording the decision-making process in determining codes, categories, and themes. In addition, we used ongoing critique of the decision-making process and consultation with an expert grounded theory researcher (Lincoln & Guba).

FINDINGS

Rural Families Creating Health

These rural families created health in an ongoing process of enduring acts of balancing in response to the inevitable transitions that occurred in family life (see Figure 8.1). The core category, *enduring acts of bal-ancing*, is demonstrated as adjustment to times of transition. Balanc-ing was needed between: (a) work and family, (b) inside and outside commitments, (c) individual and family needs, (d) resources and lack of resources, and (e) time and lack of time. Family health was inte-grated into the enduring acts of balancing in this rural sample. Family health was strengthened by the family's commitment to work through

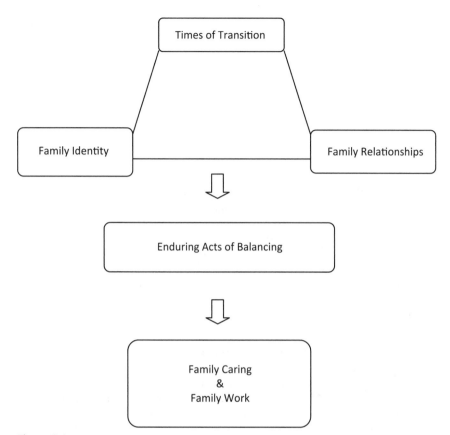

Figure 8.1. Enduring acts of balancing: Rural family health (Family Nursing Research Team—Minnesota State University–Mankato).

challenges and differences to form a safe, comfortable, caring environment of unity and uniqueness. The family was considered healthy as long as no one was taking medication. Families, with their unique and ongoing identity and relationships managed times of transition to maintain their sense of unity and integrity. Families engaged in the process of enduring acts of balancing to manage the challenge posed by specific transitions. Examples of specific balancing acts included (1) partnering and sharing essential work roles to manage the family farm, (2) being present for each other during good and bad times, (3) prioritizing family time and work time, (4) creating space for the other family member in the busy day, (5) making family decisions about economic priorities, and (6) modifying family rituals during times of transition. The outcomes of these acts of balancing were continued family work and family caring.

In the following section, selected exemplars from family interviews demonstrate aspects of the core category and its related concepts.

Enduring Acts of Balancing

The process of partnering and sharing essential work roles to manage the family farm (a uniquely rural situation) demonstrated a commitment to family of origin:

> Father: [W]e [referring to brother] had a partnership and . . . I was doing all the work with the hogs and he was there for his share of the check. . . . And I thought 'Well this is not working,' so I don't know if that fueled some resentment. I says [sic] that's it, you commit one way or the other and I had the backing of my oldest brother. He said, years later, 'Yeah it wouldn't have worked.' And I still feel that there are some of the brothers and sisters who still think they are entitled to something because their roots are here too [the family farm]. . . . And if we had been naive enough to go along with what they [the siblings] were going to decide, I don't think we would be here because we were to the point I had talked to a realtor about moving to Iowa. . . . It wasn't worth it, it was not worth it. It really has an impact on you. Not only your economics, but your family.
>
> Mother: It took awhile for some [referring to extended family members] to really be able to even talk among themselves and there was bitterness. . . . I think it has gotten better over the years.

Actively prioritizing family time over work time demonstrated commitment to family needs while recognizing individual needs:

> Mother: I just work part-time as a teacher's aide and I don't make great money, but the hours are good. I have the summer off and then I can make my family a priority. I would like to have a career, but I don't think that I would like to be stretched that way. . . . So, we kind of made that decision that we are fine to live without the two full time incomes.
>
> Father: . . . that is one of the reasons that I [changed jobs]. I [changed jobs] when she [daughter] started kindergarten . . . I just realized that it was not going to work . . . [with my previous job's] time requirements. It just did not fit into what I wanted for my family life.

A teenage son describes the benefit of creating space for the other family member in the busy day:

Son: I mean you will never be able to do that [have the perfect family] because life always throws you a curve ball and you know you have got to take the good times with the bad times. . . .

Mother: If you can do that.

Son: If you can work through it and see another person's point of view and what they are trying to bring to the family conversation. . . .

Times of Transition

Conditions that prompt the use of enduring acts of balancing in rural families included planned and unplanned *transitions* associated with family life. These transitions centered on additions and subtractions of persons and things within rural family life as well as situations affecting family security. Additions included births, growing independence of adolescents and gaining of new family members through marriage. Subtractions included deaths and losses. Family members lost jobs, functional ability, relationships through separation and divorce, and financial security through events such as crop-related disasters. Families reported facing different challenges throughout the developmental, economic, and social spectrums of their lives together. Family life followed a trajectory from formation to reformation through losses, additions, and changes in levels of dependence and interdependence.

Transitions were sometimes related to rights of passage with growth. For instance, parents of a teenager about to receive her driver's license detail feelings about their daughter's growing independence:

Mother: So, yes and no. I don't want the responsibility of having to be there [to drive their teenage daughter], but on the other hand it makes me nervous to think that she can do it [drive] on her own.

Father: And I predict that we will have several differences of opinions when, where and how.

Mother: But, she already understands, I think, her expectations are not going to be met, which then she will need to take into consideration.

Transitions were also influenced by the environment surrounding families. For instance, one father described the threat to financial security that bad weather causes and its influence on the emotional climate of the family:

Father: Oh, I think I get all stressed out [when the weather is bad and the markets react in a way that is related to family income] and am not going to show it and the ones closest are the ones who are going to feel it. They are going to hear it, it all relates back to income and providing.

Family Identity

At time of transitions, families are challenged to adjust their *family identity* within the context of their evolving world. Family identity is created through a dynamic process of internal and external feedback. Internal feedback is derived from each family's experiences of life and their perceptions. Family perception is the filter through which the family views its identity. External feedback is derived from the family's experiences of connection to the greater community. Family values, structural and qualitative family definitions, family relationships to the community, and the ability of families to seek information were all examples of identity challenge during times of transition. Children in the sample shared their impressions quite freely in response to the statement, "Describe your family for us."

A father described a situation surrounding a life-altering accident in the family's past that illuminated a conflict between family values and legal rights that challenged family identity:

> Father: [W]e didn't even go after the insurance company. We could have. I mean later when he was 21. . . . But, I didn't really feel right taking it when the Lord gave him his life . . . maybe we shouldn't. . . .

A mother and daughter shared their thoughts about how family identity adjustment was somewhat based upon relationships within the community:

> Mother: When I think of family, I think of these four and my parents . . . and sometimes it extends to people at work. . . .
> Daughter: Like older people . . . we have a lot of people that we have known over the year that we could go to . . . I don't argue with them . . . I help them around the house . . . helping them. . . .

One son described his family in comparison to other families:

> Son: I've heard some of my friends and the way their families are and I consider my family probably the best out of half the families I know. They gave me everything I needed and probably more, but we've had problems at times, too.

Other children described their families as

We are like three people renting a house together [intergenerational family].
Big, weird, argumentative, talkative, A little larger than the typical family of the Midwest. Driving to town, never home, letting the house be a mess—everyone is always coming and going. Helping with church things and community things—there's a lot . . . going on.
I guess we're all kind of flamboyant, outgoing, the family as a whole is family oriented and we like to do things together.

Family Relationships

The process of negotiating *relationships* within the family to adjust their sense of family identity was multifaceted. Families negotiated forming and reforming of relationships through communication. Connections and coalitions were realigned within the family communication process. For instance, power and control issues were negotiated and boundaries and roles were clarified. The family often came to a common view of a crisis event while working together to understand its impact. Such processes of negotiation may not have been intentional but evolved as a reflection of historic family patterns. A father described the unique family process of negotiation through communicating during a time of growing adolescent independence:

Father: We had a great conversation about two years ago, didn't we [name]? For probably an hour screaming at each other and I mean . . . we were just kind of taking shots at each other and there is nothing wrong with that because I was fueling the fire constantly. I just wanted to see how far I could get him to go and he was testing his old man to the max. . . . No violence or none of that, it was just a good scream session.

Another significant time of transition requiring active negotiation of relationships was the time of family formation. A mother described the process she went through to achieve comfort with different levels of family connections:

Mother: I've learned a lot from marrying [name] because they are very family oriented and very close . . . and my family loves each other but we never spent this much time together . . . there is always someone to turn to . . . someone always around. . . . It was hard at first because I am very independent and I felt like if it was mine then I would do it. . . . I would feel bad if someone came in and helped me, because it was mine and I was supposed to do it.

Finally, a family member described the process of negotiating care responsibilities with her sister. She and her sister were sharing the work of caring for their older mother. This process illustrates the constant formation and reformation of family that is influenced by family values.

Mother: My sister and I were taking turns keeping her [mother] and keeping her out of the nursing home as long as we possibly could . . . she has gone down hill and is in a nursing home now.

Family Caring

Through the process of enduring acts of balancing, families continue the work of *caring* for their family member in newly negotiated ways. Families reported that the work of caring involves discipline, support of each other, listening, ensuring safety, planning for the future, and monitoring member actions. Members maintained contact with each other through the work of caring by enacting coalitions, worrying about each other, and ensuring access to each other. The work of caring is also supported by extended family and employers. A family describes their attention to safety issues as a way of caring:

Mother: [B]efore we went to the county fair, my husband Billy talked to her about not talking to strangers . . . and then I think she did not want to go.
    Father: I discussed it on the way home one night, and I felt bad because then she [daughter] said that she did not want to go to the fair anymore. . . . I just wanted to have it in the back of her mind about not talking to strangers. . . . We are more worried [than our parents] because there is more of an alarm because they are our kids. . . .

A father told the story of learning the importance of holding back and working to support his son during a frightening experience. He also details the incorporation of the event into the foundation of family discipline.

Father: He says 'I rolled the pick-up in the ditch.' At that point I wanted to go right through the phone and grab him and start choking him for doing that. But, it's clicking that fast I am going 'wait a minute he is standing there talking to me telling me he just rolled this thing in the ditch,' maybe I better just mellow out here, dad, and we will go take a look and see . . . there are those scary things with kids and yet you want to react intact because, dang it, why did you do that and yet thank God, for once the brain kicked in before all the excitement did. . . . But some of those were the bad times that actually probably turn out to be good because he didn't actually get hurt and yet you're thankful that somebody . . . learned a pretty valuable lesson.

Families anticipated the inevitable letting go while acknowledging the good feelings of family times and the differences in family members. They incorporated knowledge of the influences of events in their family history on family growth. A father described a history of family counseling that has aided family growth as he stated, "We take everyone's feelings into consideration . . . about five years ago we had some family counseling on some issues and I think that has helped us a lot. . . ."

A wife described how she and her husband seek connections in everyday experiences and are influenced by their families of origin in their choice of activities, "[W]e like to watch birds, go for walks, go for hikes . . . since we come from such large families, we enjoy being together with our families and our friends."

Family Work

Essential *family work* is accomplished through shared decision-making and shared roles within the demands of rural life to facilitate getting the work of family done. Decision-making about health, priorities, and activities was accomplished by seeking information and focusing on the future. A 13-year-old boy described getting the inevitable work of cleaning done, "[Bad times are] . . . when we have to clean . . . every time something's happening. . . . It's sometimes not even that dirty."

A father describes the pull of family work and the daily grind of home maintenance integrated with childrearing tasks:

> Father: When I'm at work, I think about what all needs to be done at home, like mowing the lawn . . . it take[s] about 8 hours and I would like to be inside helping her with the dishes or washing clothes or picking up the tens of thousands of toys that are laying around. . . .

These families created health in an active process of experiencing and interacting with each other and the environment. The social process of enduring acts of balancing is an active process of creating health in the environment, evolving and changing through interactions. Enduring acts of balancing is the ongoing process of creating family health. Consequences of the process of enduring acts of balancing are the continued work of caring, getting the daily work of family done, and facilitating growth and development of individual family members.

DISCUSSION

Rural Families Creating Health

Our purpose in this study was to advance researchers' understandings of the process rural families use to create health. Rural family health is created in an ongoing process of enduring acts of balancing in response to the inevitable transitions of family life in the context of family identity and family relationships. Outcomes of this process are continued family work and family caring. Creating family health involves actively managing everyday life experiences by working together and attending to the evolving family identity.

Times of Transition

Family life theorists have done much work regarding family transitions (Bengtson & Allen, 1993). Generally, transitions in the life course of families are used as key markers of social change in family life. Transitions are viewed as normal or abnormal and are measured by the successful accomplishment of developmental tasks (Carter & McGoldrick, 1989; Duvall, 1957), with abnormally timed transitions viewed as problematic for families. Denham (1999b), for example, referred to transitional time surrounding death as a central dimension of the family's experience while caring for their dying member. Other authors have indicated that serious acute or chronic illnesses present significant transitions that challenge family coping and developmental processes (Khalili, 2007; Wright & Leahey, 1994). Families in this study indicated that transitions occur almost constantly and are related to factors beyond those traditionally identified by family life course theory: (a) exit from school, (b) entry into the labor force, (c) departure from family of origin, (d) marriage, and (e) establishment of a separate household (Modell, Furstenberg, & Hershberg, 1976). An important aspect of transition for these families included multiple examples of moving between independence and dependence within the family. Possibly their movement is significant because, according to rural nursing theory (Long & Weinert, 1989), rural families are self-reliant and more independent as groups than urban dwellers. This may lead to a family that is more interconnected, lending to a more difficult experience during evident transitions toward independence even if it does not mean separation. The highlighting of transition as an important aspect of family health is consistent with the findings of Haras (2008), thus emphasizing the relevance of the finding within the development of the science.

Family Relationships and Family Identity

Communication theorists state that family relationships, rules, and roles are worked out through interaction over time and result in the family's unique identity and creation of health (Fitzpatrick & Ritchie, 1993). In addition, through the course of family development, fundamental and enduring assumptions about the world result from significant interactions within the family and between the family and the environment. Rural families hold an identity within the greater rural community. This identification is often linked to the components of old-timer/newcomer in relationship to the length of time the family or extended family has lived and been a part of the rural community (Long & Weinert, 1989). Findings in this study suggest that the daily processes families use to create family health may be related to ongoing formation of the family paradigm being formed within the rural community context (Reiss, 1981).

Study findings support the premise that family health is inextricably intertwined with the pattern of family relations so that family health itself is part of the vital fabric of family life (Pratt, 1976). Certainly the family is more than a context for health occurrences. The family is a living, processing, adjusting, coping, and stabilizing entity. The family health experience is an active process of living in the environment, evolving and changing through interactions. These families detailed a process whereby they are conscious of their past but are constantly moving toward the future, supporting the notion that the family health experience is necessarily created through highly interactive processes considering family members and the environment, a concept similar to Newman's (1994) expanding consciousness. The participants emphasized that interactions between family members and between the family and the environment (e.g., specifically weather, extended family, and community) influence expanding consciousness.

Family Work and Family Caring

The families in the current study were able to identify a set of beliefs about the importance of getting the work of family done. Work was essential to the family and best experienced when doing the work together. This finding is consistent with that of Armer and Radina (2006) who noted that rural Amish families value work as central to health and that the ability to continue physical work activity is a most frequent health-maintaining behavior. The self-reliance of the rural family was often linked to a sense of pride in work accomplished to care for their own. Families identified being healthy until one of its family members requires taking a medication. In addition, family caring beliefs were identified.

Family caring included insuring that family members were safe and received adequate provision. The ability of each member to serve and fulfill a role within the family allows the family to grow and develop while doing the work of family. The tight bonds and intimacy of the family often challenges the individual's need for privacy, while maintaining the connected caring for family members as individuals and family as a whole.

Implications and Recommendations for Nursing

The empirically grounded framework that emerged from the data analysis in this study can serve as a framework for research in family health focused nursing. Future research is needed to consider the conceptual relationships within the framework and to test components of the framework. For instance, "Is the family's sense of the ability to get family work done related to the degree of threat to family identity?" Or "How does the closely interconnected rural family manage inevitable transitions toward independence or increased dependence in a rural community in one geographical region as compared to another?" Currently, the research team is conducting interviews with rural families to discover the processes required to attain family health within the context of chronic illness.

Nurses engaged in rural nursing practice can learn a great deal from listening to the family's discussion of their daily experiences regarding how they create health. Asking the family to respond to the following question may be helpful in initiating family-level care: "What kinds of things does your family normally do when you sense a challenge in your family life?" Nurses who are aware that their interactions with families in the rural setting are critical to evolving family identity can enhance the family's ability to create health. Nursing practice that recognizes the significance of transitions in the life of a rural family will guide families to prepare and manage their life of transitions. Nursing practice in the rural setting that acknowledges and supports the acts of balancing in a family will also foster family health. Praising the work of family, along with the individual family member's work, supports the family as a whole in the rural environment.

Pedagogy necessary to stimulate this level of practice would necessarily focus on techniques to enhance interaction between nurses
and families. Nurse educators who live and serve in rural settings can
influence the quality of care provided to rural families through the use
of frameworks and pedagogies focused specifically on rural practice.
Nursing students need continued practice with healthy families in the
rural setting to continue developing an understanding of family life and
processes in this setting.

REFERENCES

Armer, J. M., & Radina, M. E. (2006). Definition of health and health promotion behaviors among Midwestern Old Order Amish families. *Journal of Multicultural Nursing & Health, 12* (3), 44–53.

Baumann, S. L. (2000). Family nursing: Theory anemic, nursing theory-deprived.
Nursing Science Quarterly, 13 (4), 285–290.

Bengtson, V. L., & Allen, K. R. (1993). The life course perspective applied to families over
time. In P. Boss, W. J. Doherty, R. LaRossa, W. R. Shumm, & S. Steinmetz (Eds.),
Sourcebook of family theories and methods: A contextual approach. New York: Plenum.

Bigbee, J. L. (1991). The concept of hardiness as applied to rural nursing. In A. Bushy
(Ed.), *Rural Nursing* (vol. 1, pp. 39–58). Newbury Park, CA: Sage.

Blake, C., & Bisogni, C. A. (2003). Personal and family food choice schemas of rural
women in Upstate New York. *Journal of Nutrition Education & Behavior, 35* (6),
282–293.

Bushy, A. (2000). *Orientation to nursing in the rural community.* Thousand Oaks, CA:
Sage.

Carter, B., & McGoldrick, M. (1989). *The changing family life cycle.* Boston: Allyn &
Bacon.

Chesla, C. A. (2005). Articulating suffering and possibility in family life. *Journal of
Family Nursing, 11* (4), 371–387.

Cody, W. (2000). Nursing frameworks to guide practice and research with families:
Introductory remarks. *Nursing Science Quarterly, 13* (4), 277.

Denham, S. (2003). *Family health: A framework for nursing.* Philadelphia: F. A. Davis.

Denham, S. A. (1999a). Part 1: The definition and practice of family health. *Journal of
Family Nursing, 5* (2), 133–159.

Denham, S. A. (1999b). Part 2: Family health during and after death of a family member.
Journal of Family Nursing, 5 (2), 160–183.

Duvall, E. (1957). *Family development.* New York: Lippincott.

Duvall, E. (1977). *Marriage and family development* (5th ed.). New York: Lippincott.

Eggenberger, S. K., & Nelms, T. P. (2007). Being family: The family experience when
an adult is hospitalized with a critical illness. *Journal of Clinical Nursing, 16* (9),
1618–1628.

Feetham, S. L., & Meister, S. B. (1999). Nursing research of families: State of the science and
correspondence with policy. In A. S. Hinshaw, S. L. Feetham, & J. L. F. Shaver (Eds.),
Handbook of clinical nursing research (pp. 251–271). Thousand Oaks, CA: Sage.

Fitzpatrick, M. A., & Ritchie, L. D. (1993). Communication theory and the family. In P. Boss, W. J. Doherty, R. LaRossa, W. R. Schumm, & S. Steinmetz (Eds.), *Sourcebook of family theories and methods: A contextual approach*. New York: Plenum.

Gilliss, C. L., & Knafl, K. A. (1999). Nursing care of families in non-normative transitions: The state of science and practice. In A. S. Hinshaw, S. L. Feetham, & J. L. F. Shaver (Eds.), *Handbook of clinical nursing research* (pp. 231–249). Thousand Oaks, CA: Sage.

Glaser, B., & Strauss, A. (1967). *The discovery of grounded theory*. Chicago: Aldine.

Haras, M. S. (2008). Planning for a good death: A neglected but essential part of ESRD care. *Nephrology Nursing Journal, 35* (5), 451–459, 483.

Harmon Hanson, S. M., Gedaly-Duff, V., & Kaakinen, J. R. (2005). *Family health care nursing* (3rd ed.). Philadelphia: F. A. Davis.

Hauenstein, E. J. (2008). Building the rural mental health system: From De Facto system to quality care. *Annual Review of Nursing, 26,* 143–173.

Hebert, R. S., & Schulz, R. (2006). Caregiving at the end of life. *Journal of Palliative Medicine, 9* (5), 1174–1187.

Hill, R. (1949). *Families under stress: Adjustment to crisis separation and reunion*. New York: Harper & Row.

Hill, R. (1958). Social stresses on the family: Genesis features of families under stress. *Social Casework, 39,* 139–158.

Khalili, Y. (2007). Ongoing transitions: The impact of a malignant brain tumour on patient and family. *AXON, 28* (3), 5–13.

Kitrungrote, L., & Cohen, Z. (2006). Quality of life of family caregivers of patients with cancer: A literature review. *Oncology Nursing Forum, 33* (3), 625–632.

Lee, H. (1998). *Conceptual basis for rural nursing*. New York: Springer.

Lincoln, Y., & Guba, E. G. (1985). Establishing trustworthiness. *Naturalistic Inquiry*. Beverly Hills, CA: Sage.

Long, K. A., & Weinert, C. (1989). Rural nursing: Developing the theory base. *Scholarly Inquiry for Nursing Practice: An International Journal 3,* 113–127. New York: Springer.

Modell, J., Furstenberg, F., & Hershberg, T. (1976). Social change and transition to adulthood in historical perspective. *Journal of Family History, 1,* 7–32.

Newman, M. A. (1994). Paradigms of health. In M. A. Newman (Ed.), *Health as expanding consciousness* (2nd ed., pp. 1–14). New York: National League for Nursing Press.

Nightingale, F. (1855). *Letter to Lady Alicia Blackwood*. Written at Scutari. (August 6).

Nightingale, F. (1858). *Notes on matters affecting the health, efficiency, and hospital administration of the British army*. London: Harrison & Sons.

O'Brien, M. (2007). Ambiguous loss in families of children with autism spectrum disorders. *Family Relations, 56* (2), 135–146.

Office of Management and Budget. (2005). *OMB No. 05-02 Update of statistical area definitions and guidance on use of statistical area definitions*. Washington, DC: Government Printing Office.

Olson, D., Russell, C., & Sprenkle, D. (1989). *Circumplex model: Systemic assessment and treatment of families*. New York: Hawthorne.

Paavilainen, E., Seppanen, S., & Astedt-Kurki, P. (2001). Family involvement in perioperative nursing of adult patients undergoing emergency surgery. *Journal of Clinical Nursing, 10,* 230–237.

Pratt, L. (1976). *Family-structure and effective behavior: The energized family*. Boston: Houghton-Mifflin.

Ray, R. A., & Street, A. F. (2007). Non-finite loss and emotional labour: Family caregivers' experiences of living with motor neurone disease. *Journal of Nursing and Healthcare of Chronic Illness, 16* (3a), 35–43.

Reiss, D. (1981). *The family's construction of reality*. Cambridge, MA: Harvard University Press.

Rosenblatt, P. C. (1994). *Metaphors of family systems theory: Toward new construction*. New York: Guilford.

Sandelowski, M. (1995). Rigor or rigor mortis: The problem of rigor in qualitative research revisited. *Advances in Nursing Science, 16* (2), 1–8.

Strauss, A. L., & Corbin, J. (1990). *Basics of qualitative research*. Newbury Park, CA: Sage.

Walsh, F. (1993). *Normal family processes*. New York: Guilford.

Whall, A. L. (1986). The family as the unit of care in nursing: A historical review. *Public Health Nursing, 3* (4), 240–249.

Whall, A. L. & Fawcett, J. (1991). *Family theory development in nursing: State of the science and art*. Philadelphia: F. A. Davis.

Winstead-Fry, P. (1992). Family theory for rural research and practice. In P. Winstead-Fry, J. C. Tiffany, & R. V. Shippee-Rice (Eds.), *Rural health nursing* (pp. 127–147). New York: National League for Nursing Press.

Wright, L. M., & Leahey, M. (1994). *Nurses and families: A guide to family assessment and intervention* (2nd. ed.). Philadelphia: F. A. Davis.

Wright, L. M., & Leahey, M. (2005). *Nurses and families: A guide to family assessment and intervention* (3rd. ed.). Philadelphia: F. A. Davis.

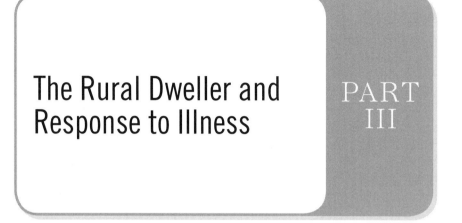

The Rural Dweller and
Response to Illness

PART
III

9

Patterns of Responses to Symptoms in Rural Residents: the Symptom–Action–Time-Line Process

JANICE A. BUEHLER, MAUREEN MALONE, and JANIS M. MAJERUS-WEGERHOFF

How people identify, evaluate, and respond to symptoms is an important determinant of their health and illness behavior (Lenz, 1984). An increasing amount of literature addresses health behaviors of rural people (Lee, 1991; Long, 1993; Long & Weinert, 1989; Moon & Graybird, 1982; Weinert & Long, 1990). However, little information is available on the patterns of responses of rural people to symptom occurrence signifying actual or potential health problems. In addition, there is a paucity of information on health behaviors of certain rural groups, specifically, women and Plains Indians.

Although actual processes of health-seeking behavior are not delineated in most research of rural health behaviors, some patterns are evident. A survey of health risk prevalence in rural Montana (Moon & Graybird, 1982) revealed that participants believed in self-responsibility for health. Lee (1991) noted that the quality of hardiness may be responsible for some rural dwellers' delay in seeking assistance from the professional health care system when symptoms of illness appear. Rural people were viewed as delaying health care until they were very ill, thus often needing hospitalization at the point care was sought (Long, 1993; Long & Weinert, 1989; Rosenblatt & Moscovice, 1982; Weinert & Long, 1990).

Studies on responses to symptom occurrence, not specific to rural people, have been conducted by behavioral and social scientists. Mechanic

(1960) stated that possible responses to illness include discretionary inaction, the use of medicines, seeking professional care, and using a lay network. Suchman (1966) described individual responses to symptom occurrence as proceeding in this sequential pattern: (a) Symptom Experience Stage, (b) Assumption of Sick Role Stage, (c) Medical Care Contact Stage, and (d) Dependent Patient Role Stage.

Segall and Goldstein (1989) noted that lay persons clearly do routinely self-evaluate and self-treat many of their health problems as a part of daily living and that the nature and extent of these self-care practices are not well understood. They concluded it is not clear whether self-care behavior is equally prevalent among different social groups, whether self-care is used for both health maintenance and the treatment of illness, and whether self-care is used only in response to selected symptomatic conditions.

METHODS

The qualitative method of grounded theory was used in this study (Glaser & Strauss, 1967). Grounded theory provides a means of understanding behavioral patterns from the perspective of the participants. It enables learning about their world and the interacting influences of personal, social, and cultural characteristics without imposing the cultural biases of the interviewer (Chenitz & Swanson, 1986). Grounded theory allows for the direct examination of the world of rural residents in a naturalistic way (Schatzman & Strauss, 1973).

The convenience sample was composed of 16 rural or frontier Montana women, 8 of whom were Native American women living on a federal reservation and 8 of whom were Caucasian farm or ranch women. Elison (1986) defined *rural* as a population density of more than 6 but less than 100 per square mile and a driving distance to a hospital of at least 30 minutes. *Frontier* is defined as a population density of less than 6 per square mile and driving time to a hospital of either 60 minutes or severe geographic and/or seasonal climatic conditions.

The eight Caucasian farm or ranch women were married and had at least two children. Six of these women were self-employed, actively farming and ranching with their husbands. Two were employed in a small city 60 miles from their homes. Four of these women lived in rural locations and four in frontier locations. Their nearest neighbors lived one-fourth mile to 8 miles away. One informant's nearest neighbor was 5 miles away but did not have a phone. For emergencies, this informant would travel 12 miles to the nearest neighbor with a telephone. The primary means of paying for health services for these women was through private pay and individual health insurance.

Of the eight Native American women, seven were classified as rural and one as frontier. Five of the informants lived on small ranches and three lived in one of two towns each with populations of less than 200 (U.S. Bureau of Census, 1987). Seven of the informants have lived on the reservation all of their lives. Three of the women were unemployed and on Aid to Families with Dependent Children, two considered themselves full-time homemakers, and the remaining three were employed in local towns. Five of the Native American women were married, two were single, and one was divorced. All informants had children, with an average number of 2.3 children per household and a range of 1–6 children per household. Five informants lived with extended family members, and three lived with only their children and husbands. All eight women used the Indian Health Service which provided free health care as entitled by treaty.

Face-to-face focused interviews were conducted in the homes of the participants. Open-ended interview questions and probes were used to stimulate free responses (Woods & Catanzaro, 1988). Topics included describing the steps used when someone in the home becomes ill, examples of when self-treatment would be used or when someone would be consulted, signs indicating illness, examples of home remedies, length of time before seeking help, and reasons for deterrence in obtaining care from professional health resources.

The grounded theory data analysis for this study revealed a basic social process (BSP) termed the *symptom–action–time-line* (SATL) *process*.

FINDINGS

Both Native American and Caucasian farm/ranch women used the SATL process to respond to symptoms of actual or potential health problems. The process consists of four stages in which symptoms are identified and actions are taken to move to a desired state of health. The stages are (a) symptom identification, (b) self-care, (c) lay resources, and (d) professional resources. Each stage has a time period (time-line) in which the participant takes actions in response to a symptom, evaluates the effectiveness of the actions in resolving the symptom, and decides whether to go on to the next stage. Time periods during stages are dependent on the intensity, duration, and amount of interference in function caused by the symptom and may be minutes, days, or years. The first stage, symptom identification, is the stimulus leading to the other stages.

Symptom Identification Stage

Symptom identification was preceded by symptom occurrence and included assessment of conditions or signs perceived as being an undesired alteration in the person's usual state of health that required actions to move the person to his or her desired state. Participants identified their desired state as being the way they were before the symptoms occurred. The symptoms had three properties: physical signs and sensations, degree of interference in the ability to function, and intensity and duration. Physical signs included "fever," "vomiting," "pain," "pulling at ears," "broken bones," "hard to breathe," and "losing blood." Interference in function included "not being able to do ordinary things like housework," "I couldn't move my finger," and "unable to eat or play." Intensity and duration of symptoms were the degree and rate of change in symptoms, the onset of new symptoms, and the length of time they persist. Examples included "temperatures over 102 degrees for 3 days" and "a bloody nose that couldn't be stopped after 2 hours." After the symptoms were assessed, they were given meaning, and a decision was made whether to take action. This was dependent on knowledge and past experience with illness, intensity and duration of the symptoms, and degree of interference with normal functioning. A Native American woman stated, "Whenever my girl pulls at her ears and is fussy, I know from before that she probably has an ear infection and we should go in [to the clinic]. . . . The first time [she was sick], I waited until she had a fever, and it went so high it really scared me." Participants in both groups stated they noticed most symptoms within minutes to a few hours after occurrence.

Variation noted between Caucasian and Native American women in symptom identification was due to meanings given to symptoms. For example, one of the Native American women, after getting no relief from headaches through use of medications prescribed by a physician, attributed her headaches to supernatural origins and sought care from a medicine man. Both groups of women described lower thresholds of tolerance for duration and intensity of symptoms in their children. This resulted in shorter SATL processes for children.

Self-Care Stage

The second stage of the SATL process was characterized by the initiation of self-care. *Self-care* involved those activities self-initiated and performed for self or family members in response to symptoms. Examples of self-care listed by respondents ranged from "getting extra rest," "slowing down," "waiting for more symptoms" to more complicated activities such as "soaking my foot three times a day." The time-line described by both groups of women for starting self-care after symptom identification was seconds for intense symptoms to a "couple of days" for minor symptoms.

The self-care stage was also characterized by using self-care tools, those items used by the respondent to resolve symptoms on their own. Both groups listed such items as nonprescription medications, leftover prescription medicine, teas, thermometers, heating pads, disinfectants, and reference books. The majority of the Native American women used traditional self-care tools to treat certain symptoms. These included sage, sweetgrass, and medicine bundles. One Native American woman used a first aid book for reference whereas half the Caucasian ranch women regularly referred to their "family health textbooks." One informant in this group stated, "I looked up symptoms my daughter had, and the book told me what I could do for her at home or if I needed to see a doctor." Another informant added, "Everyone in my family knows how to look up their illnesses in our health book." All of these informants live in the frontier area. Another self-care tool mentioned only by these frontier women was "animal" ointments to treat hand rashes resulting from feeding lambs.

Actions for this stage included initiating self-care; evaluating its effectiveness based on a decrease in the duration, intensity, or the amount of interference in the ability to function; and deciding to seek help if self-care was ineffective. A typical response, for both Native American and Caucasian informants, regarding the decision to seek help was, "I tried taking Tylenol but after two days I still had a fever, so I called my mother for advice."

Lay Resources Stage

In this third stage, the participants involved their informal network of family, friends, and neighbors, that is, their *lay resources*, by describing the symptoms and obtaining assistance to alleviate symptoms. Properties of this stage included symptom validation, asking advice for self-care or self-care tools, receiving physical care, or seeking emotional support—particularly for deciding to go to a physician. Time-lines for consulting lay resources after symptom identification ranged from 1–3 days for both groups. Both groups had usually initiated a self-care activity before they consulted their lay resources.

Ranch women stated their most frequently used lay resources were their mothers, but they also consulted with neighbors. Two frontier ranch women described how they had become aware of each other having similar joint pain of the great toe. They compared their symptoms over the phone while referring to their health textbooks that guided them to diagnosing themselves as having gout. They then verified these symptoms and information with another lay resource, a neighbor who was a registered nurse (RN). Ranch women also described an organized informal lay network of volunteer farmers and ranchers who acted as first responders to emergencies. They were called for such symptoms as "chest pain," "losing blood," and "broken bones."

Organized volunteer networks of lay resources were not described by Native American women. The majority identified their mothers as their primary source of help. A few consulted only with their husbands, stating that they had no relatives or friends living in the area for them to contact. Participants stated they would usually consult a relative before they would consult a neighbor who was not a relative. The majority of the Native American women also consulted their lay network for advice on the use of traditional healing practices. The following described this use of a lay resource.

> My son (9-months-old) had been fussy for two days; he was not taking his bottle and had cold sweats. Tylenol didn't seem to be helping, so my mother suggested that I take him to my aunt because he might have colic. My aunt massaged him and blew smoke in his ear. He went to sleep and was O.K. after that.

Actions for this stage included contacting a lay resource; evaluating whether there was a decrease in the symptom's intensity, duration, or interference with function; and deciding whether to take further action. Varying degrees of self-care continued throughout this stage.

Professional Resources Stage

Seeking help from *professional resources* occurred when there was failure to alleviate symptoms through the use of self-care or lay resources, or when symptoms intensified, or when new symptoms developed.

Professional resources listed by both groups included physicians, RNs, dentists, and chiropractors. Both groups stated they consulted professional help when "nothing else helped," "there wasn't anything I could do," or "for emergencies." Nurses were sometimes consulted for advice about whether symptoms required immediate attention or could wait awhile longer. Nurses were frequently used as lay resources in this instance, since they were called at their homes when off duty. Physicians were usually not called at home unless the participant had been under physician care for a specific condition.

Time-lines, from the symptom identification stage to the professional resource stage in situations other than emergencies, were 4–7 days for rural women and 1–2 weeks for frontier women. Time-lines for Native American women ranged from 2–5 days in both rural and frontier areas.

Time-line variations occurred for children and in emergencies. For children, total time-line durations were much shorter, ranging from less than 1 day to 3 days. Each stage within the time-line process was shorter; lay resources were consulted sooner and often used only to help transport the child to the professional resource. Barriers to seeking professional care were minimized so that time and distance became less important for children than for adults. In emergencies, individuals tended to bypass self-care and lay resources and go directly to professionals. Barriers were minimized according to the urgency of symptom occurrence.

If symptoms were not alleviated after going to a professional resource, participants either returned to the same professional or went to a different professional. At times, symptoms were simply "tolerated." Several Native American women sought alternative care by contacting a medicine man. This occurred because they believed physicians had not helped. The medicine man was described by these participants as another type of professional. The most frequently identified barriers to professional resources were distance and transportation. Other barriers mentioned were fear of "bad news," a lack of women doctors, and the time required to see a professional, especially time spent in waiting rooms.

Implications

The SATL process clarifies response patterns rural women display when confronted with symptoms of actual or potential health problems. The process provides a framework for health care professionals that is client centered, and, therefore, has powerful implications for intervention and health education; promotes culturally sensitive planning and provision of health services; and adds to the body of literature on rural use of health resources.

The SATL process provides a systematic framework for health care providers to assess patterns of response to symptoms and to develop interventions to facilitate rural residents' responses to their symptoms. For a full understanding of what actions a rural client will use to alleviate a health problem, each stage in the process must be carefully assessed on an individual basis.

CONCLUSION

Findings in this study suggest that rural residents use several indicators to identify and evaluate their symptoms. These indicators can be clarified by using the properties of the symptom identification stage as an assessment guide. It will yield information on what signs and sensations prompted symptom identification, tolerance levels for symptoms, amount of interference caused by symptoms, knowledge levels about symptoms, meanings of symptoms, and the time-line and conditions necessary for taking further actions. With these baseline data, health care providers can determine a client's capability to accurately interpret a symptom and take appropriate actions. Corresponding interventions may be aimed at increasing the client's knowledge of indicators of disease processes and the preferable time period in which to initiate an action.

Through assessment of the self-care stage of a client's SATL, information can be elicited regarding the client's self-care patterns. This includes the conditions under which self-care is activated and the variety of self-care tools that are available and employed by the client. Interventions can be directed at expanding a person's access to more effective self-care tools or adapting health care to the tools already available to the person. Findings in this study suggest that assessment of self-care resources leads to an evaluation of a client's lay resources, since self-care tools are often shared with a network of relatives or neighbors. Knowing whom a rural client most often relies on for symptom validation provides valuable information about functional support systems actively used by rural/frontier people. Interventions with a rural client may be more effective if key people in these networks are included.

Assessment of the professional resource stage provides information about the conditions necessary for an individual to seek professional care, appropriateness of time-lines, and barriers that prevent access to care. For example, if clients are seeking professional care for conditions that could be handled at home, interventions can be aimed at making a client's response pattern clear to both the provider and the client by using the SATL process. With this information, the client and provider can identify which response in the process is deficient and mutually determine a more appropriate response.

The multidimensionality of the SATL process increases health professionals' awareness of the dimensions and complexities involved in caring for people from diverse cultural and geographical backgrounds. A health care provider can identify cultural views of health and illness by using the SATL process. These beliefs are deeply entwined within traditional customs and culture. By gaining insight into the traditional attitudes that people have toward health and illness, health care providers can become more sensitive to the issues surrounding health care and the cultural health beliefs of the consumer, thereby providing more comprehensive health care.

Finally, the SATL process has important implications for research. Although research studies appear in the literature on self-care, use of lay or informal health resources, and use of formal health services, these studies tend to focus on single health resource utilization. The SATL process begins to explicate how various types of health resources are used in an integrated manner by actual rural/frontier residents. Furthermore, the preponderance of literature on consumer use of health resources focuses on urban rather than rural populations. Further research is needed to validate the use of the SATL process among rural and urban subpopulations.

REFERENCES

Chenitz, W., & Swanson, J. (1986). *From practice to grounded theory.* Menlo Park, CA: Addison-Wesley.

Elison, G. (1986). Frontier areas: Problems for delivery of health care services. *Rural Health Care, 8* (5), 1, 3.

Glaser, B., & Strauss, A. (1967). *Discovery of grounded theory.* Chicago: Aldine.

Lee, H. J. (1991). Relationship of hardiness and current life events to perceived health in rural adults. *Research in Nursing and Health, 14,* 351–359.

Lenz, E. (1984). Information seeking: A component of client decisions and health behavior. *Advances in Nursing Science, 6* (3), 59–72.

Long, K. A. (1993). The concept of health: Rural perspectives. *Nursing Clinics of North America, 28* (1), 123–130.

Long, K. A., & Weinert, C. (1989). Rural nursing: Developing the theory base. *Scholarly Inquiry for Nursing Practice: An International Journal, 3* (2), 113–131.

Mechanic, D. (1960). Illness behavior and medical diagnosis. *Journal of Health Social Behavior, 1,* 86–94.

Moon, R., & Graybird, D. (1982). *High risk prevalence: A report card for Montana.* Helena: Montana Department of Health and Environmental Sciences.

Rosenblatt, R., & Moscovice, I. (1982). *Rural health care.* New York: Wiley.

Schatzman, L., & Strauss, A. (1973). *Field research.* Englewood Cliffs, NJ: Prentice-Hall.

Segall, A., & Goldstein, J. (1989). Exploring the correlates of self-provided health care behavior. *Social Science Medicine, 29* (2), 153–161.

Suchman, E. (1966). Health orientation and medical care. *American Journal of Public Health, 56* (1), 97–105.

U. S. Bureau of Census. (1987). *Statistical Abstract of the United States: 1988* (108th ed.). Washington, DC: U.S. Government Printing Office.

Weinert, C., & Long, K. A. (1990). Rural families and health care: Refining the knowledge base. *The Journal of Marriage and Family Review, 15* (1–2), 57–75.

Woods, N. F., & Catanzaro, M. (1988). *Nursing research: Theory and practice.* St. Louis, MO: Mosby.

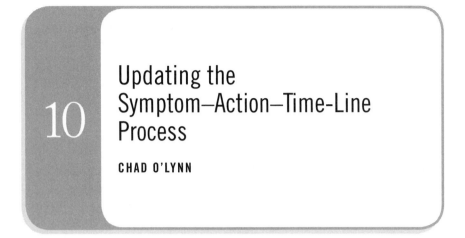

10

Updating the Symptom–Action–Time-Line Process

CHAD O'LYNN

In Chapter 9, an important study was reprinted from the first edition of this book. The Buehler, Malone, and Majerus (1998) study is important because the authors proposed an initial model detailing how rural dwellers recognize health symptoms and the process rural dwellers go through in relieving those symptoms. As Buehler et al. noted, the significance of such a model is the provision of a framework from which health care providers can better assess an individual's interpretation and response to symptoms. Health care providers can work with individuals to more accurately interpret symptoms and choose responses that optimize health outcomes. In addition, the model provides health care providers a framework to better assess all resources available to individuals (such as self-care or lay resources) that might be tapped to resolve health problems and provide emotional support during illness. Buehler et al. recommended that further research be completed to validate the use of their Symptom–Action–Time-Line (SATL) process model for rural dwellers.

The study completed by Buehler et al. (1998) was small in scope and limited to a small group of rural Montana women. To appropriately transfer the model for use in other studies, further examination of the model is warranted. My purpose in this chapter is to provide part of this examination. In this chapter, I report the findings of a recent literature review designed to examine the level of support for the SATL process model. Based on these findings and a discussion of the model's limitations, I recommend revisions to the SATL process model. The revisions may enable the model to be used with other populations.

REVIEW OF THE SATL PROCESS

I refer the reader to Chapter 9 for details on the derivation of the SATL process through grounded theory methodology. However, I present a brief review and graphic depiction of the SATL in this section.

The SATL process comprises four phases: (a) symptom identification, (b) self-care, (c) lay resources, and (d) professional resources. The process is preceded by the occurrence of a symptom, and unless that symptom is recognized by an individual (symptom identification), the process does not continue. It is important to note that Buehler et al. (1998) defined a *symptom* as a negative entity (e.g., a person identifies a symptom as an alteration in the usual state of health that requires some sort of action). This definition is crucial in prefacing the SATL process as one of resolving a problem.

Symptoms have three general components: (a) physical signs and sensations, (b) degree of interference with the person's usual or desired level of functioning, and (c) intensity and duration of the symptom (Buehler et al., 1998). These three components, in addition to an individual's prior experience and knowledge of the symptom, are used in developing meaning of the symptom for the individual. Based on this meaning, an individual will decide whether to take action. Generally, the first action taken after identifying a symptom is one of self-care.

Self-care includes activities that are initiated and performed by the individual experiencing the symptom in the hope of alleviating the symptom (Buehler et al., 1998). For individuals dependent upon others for health needs (e.g., children, dependent elders), family members would be responsible for initiating activities to address an identified symptom. Self-care activities are variable and include taking over-the-counter medications, taking home and herbal remedies, or reading reference books to learn more about the symptom and symptom resolution. Self-care activities, as well as all other actions taken in the SATL process, are evaluated by the individual in terms of efficacy, and a decision is made whether to proceed or not through the SATL process, alter actions, or cease activities.

If self-care activities do not resolve a symptom to the individual's satisfaction, or if assistance is needed, lay resources are tapped. Lay resources comprise family, friends, neighbors, or support persons and are used to provide (a) validation of symptom interpretation, (b) advice and emotional support, and (c) physical care (Buehler et al., 1998). Although not specifically defined by Buehler et al., lay resources differ from professional resources in that lay resources are not financially reimbursed for their services. If symptoms do not resolve, if symptoms intensify, or additional symptoms occur, professional resources are then sought. If professional resources do not lead to symptom resolution, individuals may seek other professional resources.

The time one takes to progress through the SATL process is variable (Buehler et al., 1998). The amount of time to act generally depends upon the intensity and duration of a symptom and how much the symptom interferes with usual functioning. When a symptom is particularly intense or greatly interferes with usual functioning, actions occur more quickly. In addition, if children are involved, or if the symptom is interpreted to constitute an emergency, actions occur relatively quickly and may bypass phases of the SATL process altogether, prompting the individual to use a professional resource immediately upon identifying a symptom. However, if one progresses through the SATL process completely, the time taken to go from symptom identification to self-care can take up to 2 days, from symptom identification to lay resources can take from 1–3 days, and from symptom identification to professional resources can take from 4–14 days. Decision points within the SATL process and how individuals progress through the SATL process have great implications for health care providers and researchers. A graphic depiction of the SATL process is located in Figure 10.1.

METHOD FOR LITERATURE REVIEW

Much of the literature pertaining to rural health care focuses on disparities in health for rural dwellers as compared with nonrural dwellers, description of the health of rural dwellers, barriers to accessing health care services for rural dwellers, and the experiences and demographics of health care providers in rural areas. None of these broad areas of literature addresses directly the SATL process of identifying symptoms and actions to resolve them, with the possible exception of access barriers. Buehler et al. (1998) discussed access barriers only secondarily; more

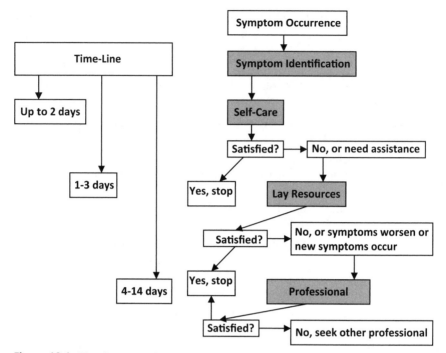

Figure 10.1. The Symptom–Action–Time-Line (SATL) process (adapted from Buehler, Malone, & Majerus, 1998).

specifically in that additional effort is made to overcome access barriers if symptoms involved children or were deemed emergent. This secondary focus is reasonable in that access barriers more than likely modulate the SATL process rather than serve as foundational antecedents in determining the components of the process itself. As such, literature examining specific barriers for rural dwellers in accessing health services was not deemed appropriate for inclusion in the literature review.

In July 2004, I conducted a search of peer-reviewed resources contained in the Cumulative Index to Nursing & Allied Health Literature (CINAHL) (1982 through July 2004), MedLine (1966 through July 2004), and PsychInfo databases (1985 through July 2004) to locate research-based support for the SATL process model, using the keyword of *rural* and its associated keywords of *rural health, rural environment,* and *rural populations.* Rural keywords were the primary sorting category to ensure that the literature would be salient to rural dwellers, although use of the SATL process may be present in nonrural populations as well. I then combined the rural keywords with other keywords suggestive of the SATL process including *self-care, decision-making, self-assessment, alternative therapies, complimentary medicine,* and *home remedies* based on available keyword search options within each database. I excluded dissertation abstracts because of the difficulty of obtaining full texts of multiple dissertations. The search yielded a total of 155 journal articles.

From this yield, I excluded review articles, case studies, and anecdotal reports resulting in a new pool of research-only reports. In addition, I excluded all articles reporting studies occurring outside the United States. This latter exclusion is reasonable because the study by Buehler et al. (1998) occurred in the United States where health care is so heavily financed by nongovernmental sources compared with most other developed countries. These steps resulted in 60 articles available for review.

Following a critical review of the 60 articles, I made further exclusions. I excluded intervention and correlation studies that did not address components relevant to the SATL process. Furthermore, I excluded studies that focused only on health care providers. The final sample of articles for review included 36 research reports.

FINDINGS FROM THE LITERATURE REVIEW

The 36 studies included in this review were published between 1991 and 2004. Participants in these studies represented all regional areas of the continental United States except the desert Southwest and California. All of the studies included rural dwellers, although 6 studies (17%) included urban participants as a comparison group. Table 10.1 shows the gender and racial or ethnic characteristics of the participants. Notably absent in the studies were Asian or Pacific Islander participants. Otherwise, non-Hispanic Caucasian, African American, Native American, and Hispanic participants were represented.

Buehler et al. (1998) noted a paucity in the literature of resources that describe the process rural individuals undertake in managing symptoms once they have been identified. Generally, I confirmed this paucity in the present literature review. Of the 36 studies reviewed, 8 (22%) minimally supported the tendency to use self-care and lay resources before going to a health professional for nonemergent symptoms experienced by adults (Congdon & Magilvy, 2001; Davis, Henderson, Boothe, et al., 1992; Grubbs & Frank, 2004; Horner, Ambrogne, Coleman, et al., 1994; Johnson, 1994; Lee & Winters, 2004; Roberto & Reynolds, 2002; Sellers, Poduska Propp,

Table 10.1

PARTICIPANTS' GENDER AND RACIAL/ETHNIC CHARACTERISTICS
(*n* = 36 STUDIES)

CHARACTERISTIC	*n*	%
Gender		
All female	10	28
Mixed	25	70
All male	1	3
Race/Ethnicity		
All non-Hispanic White	4	11
Mixed	27	75
All minority	2	6
Unknown	3	9

& White, 1999). However, none of these studies described or tested a comprehensive process of symptom identification and action.

The majority of the studies I reviewed confirmed the use of self-care strategies to treat symptoms (Arcury, Quandt, McDonald, & Bell, 2000; Arcury, Quandt, Bell, & Vitolins, 2002; Armer, 1996; Bennett & Lengacher, 1999; Boyd, Taylor, Shimp, & Semler, 2000; Burman, 2001; Canales & Geller, 2003; Congdon & Magilvy, 2001; Davis et al., 1992; Engberg, McDowell, Burgio, Watson, & Belle, 1995; Ganther, Wiederholt, & Kreling, 2001; Gaskins & Lyons, 2000; Grubbs & Frank, 2004; Horner et al., 1994; Johnson, 1994; Lee & Winters, 2004; Long & Curry, 1998; Moore & Johnson, 1993; Rabiner, Konrad, DeFriese, et al., 1997; Roberto & Reynolds, 2001, 2002; Rohrer, Kruse, Borders, & Kupersmith, 2003; Sellers et al., 1999; Stoller, Gilbert, Pyle, & Duncan, 2001; Sullivan, Weinert, & Cudney, 2003; Vallerand, Fouladbakhsh, & Templin, 2003, 2004; Vitolins, Quandt, Case, et al., 2000; Wallace, Tuck, Boland, & Witucki, 2002). Many of these studies supported the self-care strategies described by Buehler et al. (1998), including taking over-the-counter medications, herbal remedies, and family remedies; referring to health information sources, such as books and television; and using physical treatments, for example, heating pads, stretching, or yoga. However, a number of authors discussed the value of prayer and spirituality as self-care strategies (Arcury, Bernard, Jordan, & Cook, 1996; Arcury et al., 2000; Bennett & Lengacher, 1999; Congdon & Magilvy, 2001; Gaskins & Lyons, 2000; Johnson, 1999; Roberto & Reynolds, 2002; Wallace et al., 2002). Buehler et al. did not discuss these strategies. In some of the studies that compared rural and nonrural dwellers, researchers noted that rural dwellers were more likely to use self-care strategies to treat symptoms than nonrural dwellers (Boyd et al., 2000; Ganther et al., 2001; Moore & Johnson, 1993; Rabiner, et al., 1997).

I also found support for the use of lay resources in managing symptoms in the studies reviewed. Primarily, researchers reported the strategies of soliciting the assistance and support of friends and family in managing symptoms and in using formal support groups (Arcury et al., 2002; Bennett & Lengacher, 1999; Boyd et al., 2000; Burman, 2001; Canales & Geller, 2003; Congdon & Magilvy, 2001; Gaskins & Lyons, 2000; Gross & Howard, 2001; Grubbs & Frank, 2004; Hines et al., 1999; Horner et al., 1994; Johnson, 1998; Long & Curry, 1998; Roberto & Reynolds, 2001, 2002; Stafford, Szczys, Becker, Anderson, & Bushfield, 1998; Sullivan et al., 2003; Vallerand et al., 2004; Wallace et al., 2002). However, in only a few of the studies I reviewed did researchers discuss the progression to lay resource use after self-care had failed or the use of lay resources prior to the use of professional resources (Davis et al., 1992; Horner et al., 1994; Lee & Winters, 2004; Roberto & Reynolds, 2002; Sellers et al., 1999).

Generally, the results of the studies support the finding from Buehler et al. (1998) that professional resources are utilized after self-care or lay resources are used. Some of the studies I reviewed included the use of complementary or alternative therapies to manage symptoms (Arcury et al., 1996; Arcury et al., 2000; Arcury, et al., 2002; Bennett & Lengacher, 1999; Canales & Geller, 2003; Congdon & Magilvy, 2001; Gaskins & Lyons, 2000; Johnson, 1999; Long & Curry, 1998; Vallerand, et al., 2003; Wallace et al., 2002). Complementary therapies included spiritual interventions as noted earlier, but also included the use of professional resources such as those provided by a masseuse, acupuncturist, naturopath, chiropractor, and herbalist. Other results supported the finding that professional resources are utilized if symptoms persisted (Horner et al., 1994; Roberto & Reynolds, 2002).

None of the researchers of the studies I reviewed provided specific time frames for utilizing resources as described by Buehler et al. (1998). However, research results did support basic time-line tenets within the SATL process, particularly those referring to the use of professional resources: Progression to and direct utilization of professional resources was quicker if symptoms involved children (Gross & Howard, 2001; Strickland & Strickland, 1996) or were perceived as emergent or crisis in nature (Congdon & Magilvy, 2001; Lee & Winters, 2004; Long & Curry, 1998; Sullivan et al., 2003). In addition to these situations, some researchers noted that the progression to professional resource utilization was quicker if the individual perceived a need for a prescription to treat the symptom (Johnson, 1994; Lee & Winters, 2004) or if the symptom would result in the individual missing work (Lee & Winters; Sullivan et al.) Buehler et al. did not note these latter two situations.

Buehler et al. (1998) reported that if professional resources were not effective in relieving symptoms, participants continued to work with the professional, seek another professional (particularly a provider of alternative therapy), or accept the symptom's nonresolution. In the studies I reviewed, researchers did not address this specific decision point in the same fashion. However, a number of researchers reported that participants used multiple strategies concurrently (Arcury et al., 1996; Bennett & Lengacher, 1999; Burman, 2001; Canales & Geller, 2003; Johnson, 1999; Roberto & Reynolds, 2001; Stafford et al., 1998; Vallerand et al., 2004). Many of these studies pertained specifically to the use of complementary or alternative therapies.

DISCUSSION

The literature reviewed supports aspects of the SATL process used by rural dwellers. Although none of the researchers contradicted the model proposed by Buehler et al. (1998), no researcher discussed or tested a comprehensive process for symptom identification and action. It should be noted, however, that the number of studies I reviewed was small. Most of the studies were cross-sectional and descriptive in design, limiting the ability to confirm the SATL process model within individuals over time. Moreover, most of the studies I reviewed had small sample sizes, focused on older populations, and did not include participants residing outside the United States.

With the exception of the Asian or Pacific Islander communities, the literature I reviewed represented racial or ethnic diversity. In addition, the literature represented geographic diversity. I recommend that studies examining rural Alaskan, Hawaiian, and Southwest communities be conducted to provide additional information about the SATL process.

In terms of gender, women were well represented in the sample of studies I reviewed, including 10 studies in which women were studied exclusively. In only one study (Sellers et al., 1999) researchers examined men or men's health exclusively. This limitation is significant because Sellers et al. noted that although both men and women may rely on self-care and lay resources before utilizing professional resources, men may interpret symptoms very differently and delay use of professional resources as long as possible (Levant & Habben, 2003; Sabo & Gordon, 1995; Sellers et al.). Consequently, men may incorporate very different time frames for actions. I recommend that additional men's studies in rural communities be conducted to validate the SATL process.

Despite the general support in the literature for the SATL process as described by Buehler, et al. (1998), the SATL process model has some limitations. Foremost is its difficulty in describing actions taken for multiple symptoms, particularly those associated with chronic illnesses. The model, with its emphasis on sequential progression through the SATL phases, is best suited for single problems or injuries, such as a fever, flu, or fractured bone. Such problems are readily identified, given meaning, and subjected to treatment. Chronic conditions, such as diabetes or congestive heart failure, are characterized by recurring and multiple symptoms with varying degrees of intensity and duration. Initial presentation of symptoms may indeed lead an individual through the customary SATL process. However, as individuals become more familiar and educated regarding how to interpret symptoms when they recur, previous experiences may influence whether or not they bypass self-care and lay resources completely and proceed directly to utilizing professional resources.

Although not stated by Buehler et al. (1998), one may infer from the model that when one progresses linearly through the SATL process, previous strategies may be abandoned because of unsatisfactory outcomes. The literature I reviewed did not support this inference. On the contrary, researchers described the concurrent use of multiple modes of symptom treatment. This concurrent use of strategies suggests a more circular model. With a more circular model, one can more readily explain how an individual might use prayer, hot packs, support from friends, prescription drugs, and physical therapy concurrently to manage an illness or injury, with varying use of these strategies over time as symptoms wax and wane.

Another limitation of the SATL process model is Buehler et al.'s (1998) failure to discuss symptoms that are recognized as problematic but ignored. For example, one may recognize a self-limiting symptom such as a strained muscle, but choose no action to relieve the strain. One could consider the act of ignoring a recognized symptom as a type of self-care action. The act of ignoring symptoms may be characteristic of rural men (Levant & Habben, 2003; Sellers et al., 1999). In addition, Buehler et al. described a symptom as a physical sign or sensation. This definition excludes psychological symptoms, such as those typically seen in depressive and anxiety disorders that may be readily recognized by the individuals experiencing them. Inclusion of these symptoms is key because mental health services are often unavailable or poorly implemented in rural communities (DeLeon, Wakefield, & Hagglund, 2003; Dobalian, Tsao, & Radcliff, 2003; Haard & Anderson, 2004; Kane & Ennis, 1996; National Institute of Nursing Research, 1995).

The emphasis on the time-line aspect of the SATL process model is problematic, in that it suggests a rather linear progression through phases of symptom identification and resultant actions. Buehler et al. (1998) noted that time frames for action were influenced by whether or not the symptoms were associated with children or with emergent conditions. As noted previously, others have suggested that time frames for action are also influenced by whether or not symptoms required a prescription or caused one to miss work (Johnson, 1994; Lee & Winters, 2004; Sullivan et al., 2003). In addition, it is reasonable to assume that barriers in accessing health resources for rural dwellers as described widely in the literature will influence how quickly or slowly one may adopt actions to address symptoms. As such, time frames are descriptive outcomes resulting from contextual variables. In one of the studies I reviewed (Strickland & Strickland, 1996), the researchers wondered whether self-care and lay resources were used based on preference and efficacy or whether access barriers slowed or prevented the utilization of professional resources. Consequently, time frames should be discussed in terms of how contextual variables for rural dwellers influence actions responsive to symptoms, rather than presented as a fundamental component of an action process itself.

Still another limitation of the SATL model is that it focuses on problem solving and does not account for activities to prevent problem occurrence. In other words, the model does not explain actions taken to prevent illness and promote health. These actions constitute a growing proportion of health activities and expenditures and form the foundation for a variety of health initiatives. In addition, rural people find these activities important and engage in them (Davis et al., 1992; Meadows, Thurston, & Berenson, 2001; Pullen, Walker, & Fiandt, 2001; Vitolins et al., 2000).

RECOMMENDATIONS FOR REVISION OF THE SATL PROCESS MODEL

To address the limitations of the existing SATL process model and better reflect the literature reviewed, I make the following recommendations for revision:

1. Expand the definition of symptom to include psychological symptoms.
2. Expand the definition of symptom to be more reflective of a *health need* so that measures one takes to prevent illness or promote health are included.
3. Recognize that intentional disregard of a symptom is a type of self-care action.
4. Embed the model within an environmental context external to the decision tree to account for variables such as gender, culture, race or ethnicity, socioeconomic status, family or social role, residential location, barriers in accessing resources, and so forth.
5. Reassign the time-line aspect of the process to a descriptive outcome, rather than a component of the action process itself.
6. Design the model to be more circular in nature.
7. Rename the model, The Symptom-Action Process (SAP).

Figure 10.2 shows a graphic depiction of the revised model.

In the revised model, the action process is embedded in an external context. After symptoms are identified, individuals may incorporate various types of actions: (a) self-care, (b) lay resources, or (c) professional resources in a sequential or concurrent fashion. The context will influence which action, or combination of actions, is taken. The sloping nature of the action types reflects the propensity to progress from self-care to lay resource use to professional resource use. The double arrows between action types account for fluid movement among aspects of the model and concurrent use of types of actions. New to this model are the arrows leading from the action types back to the symptom occurrence aspect of the model. These arrows close the circle of the process and account for symptoms that might recur, new symptoms that develop, or new information requiring new action resulting from previous actions taken by an individual.

Both the SATL process model and the revised SAP model describe a process in which an individual identifies a problem or need and takes

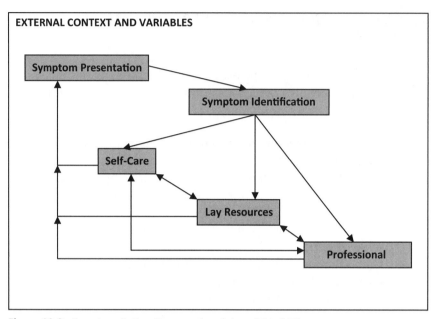

Figure 10.2. Symptom-Action Process: A revision of the SATL process.

action(s) to address it. As such, these models may describe the behaviors of all individuals, including nonrural dwellers, although how actions are taken may differ across populations. I recommend that research be conducted to evaluate how well the revised model is empirically supported. If the revised model is well supported, then it may serve as an ideal framework for comparison studies examining health behaviors across participant demographic variables.

CONCLUSION

Buehler et al. (1998) derived the SATL process model from a grounded theory study in which they described the process a group of rural Montana women used to respond to health symptoms. I conducted a current literature review to determine the level of support for this model. I reviewed 36 research studies located in the CINAHL, MedLine, and PsychInfo databases that focused on the process rural dwellers use to respond to health symptoms. Those studies provide general support for

aspects of the SATL process model, although in only 8 studies researchers described a sequential process of how rural dwellers respond to
health symptoms.

Despite the general support for the SATL process model, I noted
several limitations of the model. To address these limitations and maintain support from the reviewed literature, I proposed a revised model
titled SAP. The revised model may provide a better framework in examining the health behaviors of various subgroups of rural dwellers, as
well as assist in comparing the behaviors between rural and nonrural
dwellers. Examination of how and why these health behaviors are manifested may enhance the understanding among health professionals and
policy makers. The SAP model will aid professionals in assessing the
health needs of rural dwellers and in planning how best to meet those
needs with policies and services. I recommend further research with
rural men and rural Asian or Pacific Islander participants to determine
the support for the revised model. In addition, examination of studies
completed outside the continental United States should occur to determine whether the revised model has broader relevance to rural dwellers
across the globe.

REFERENCES

Arcury, T. A., Bernard, S. L., Jordan, J. M., & Cook, H. L. (1996). Gender and ethnic
differences in alternative and conventional arthritis remedy use among community-
dwelling rural adults with arthritis. *Arthritis Care Research, 9,* 384–390.

Arcury, T. A., Quandt, S. A., Bell, R. A., & Vitolins, M. Z. (2002). Complementary and
alternative medicine among rural older adults. *Complementary Health Practice
Review, 7,* 167–186.

Arcury, T. A., Quandt, S. A., McDonald, J., & Bell, R. A. (2000). Faith and health self-
management of rural older adults. *Journal of Cross Cultural Gerontology, 15* (1),
55–74.

Armer, J. M. (1996). An exploration of factors influencing adjustment among relocating
rural elders. *Image: Journal of Nursing Scholarship, 28,* 35–39.

Bennett, M., & Lengacher, C. (1999). Use of complementary therapies in a rural cancer
population. *Oncology Nursing Forum, 26,* 1287–1294.

Boyd, E. L., Taylor, S. D., Shimp, L. A., & Semler, C. R. (2000). An assessment of home
remedy use by African Americans. *Journal of the National Medical Association,
92* (7), 341–353.

Buehler, J., Malone, M., & Majerus, J. (1998). Patterns of responses to symptoms in
rural residents: The Symptom-Action-Time-Line process. In H. Lee (Ed.), *Conceptual basis for rural nursing* (pp. 318–328). New York: Springer.

Burman, M. E. (2001). Family caregiver expectations and management of the stroke
trajectory. *Rehabilitation Nursing, 26,* 94–99.

Canales, M. K., & Geller, B. M. (2003). Surviving breast cancer: The role of complementary therapies. *Family & Community Health, 26,* 11–24.

Congdon, J. G., & Magilvy, J. K. (2001). Themes of rural health and aging from a program of research. *Geriatric Nursing, 22,* 234–238.

Davis, D. C., Henderson, M. C., Boothe, A., Douglass, M., Faria, S., Kennedy, D., et al. (1992). Health beliefs and practices of rural elders. *Caring, 11* (2), 22–28.

DeLeon, P., Wakefield, M., & Hagglund, K. (2003). The behavioral health care needs of rural communities in the 21st century. In B. Stamm (Ed.), *Rural behavioral health care: An interdisciplinary guide* (pp. 23–32). Washington, DC: American Psychological Association.

Dobalian, A., Tsao, J. C., & Radcliff, T. A. (2003). Diagnosed mental and physical health conditions in the United States nursing home population: Differences between urban and rural facilities. *Journal of Rural Health, 19,* 477–483.

Engberg, S. J., McDowell, B. J., Burgio, K. L., Watson, J. E., & Belle, S. (1995). Self-care behaviors of older women with urinary incontinence. *Journal of Gerontological Nursing, 21* (8), 7–14.

Ganther, J. M., Wiederholt, J. B., & Kreling, D. H. (2001). Measuring patients' medical care preferences: Care seeking versus self-treating. *Medical Decision Making, 21* (2), 133–140.

Gaskins, S., & Lyons, M. A. (2000). Self-care practices of rural people with HIV disease. *Online Journal of Rural Nursing and Health Care, 1* (1). Retrieved June 1, 2004, from http://www.rno.org

Gross, G. J., & Howard, M. (2001). Mothers' decision-making processes regarding health care for their children. *Public Health Nursing, 18,* 157–168.

Grubbs, L., & Frank, D. (2004). Self-care practices related to symptom responses in African-American and Hispanic adults. *Self-Care, Dependent-Care, and Nursing, 12* (1), 4–9.

Haard, L., & Anderson, E. (2004). Factors related to depression in rural and urban non-custodial, low-income fathers. *Journal of Community Psychology, 32* (1), 103–119.

Hines, S. C., Glover, J. J., Holley, J. L., Babrow, A. S., Badzek, L. A., & Moss, A. H. (1999). Dialysis patients' preferences for family-based advance care planning. *Annals of Internal Medicine, 130,* 825–828.

Horner, S. D., Ambrogne, J., Coleman, M. A., Hanson, C., Hodnicki, D., Lopez, S. A., et al. (1994). Traveling for care: Factors influencing health care access for rural dwellers. *Public Health Nursing, 11,* 145–149.

Johnson, J. E. (1994). Sleep and alcohol use in rural old-old women. *Journal of Community Health Nursing, 11,* 211–218.

———. (1998). Older rural adults and the decision to stop driving: The influence of family and friends. *Journal of Community Health Nursing, 15,* 205–216.

———. (1999). Older rural women and the use of complementary therapies. *Journal of Community Health Nursing, 16,* 223–232.

Kane, C. F., & Ennis, J. M. (1996). Health care reform and rural mental health: Severe mental illness. *Community Mental Health Journal, 32,* 445–462.

Lee, H. J., & Winters, C. A. (2004). Testing rural nursing theory: Perceptions and needs of service providers. *Online Journal of Rural Nursing and Health Care, 4* (1). Retrieved June 1, 2004, from http://www.rno.org/

Levant, R., & Habben, C. (2003). The new psychology of men: Application to rural men. In B. Stamm (Ed.), *Rural behavioral health care: An interdisciplinary guide* (pp. 171–180). Washington, DC: American Psychological Association.

Long, C. R., & Curry, M. A. (1998). Living in two worlds: Native American women and prenatal care. *Health Care for Women International, 19*, 205–215.

Meadows, L. M., Thurston, W. E., & Berenson, C. A. (2001). Health promotion and preventive measures: Interpreting messages at midlife. *Qualitative Health Research, 11*, 450–463.

Moore, J. F., & Johnson, J. E. (1993). Over-the-counter drug use by the rural elderly. *Geriatric Nursing, 14*, 190–191.

National Institute of Nursing Research. (1995). *Chapter 2: Rural America: Challenges and opportunities*. Retrieved April 9, 2003, from ninr.nih.gov/ninr/research/vol7/chapter2.html

Pullen, C., Walker, S. N., & Fiandt, K. (2001). Determinants of health-promoting lifestyle behaviors in rural older women. *Family & Community Health, 24*, 49–72.

Rabiner, D. J., Konrad, T. R., DeFriese, G. H., Kincade, J., Bernard, S. L., Woomert, A., et al. (1997). Metropolitan versus nonmetropolitan differences in functional status and self-care practice: Findings from a national sample of community-dwelling older adults. *Journal of Rural Health, 13*, 14–28.

Roberto, K. A., & Reynolds, S. G. (2001). The meaning of osteoporosis in the lives of rural older women. *Health Care for Women International, 22*, 599–611.

Roberto, K. A., & Reynolds, S. G. (2002). Older women's experiences with chronic pain: Daily challenges and self-care practices. *Journal of Women & Aging, 14* (3–4), 5–23.

Rohrer, J. E., Kruse, G., Borders, T., & Kupersmith, J. (2003). Realized access to physician services among the elderly in West Texas. *Journal of Rural Health, 19*, 72–78.

Sabo, D., & Gordon, D. F. (1995). Rethinking men's health and illness. In D. Sabo & D. F. Gordon (Eds.), *Men's health and illness: Gender, power, and the body* (pp. 1–22). Thousand Oaks, CA: Sage.

Sellers, S. C., Poduska, M. D., Propp, L. H., & White, S. I. (1999). The health care meanings, values, and practices of Anglo-American males in the rural Midwest. *Journal of Transcultural Nursing, 10*, 320–330.

Stafford, D., Szczys, R., Becker, R., Anderson, J., & Bushfield, S. (1998). How breast cancer treatment decisions are made by women in North Dakota. *American Journal of Surgery, 176*, 515–519.

Stoller, E. P., Gilbert, G. H., Pyle, M. A., & Duncan, R. P. (2001). Coping with tooth pain: A qualitative study of lay management strategies and professional consultation. *Special Care in Dentistry, 21*, 208–215.

Strickland, J., & Strickland, D. L. (1996). Barriers to preventive health services for minority households in the rural south. *Journal of Rural Health, 12*, 206–217.

Sullivan, T., Weinert, C., & Cudney, S. (2003). Management of chronic illness: Voices of rural women. *Journal of Advanced Nursing, 44*, 566–574.

Vallerand, A. H., Fouladbakhsh, J. M., & Templin, T. (2003). The use of complementary/alternative medicine therapies for the self-treatment of pain among residents of urban, suburban, and rural communities. *American Journal of Public Health, 93* (6), 923–925.

Vallerand, A. H., Fouladbakhsh, J. M., & Templin, T. (2004). Self-treatment of pain in a rural area. *Journal of Rural Health, 20,* 166–172.

Vitolins, M. Z., Quandt, S. A., Case, L. D., Bell, R. A., Arcury, T. A., & McDonald, J. (2000). Vitamin and mineral supplement use by older rural adults. *Journal of Gerontology: Medical Sciences, 55A* (10), M613–M617.

Wallace, D. C., Tuck, I., Boland, C. S., & Witucki, J. M. (2002). Client perceptions of parish nursing. *Public Health Nursing, 19,* 128–135.

11

The Chronic Illness Experience of Isolated Rural Women: Use of an Online Support Group Intervention

CHARLENE A. WINTERS and THERESE SULLIVAN

Chronic illness is a major public health problem (Marks, 2003) affecting more than 113 million Americans in 2005 (Centers for Disease Control [CDC], 2008; Husaine & Moore, 1990; Jensen, 1991; Stuifbergen, 1995). Seven of every 10 Americans who die each year, or more than 1.7 million people, die of a chronic disease (CDC, 2008). Effective self-management is instrumental to a person's ability to adapt successfully to his or her illness and maintain a quality life. Education; support from family, friends, and health care providers; and the ability to manage uncertainty are important factors in chronic illness self-management (Strauss, Corbin, Fagerhaugh, et al., 1984).

The context within which chronic illness occurs has a significant impact on how the chronically ill arrange for services and support. Persons living in sparsely populated rural areas have few health care providers, hospitals, and other resources (Gesler, Hartwell, Ricketts, & Rosenberg, 1992; Agency for Health Care Policy & Research, 1996). Living in rural areas with few health care resources may complicate an individual's ability to manage his or her illness. More than one-fifth of America's population lives in rural areas (United States Census Bureau, 2000), yet little is known about how rural persons experience chronic illness (Scott, 2000). Our purpose in the study reported in this chapter was to explore the chronic illness experience of isolated rural women living with arthritis, fibromyalgia, cancer, diabetes, and multiple sclerosis (MS).

Arthritis and other rheumatic conditions, cancer, diabetes, and MS are common among Americans, affecting more than 75 million persons. Recent national figures indicate that arthritis and other rheumatic conditions alone affect nearly 46 million Americans and continue to be the leading causes of disability (Hootman, Bolen, Helmick, & Langmaid, 2006). Cancer continues to be the second leading cause of death in the United States, and more than 11 million people are living with a history of cancer (Ries, Melbert, Krapcho, et al., 2008). Diabetes mellitus (DM) affects 18 million Americans and is the leading cause of new cases of blindness, kidney failure, and lower extremity amputations. Just having DM greatly increases a person's risk for heart attack or stroke (Albright, 2008). In 2004, more than 400,000 persons living in the United States had MS and 200 new cases were diagnosed each week (*About MS*, 2004). MS is most common in the northern states and occurs mostly in women of northern European ancestry aged 20–50 years.

Disparities in health among rural dwellers are well documented. Living in sparsely populated rural areas is in itself a health risk factor because of numerous conditions that can negatively influence health (Eberhardt, Ingram, Makuc, et al., 2001). Rural residents tend to have more chronic illnesses, have lower rates of health insurance, and have limited access to health care services and health care providers (Meit, 2004). For example, in Montana, a person may need to travel 120 miles one-way to a health care specialist (Winters, 1999) or 320 miles round-trip to an illness-related support group; and in many areas public transportation is inadequate or nonexistent.

Management of chronic illness requires persons to recognize and control symptoms; implement prescribed treatments; adjust to changes in the course of the disease; prevent medical crises; attempt to normalize daily life; fund medical care; and confront emotional, marital, and family problems (Benet, 1996; Hwu, 1995; Robinson, 1993; Strauss et al., 1984; Winters, 1997, 1999). An individual's adaptive behaviors, psychosocial outcomes, and ability to provide self-care are influenced by uncertainty about the meaning of symptoms and treatment outcomes (Mast, 1995; Mishel, 1993; Strauss et al., 1984; Weiner, 1975). Uncertainty occurs when people lack the information or knowledge needed to understand their illness and is influenced by resources available to assist persons in the interpretation of illness-related events. Resources include relationships individuals have with their health care providers, cognitive ability, and social support (Mast, 1995; Mishel, 1984). How rural persons experience chronic illness in the face of limited access to resources is not fully known. We designed this qualitative descriptive study to explore the illness experiences of chronically ill isolated rural women.

METHODS

We conducted a secondary analysis of existing data from one cohort of participants in the Women to Women Project (WTW). WTW is a large-scale, multiphase intervention study that provides online peer support and health education via computer and the Internet to isolated rural women living with chronic illness. The overall goal of WTW is to evaluate the impact of participation on psychosocial health. In Phase I of WTW, a purposive sample of 120 chronically ill women from one western American state was randomized into four cohorts of 30 women. Each cohort had 15 women with computers and 15 women without computers. The computer groups participated in an online support group using an asynchronous chat room and structured education sessions spanning a period of 5 months. The groups without computers did not participate in the computer-based activities and continued to use their usual sources of support and information. All participants received a three-ring binder containing a description of the study and articles on a variety of health issues pertinent to women with chronic illness. Each participant completed written questionnaires to measure psychosocial outcomes over a 10-month period (Sullivan, Weinert, & Cudney, 2003; Weinert, 2000). Although WTW addressed psychosocial health, the study we describe in this chapter specifically focused on the experiences of living with chronic illness shared by the women in one computer group. The Montana State University–Bozeman Human Subjects Committee approved this study.

Sample

Eligible participants in WTW were women diagnosed with cancer, DM, rheumatoid diseases, or MS who lived at least 25 miles from an urbanized area (12,500 persons or more). All women in WTW were required to read and speak English, have sufficient dexterity to communicate using a computer keyboard, and have a telephone in their home. The women were recruited to participate via word-of-mouth and with the help of voluntary agencies, state agricultural extension services, schools of nursing, parish nurses, nursing students, health professionals, public and professional libraries, newspapers, and public television announcements.

Participants in the study we report in this chapter came from one computer group (n = 15). We chose this cohort because it was the first cohort to complete WTW. We included all women in the computer group in the sample. Fourteen of the women were Caucasian and one was Native American. All the women were from rural areas and lived on farms or in small towns. Eight of the women worked full-time outside the home; two were full-time homemakers; five were unemployed. The women reported their primary health problem to be cancer (n = 2), MS (n = 5), rheumatoid arthritis or fibromyalgia (n = 5), and DM (n = 3). Mean age was 47.2 years and the average time between illness diagnosis and the beginning of the study was 5.29 years.

Data Collection

We analyzed qualitative and demographic data collected for WTW and made no direct or indirect contact with the participants during this study. The qualitative data consisted of 453 messages posted to the online support group chat room by the women over a 22-week period. The messages were conversations held between group members on topics of their choice. They had been stored verbatim in the end-user database then downloaded by the WTW research assistant for analysis. Although all the women participated in the discussions, the number of messages posted and their lengths varied. The number of postings ranged from 4–118 (m = 57.18; sd = 39.30) and the time spent online ranged from 346–3,239 minutes (m = 1,370.23; sd = 873.37) indicating that women were spending time online even if they were not posting.

The quantitative data analyzed for the study consisted of demographic information. The data were collected as part of the screening interview to determine eligibility for participation in WTW. Electronic and printed copies of the data were provided to us by the WTW project manager under the direction of the principal investigator for WTW.

Data Analysis

We checked a printed copy of each chat room conversation for accuracy with the electronic data, then analyzed the conversations for common themes using methods described by Miles and Huberman (1994). We analyzed chat room conversations specifically by (a) reading each conversation completely to get a sense of the whole, (b) dividing conversations into units denoted by a change in subject matter or activities described, and (c) labeling individual units from each conversation using a word or words that represented the unit topic (descriptive codes) and writing them in the margins of each printed copy. We also wrote theoretic memos (thoughts about the connections between the codes) in the margins. We continued coding until we classified all of the data. After coding by hand on the hard copy, we entered the electronic file of each conversation into QSR NUD*IST (Version 4), a software program designed to manage qualitative data. We then entered the codes for each conversation and compared them with other coded conversations to identify common themes among them. To confirm and validate findings, we linked all initial codes, theoretic memos, and the emerging themes to primary data sources. We discussed emerging themes until we achieved consensus.

We analyzed quantitative data to provide a description of the participants and to provide context for the qualitative findings. We displayed all data using Statistical Package for the Social Sciences (Version 11.5) and analyzed the data using descriptive statistics to determine item frequencies and measures of central tendency.

FINDINGS

It was clear from the qualitative data that the women in the computer group felt positive about the intervention. They were pleased to have access to information about their illness and to other women facing similar challenges. Many expressed feeling a "connection" with group members. Some women referred to the group as their "cyber friends," exchanged phone numbers, and made plans to meet off-line. In addition to talking about their illnesses, the women shared stories about their families, exchanged recipes, described vacations, and told jokes. They offered words of support, prayer, and hope for "better times" for their online peers and their family members. As the computer intervention was nearing conclusion, the women expressed sadness about losing the connection with their newly made friends. They spoke of "going through withdrawal" and having a "hard time" giving up the program. One participant wrote,

I will miss visiting with you all. There have been times when I felt too crummy to type anything, but I could always read. My last exacerbation would have been ten times worse if I had not been able to hear your words of wisdom, jokes, and suggestions for better health.

Common Themes

We identified six common themes from analyzing the online support group conversations.

1. Uncertainty/searching for answers
2. Physical and emotional isolation
3. Maintaining balance
4. Others first
5. Vigilance: Financial, physical, emotional
6. Ways of coping

Uncertainty/Searching for Answers

The women experienced uncertainty throughout their illness experiences. Before diagnosis, uncertainty was related to not knowing what was happening to them and the inability of their health care providers to provide an immediate explanation of their symptoms. A long diagnostic process was common requiring trips to more than one health care provider before the correct diagnosis was made. One woman wrote, "I can't even count how many things I went to the doctor for over the years that I am now told are symptoms of this hateful illness." The average time from onset of symptoms to diagnosis was 9.7 years (range = <1–32 years). Frustration and an erosion of trust in their physician's judgment accompanied uncertainty, while women who were quickly diagnosed thought of their health care provider as "good."

Diagnosis did not put an end to the uncertainty. New or changing symptoms were common as were new treatments with unfamiliar outcomes and side effects. Uncertainty prompted a search for information, explanations, and answers. The women read about their illnesses and asked questions of their health care providers. During the intervention, the women asked others in the group if they had similar experiences to their own and were relieved to hear that they did. One woman expressed surprise and relief at the similarities of the experiences described by the women. She had felt alone and doubted her "stability" thinking that she must have been "making things up in her head" because "doctors couldn't seem to find a reason" for her symptoms.

Physical and Emotional Isolation

The women lived in rural communities or on farms, in areas of few health care resources and had little contact with other chronically ill women. The women felt emotionally isolated, afraid to talk about their illnesses with persons who were not ill for fear of alienating them and straining their relationships. They wrote of not being able to tell non-ill persons how they really felt for fear they would tire of hearing from them and "walk away." Although they had the support of family and friends, not being able to share feelings about their illnesses with others who were not ill potentially decreased the support they received and promoted their sense of emotional isolation. As one woman wrote, "This disease accomplishes one thing. It isolates."

Maintaining Balance

This theme referred to the women's roles, responsibilities, and need to balance activities and energies to maintain each role. Eight of the 15 women worked full-time outside the home. One commented, "I need to say NO to more things and not get so upset over things that haven't gotten done. I know this but I need to remember it." Limited or no access to health care providers, pharmacies, and other health care services sometimes strained the women's ability to maintain balance. The need to travel to distant cities for specialized health care sometimes required an overnight stay and the driving assistance of a family member or friend. Time away from home and work affected the delicate balance the women were trying to achieve.

Others First

The women in this study put the needs of their communities, employers, and families before their own. They found time to provide community service and participate in civic activities, spend time with friends, and assist neighbors in need. The women worked long hours at home, and for employers, while still finding time to see to the needs of their spouses and children, whether the children were living at home or not. The women wrote about accompanying family members and friends to various activities that often involved long hours in the car. Putting others first affected their ability to maintain balance in their lives by draining their energy and exacerbating their symptoms. Although sometimes uncertain about how their activities would affect them, over time the women learned that they would "pay the price" if they did too much. However, knowing this did not guarantee that they would pull back. Often times they would continue their activities and suffer the consequences.

> I need to share with you . . . maybe it is like true confessions . . . how I didn't accept responsibility for my recent exacerbation. My employer needed . . . my church needed . . . my students needed . . . and all the time I was getting more tired and nauseated but I kept on going until I was really sick.

Vigilance

We used this theme to describe the alert watchfulness the women displayed toward their physical, emotional, and financial health. Prior to diagnosis, the women actively sought meaning for their symptoms. After diagnosis, the women were alert for any changes that might indicate improvement or deterioration in their conditions, the onset of new problems, or treatment side effects. During the intervention, the women discussed at length their symptoms, queried others to see if they were experiencing similar problems, and shared strategies used to manage them. The most common physical symptoms discussed were pain, sleeplessness, and fatigue. The most common emotions expressed were frustration, depression, and stress.

The cost of care was a frequent topic of discussion among the women. Many shared that they were stressed by the financial burden of health care and uncertain about how they would pay for their care. The women spent a considerable amount of their time dealing with this issue. Online, the women shared strategies to cut costs, finance care, and navigate the bureaucratic red tape of the programs that assist persons with chronic illness. Some expressed their appreciation for health insurance and concern for those who did not have coverage. They welcomed assistance from husbands who would "handle all that."

Ways of Coping

We used this theme to describe several methods used by the women to cope with their illnesses. Common methods included information gathering and self-care. The women took active roles caring for themselves by learning about their illnesses through reading, attending informational sessions presented by experts in the field, and asking questions of their health care providers. As one woman wrote, taking an active role in her health care and not waiting for the doctors to "tell her what to think and do" provided a sense of "control over her illness." The women participated in their prescribed treatments but also tried new things, such as herbs and special diets, with the hope of improving their well-being. They frequently shared self-care strategies with their online peers. Good communication and positive relationships with their health care providers were viewed as essential to their ability to cope with their illnesses. Women who felt that they were "heard" by their health care provider evaluated them as "good" and "caring." A good relationship with their health care providers was important enough to prompt some women to change doctors.

Faith and humor were frequently used as coping mechanisms. The women's conversations frequently included references to scripture, prayer, and faith. Funny stories, anecdotes, and jokes were also common and well received. The women commented on several occasions how good it was for them to laugh and asked their peers to "Keep the jokes coming."

Keeping busy, even though activity could exacerbate their symptoms, was a common strategy used by the women. Participants attempted to maintain normalcy in their lives by maintaining their usual routines and activities. The women tried to balance their activities with rest periods but often did more than they should have done. Maintaining normalcy also involved not talking about their illness with persons who were not ill.

The support network of family and friends was an important coping mechanism. Although persons without illness may not fully understand what the women were going through, their help was needed and appreciated. Contact with other chronically ill persons was seen as especially helpful. The women expressed a great deal of appreciation for their online peers. One woman wrote, "I have gotten so used to talking to all of you! It's different than talking to anyone else, because we can 'let it all hang out' and everyone understands. Thanks for listening to me and encouraging me." Reaching out and providing support to others was also important. The women shared information, gave advice, and demonstrated concern and compassion for members of the online group and their families.

DISCUSSION AND IMPLICATIONS

The findings from the qualitative data support what is already known about chronic illness and adds knowledge specific to living with chronic illness in a rural setting. The data confirmed that chronically ill persons strive to understand their illnesses, recognize and control symptoms, implement prescribed treatments, adjust to changes in the course of the diseases, deal with uncertainty, attempt to normalize daily life, find ways to fund medical care, and confront emotional and physical problems (Strauss et al., 1984). The findings also corroborate that difficulty in achieving a diagnosis can lead to uncertainty and an erosion of faith in the physician (Mishel, 1988, 1993; Mishel & Braden, 1988). The findings support the emotional isolation commonly felt by persons with chronic illnesses (Davies & Sque, 2002) and the importance of support, understanding, and a sense of collaboration between patient and health care provider (FitzGerald, Pearson, & McCutcheon, 2001).

The findings specific to managing chronic illness in a rural setting were experiences related to physical isolation and limited access to others with a similar condition. The emotional isolation the women in this study experienced may have been complicated by their physical isolation. Distance, weather conditions, and geographical constraints affected the women's access to health care providers and health care resources and potentially decreased the support available to them. For example, some of the women in this study traveled hundreds of miles to reach the closest health care specialists, not because they were the "best" but because they were the closest to them. It was also common for those who attended presentations by health experts to have to travel 3 or more hours to a distant city to attend the seminar.

Distance is an accepted part of rural living (Long & Weinert, 1989). However, traveling can be arduous for ill persons, physically and financially, and often involves careful planning. A trip to the specialist sometimes meant an overnight stay, required the driving assistance of a family member or friend, as well as additional trips for diagnostic testing and follow-up care. Effective time management and advanced planning were essential components of the women's illness management strategies. Health care specialists can help decrease the physical and financial burden of chronic illness with thoughtful scheduling, effective communication, and careful collaboration with the women's local health care providers when appropriate. In some circumstances, the use of telemedicine may be an appropriate alternative to a trip to a distant health care specialist.

The women had the support of family members; however, some lived a distance away. They were also physically isolated from other persons living with similar health problems. The women believed that persons who were not ill were less able to understand what they were going through. They also worried that "compassion fatigue" would become a problem for family and friends who were nearby. As a result, the women "put on a happy face" and "didn't let others know how they felt" and experienced emotional isolation. Health care providers can help their patients cope with their illness by encouraging what has worked; in this case, faith, humor, and keeping busy. Facilitating a phone number or e-mail exchange between interested patients or recommending one of the many professional organizations that have online support groups can be empowering (Burrows, Nettleton, Pleace, Loader, & Muncer, 2000) and should be considered. Given the positive experiences of the 15 women in this study, an online chronic illness support group appears to be a viable solution to the problem of isolation. However, additional research is needed to examine the value and health benefits of virtual communities (Eysenbach, Powell, Englesakis, Rizo, & Stern, 2004).

The women were frustrated by delayed or difficult diagnoses, professionals who "didn't listen," and the high costs of care. The women desired to be understood, to understand what was happening to them, and to be able to implement appropriate self-care strategies. Clear, open, and frequent communication with clients may help to decrease frustration and uncertainty while providing the basis for a positive relationship. Health care providers can help their patients to implement self-care strategies by providing both verbal and written information and recommending reputable online information resources. Providing "virtual office hours" where rural patients can contact their health care providers via e-mail might also be helpful. Although information can decrease uncertainty (Mishel, 1993), health care providers should remind their patients that uncertainty is part of chronic illness.

Although the findings add to our understanding of the chronic illness experiences of rural women, questions remain. For example, do isolated rural women with other diagnoses experience chronic illness differently? Do younger or older women and teens manage their illnesses differently than middle-aged women? Furthermore, more research is needed regarding the role nurses play in the experiences of chronically ill rural women. The women were referring to physician providers in their chat room conversations and never mentioned nurses in their postings. More research is needed to understand the role nurses play in the illness experiences of rural women.

CONCLUSION

Using a computer and the Internet was a manageable and accepted method of providing peer-support to a group of isolated rural women with chronic illness. With proper instruction and assistance, even the most novice computer user was able to navigate the computer and participate in online conversations with a group of their peers. The women's illness experiences support the findings of others and illustrate commonalities found among persons living in rural areas. Recognizing the common problems and uncertainties experienced by these women is an important step in planning effective care. Further exploration is needed to understand the complex and multifaceted chronic illness experiences of isolated rural women.

ACKNOWLEDGMENTS

This research was funded by the Center for Research on Chronic Health Conditions in Rural Dwellers (Grant NIH/NINR IP20 NR 07790-01). The authors acknowledge Dr. Clarann Weinert for her assistance with this study.

REFERENCES

About MS. (2004). Retrieved July 2, 2004, from http://www.nationalmssociety.org/about%20ms.asp

Agency for Health Care Policy & Research. (1996). *Improving health care for rural populations. Research in Action fact sheet.* (AHCPR Publication No. 96–P040). Washington, DC: U.S. Government Printing Office.

Albright, A. (2008). *Diabetes: 2008 at a Glance.* Retrieved October 16, 2008, from http://www.cdc.gov/nccdphp/publications/aag/ddt.htm

Benet, A. (1996). A portrait of chronic illness: Inspecting the canvas, reframing the issues. *American Behavioral Scientist, 39,* 767–776.

Burrows, R., Nettleton, S., Pleace, N., Loader, B., & Muncer, S. (2000). Virtual community care? Social policy and the emergence of computer mediated social support. *Information, Communication and Society, 3* (1), 95–121.

Centers for Disease Control (CDC). (2008, March 20). *Chronic disease overview.* Retrieved October 16, 2008, from http://www.cdc.gov/nccdphp/overview.htm

Davies, M., & Sque, M. (2002). Living on the outside looking in: A theory of living with advanced breast cancer. *International Journal of Palliative Nursing, 8,* 583–584, 586–590.

Eberhardt, M. S., Ingram, D. D., Makuc, D. M., Pamuk, E. R., Freid, V. M., Harper, S. B., et al. (2001). *Urban and rural health chartbook. Health, United States, 2001 with rural and urban chartbook* (NCHS Publication No. PHS 01–1232). Hyattsville, MD: National Center for Health Statistics.

Eysenbach, G., Powell, J., Englesakis, M., Rizo, C., & Stern, A. (2004). Health related virtual communities and electronic support groups: Systematic review of the effects of online peer to peer interactions. *British Medical Journal, 328* (7449), 1166–1170.

FitzGerald, M., Pearson, A., & McCutcheon, H. (2001). Impact of rural living on the experience of chronic illness. *Australian Journal of Rural Health, 9,* 235–240.

Gesler, W., Hartwell, S., Ricketts, T., & Rosenberg, M. (1992). Introduction. In W. Gesler & T. Ricketts (Eds.), *Health in rural North America* (pp. 1–22). New Brunswick, NJ: Rutgers University Press.

Hootman, J., Bolen, J., Helmick, C., & Langmaid, G. (2006). Prevalence of doctor-diagnosed arthritis and arthritis-attributable activity limitation—United States, 2003–2005. *MMWR, 55* (40), 1089–1092.

Husaine, B., & Moore, S. (1990). Arthritis disability, depression, and life satisfaction among black elderly people. *Health and Social Work, 15,* 253–259.

Hwu, Y. J. (1995). The impact of chronic illness on patients. *Rehabilitation Nursing, 20,* 221–225.

Jensen, A. (1991). Psychosocial factors in breast cancer and their possible impact upon prognosis. *Cancer Treatment Reviews, 18,* 191–210.

Long, K. A., & Weinert, C. (1989). Rural nursing: Developing the theory base. *Scholarly Inquiry for Nursing Practice, 3,* 113–127.

Marks, J. S. (2003). *The burden of chronic disease and the future of public health.* Retrieved June 28, 2004, from http://www.cdc.gov/nccdphp/burden_pres/

Mast, M. E. (1995). Adult uncertainty in illness: A critical review of research. *Scholarly Inquiry for Nursing Practice, 9,* 3–24; discussion 25–29.

Meit, M. (2004). *Bridging the health divide: The rural public health research agenda.* Pittsburgh, PA: University of Pittsburgh Center for Rural Health Practice.

Miles, M. B., & Huberman, A. M. (1994). *Qualitative data analysis* (2nd ed.). Thousand Oaks, CA: Sage.

Mishel, M. H. (1984). Perceived uncertainty and stress in illness. *Research in Nursing & Health, 7,* 163–171.

Mishel, M. H. (1988). Uncertainty in illness. *Image: Journal of Nursing Scholarship, 20,* 225–232.

Mishel, M. H. (1993). Living with chronic illness: Living with uncertainty. In S. Funk, E. Tornquist, M. Champagne, & R. Wiese (Eds.), *Key aspects of caring for the chronically ill: Hospital and home* (pp. 46–58). New York: Springer.

Mishel, M. H., & Braden, C. J. (1988). Finding meaning: Antecedents of uncertainty in illness. *Nursing Research, 37,* 98–103, 127.

QSR NUD°IST. (1998). Version 4. QSR International Pty Ltd, Melbourne, Australia.

Ries, L.A.G., Melbert, D., Krapcho, M., Stinchcomb, D.G., Howlader, N., Horner, M. J., et al. (2008). SEER Stat Fact Sheets. Retrieved October 16, 2008, from http://seer.cancer.gov/statfacts/html/all.html

Robinson, C. A. (1993). Managing life with a chronic condition: The story of normalization. *Qualitative Health Research, 3* (1), 6–28.

Scott, J. (2000). A nursing leadership challenge: Managing the chronically ill in rural settings. *Nursing Administration Quarterly, 24* (3), 21–32.

Strauss, A., Corbin, J., Fagerhaugh, S., Glaser, B., Maines, D., Suczek, B., et al. (1984). *Chronic illness and the quality of life* (2nd ed.). St. Louis: Mosby.

Stuifbergen, A. (1995). Health-promoting behaviors and quality of life among individuals with multiple sclerosis. *Scholarly Inquiry for Nursing Practice, 9,* 31–50.

Sullivan, T., Weinert, C., & Cudney, S. (2003). Management of chronic illness: Voices of rural women. *Journal of Advanced Nursing, 44,* 566–574.

United States Census Bureau. (2000). *United States—Urban/Rural and Inside/Outside Metropolitan Area.* Retrieved June 15, 2009, from http://www.census.gov

Weiner, C. (1975). The burden of rheumatoid arthritis: Tolerating the uncertainty. *Social Science and Medicine, 9,* 97–104.

Weinert, C. (2000). Social support in cyberspace for women with chronic illness. *Rehabilitation Nursing, 25,* 129–135.

Winters, C. A. (1997). *Living with chronic heart disease: A pilot study.* Retrieved March 31, 2004, from http://www.nova.edu/ssss/QR/QR3–4/winters.html

Winters, C. A. (1999). Heart failure: Living with uncertainty. *Progress in Cardiovascular Nursing, 14,* 85–91.

Negotiation of Constructed Gender Among Rural Male Caregivers

12

CHAD O'LYNN

Nearly 20% of all Americans will be over age 65 by 2030 (U.S. Census Bureau, 2004). Associated with increased age is the increased incidence of chronic health conditions requiring caregiving services. Many aspects of caregiving have been studied; however, family caregiving in rural communities remains poorly understood. In addition, health care resources and support in rural communities are stretched thinly compared to urbanized communities. Consequently, the growing number of intervention studies based on current descriptions, theoretical models, and urban assumptions of caregiving may not apply to rural caregivers. Additional research is needed to explore the unique needs of rural caregivers. Among rural caregivers, men have been particularly ignored by researchers and policy makers.

SIGNIFICANCE OF THE PROPOSED STUDY

The reported percentage of family caregivers who are male ranges between 30% (Marks, 1996; National Alliance for Caregiving & American Association of Retired Persons [NAC & AARP], 1997, 2004) and 44% (Opinion Research Corporation [ORC], 2005). Conservatively, over 12.5 million American men are caring for dependent adults (U.S. Census

Bureau, 2002). The number of male caregivers is expected to increase as the number of older Americans increases and the number of female family members who have traditionally filled caregiver roles decreases (Kramer, 2002). Just as with women, caregiving is associated with negative health changes for men (Vitaliano, Zhang, & Scanlan, 2003). Consequently, increasing numbers of men providing caregiving may present a growing men's health concern.

Few rural studies have included male caregivers in their samples; yet knowledge of their needs and perspectives is essential to optimize their health and success as caregivers. It is hypothesized that healthy and successful rural male caregivers will provide better care to their care recipients, and thus reduce morbidity and premature institutionalization of dependent elders. The specific aims of this study were to

1. Explore the meanings and experiences of caregiving from the perspectives of rural male caregivers;
2. Explore the processes used by rural male caregivers as they progress through the caregiving experience;
3. Explore the effects of caregiving on rural male caregiver health and caregiver success; and
4. Develop a theoretical understanding of how male gender and rurality affect caregiving.

LITERATURE REVIEW

Caregiving

The experience of caring for family members has been correlated with numerous negative and positive psychological and physical health consequences, although greater attention has been given to negative consequences. Researchers' tendency to examine negative aspects of caregiving has been criticized (Acton & Winter, 2002; Archbold, Stewart, Greenlick, & Harvath, 1992; Kramer, 1997); however, the evidence for negative consequences of caregiving is strong and unequivocal (National Institute of Nursing Research [NINR], 1994; Pinquart & Sorenson, 2006; Vitaliano, Zhang, & Scanlan, 2003; Yee & Schulz, 2000). Commonly, aspects of caregiving that yield negative health consequences include limitations placed upon the caregiver's life, competing roles and time demands for caregivers, and demands placed on caregivers stemming from the care recipient's emotional and physical needs (NAC & AARP, 2004; NINR, 1994). Less documented aspects include lack of social support and deterioration of the relationship between caregiver and recipient. In sum, these aspects lead to increased caregiver burden and caregiver strain, which in turn elevate levels of stress among caregivers to the point of threatening caregiver health.

Caregiver burden and caregiver strain are constructs that have been poorly defined and variably operationalized among researchers. Burden refers to the distress experienced by caregivers and has been operationalized in tools such as the Zarit Burden Inventory (Zarit, Reever, & Bach-Peterson, 1980). Using Lazarus' Stress Theory as a foundation, caregiver strain is a state that results from enduring problems that are appraised as threats to caregiver well-being and require a coping response (Lawton, Kleban, Moss, Rovine, & Glicksman, 1989; Pearlin & Schooler, 1978; Robinson, 1983). Caregiver strain is categorized as emotional, physical, financial, or familial in nature. Emotional strain is the category best supported in the literature and has been most frequently operationalized as caregiver depression (NINR, 1994). It is estimated that the stress of caregiving can reduce a caregiver's life by as many as ten years (Arno, 2006).

Positive aspects of caregiving reported in the literature include feeling useful and needed and achieving a sense of personal affirmation (operationalized as caregiver satisfaction) and personal meaning (operationalized as reciprocity, mutuality, affection, or attachment) (NINR, 1994). Theoretically, positive affirmation and meaning may ameliorate negative health consequences of caregiving.

The literature of male caregiving primarily focuses on quantitatively measured differences between male and female caregivers. A number of researchers reported that male caregivers have less depression, fewer role conflicts, less caregiver burden and strain, and greater satisfaction than their female counterparts (Carpenter & Miller, 2002; Gitlin, Belle, Burgio, et al., 2003; Pinquart & Sorenson, 2006; Yee & Schulz, 2000). However, several researchers provided opposing findings or reported no significant differences between male and female caregivers on selected measures (Baillie, Norbeck, & Barnes, 1988; Ladner & Cuellar, 2002; Schulz, Beach, Lind, et al., 2001). Explanations for variable findings illuminate methodological limitations of these studies, such as an over-reliance upon cross-sectional designs (Bookwala, Newman, & Schulz, 2002; Carpenter & Miller, 2002); lack of reporting effects sizes or clinical significance of findings (Miller & Cafasso, 1992); or sampling procedures that hide unique findings for men or for subcategories of male caregivers (Harris, 2002; Houde, 2002; Thompson, 2002). Theoretical limitations in which findings unique to male subjects are compared to normative female data are also prevalent in the literature (Kramer, 2002; Miller & Cafasso, 1992; Thompson; Young & Kahana, 1989). These limitations have promoted, at worst, the invisibility of male caregivers, and at best, an unreliable understanding of male caregivers (Stoller, 2002; Thompson). As such, the knowledge base from these studies is not sufficient to develop support strategies and interventions that are applicable and acceptable to male caregivers (Gwyther, 1992; Thompson).

Rural Health and Rurality

A lack of agreement on the definition of *rural* among researchers has led to great variation in study samples, thus making comparison among studies difficult. However, the term *frontier* is consistently used to describe the most rural of areas, generally considered to have a population density of less than six persons per square mile (Hewitt, 1992; Wagenfeld, 2000, 2003). Frontier areas may exemplify commonly reported barriers to health services in rural communities and the unique cultural aspects of rural dwellers (Hewitt; Lee, 1998b; Wagenfeld). Studies using frontier samples may yield findings most applicable to rural communities as a whole.

Despite great variation among rural communities, health disparities for rural dwellers are well-documented. Published reviews have noted that rural dwellers have higher rates of chronic illness, mental illness, obesity, social and physical limitations, death from motor vehicle accidents, and smoking and alcohol consumption than their urban counterparts (Center on an Aging Society, 2003; Eberhardt, Ingram, & Makuc, 2001; NINR, 1995). In addition, rural dwellers pay more out-of-pocket expenses for health services, use preventative health services less frequently, and for elders, report a lower quality of life (Ballantyne & Buehler, 1998; Center on an Aging Society; Goins & Mitchell, 1999; Kumar, Acanfora, Hennessy, & Kalache, 2001; Lishner, Richardson, Levine, & Patrick, 1996; Morgan, Semchuk, Stewart, & D'Arcy, 2002; NINR; National Rural Health Association [NRHA], 2007). Chief explanatory factors for these disparities include a lack of accessible, affordable, available, and diverse health services in rural areas; increased distance to services; inadequate transportation; concerns about privacy; and increased poverty rates for rural dwellers (Ballantyne & Buehler; Center on an Aging Society; Lishner et al., 1996; Morgan et al., 2002; NINR; NRHA, 2007). Unfortunately, many social and governmental programs implemented to address disparities are founded on knowledge derived from urban-based research models, often rendering these programs unacceptable to rural dwellers and inappropriate to the unique needs and realities of rural communities (Bull, Krout, Rathbone-McCuan, & Shreffler, 2001; Ryan-Nicholls, 2004). Rural disparities combined with poorly suited services provide a context in which rural caregivers are likely to experience greater challenges and health risks than their urban counterparts.

Bigbee (1993) identified literature support for the existence of a rural culture. Rural culture is characterized by relatively close and long-term relationships with family and neighbors that result in a lack of anonymity and a blurring of social roles. Rural dwellers tend to be more morally and politically conservative and traditional in their values than urban dwellers. Rural dwellers value individualism, hard work, independence, and self-sufficiency. Bigbee reported that geographical isolation substantially shapes rural culture and enhances the visibility of other rural attributes, such as a keen perception of and distrust of outsiders (Bailey, 1998; Lee, 1998a), ethnocentrism (Dybbro, 1998), and an increased reliance upon nonformal health resources to manage health and illness (Buehler, Malone, & Majerus, 1998; O'Lynn, 2006). However, Wagenfeld (2003) indicated that the cultural divide between urban and rural dwellers is narrowing, especially as communication technology and migration patterns change. This narrowing is not uniform and is likely to be slower in more isolated or frontier rural communities. It is the nexus of rural demographics and rural culture that defines the construct rurality, in that rural residence alone does not account for the unique context and experiences of rural dwellers (Wagenfeld). Wagenfeld questioned whether an urban individual who relocates to a rural area is truly rural, a consideration that is congruent with the perspective of insider/outsider status common among rural dwellers (Lee).

Rural Masculinity

Minimal research has been published on how masculinity is manifested in rural communities, yet a consistent portrayal of rural masculinity is found in popular literature and films. Although cognizant of the complexity of gender and multiple masculinities within subgroups of men, Levant and Habben (2003) proposed that rural men are likely more traditional in their masculine ideology than are urban men, an ideology characterized by toughness, self-reliance, homophobia, avoidance of feminine behaviors and emotionality, and a high value placed on accomplishment and work. In addition, due to the lack of anonymity typical in rural communities, the actions and reputations of rural men are highly visible and carry much weight. "As a result, rural men are more likely to try to adhere to a higher moral code or else keep their problems very private" (p. 177). Adherence to a more traditional masculine ideology may encourage rural men to avoid assistance from others, especially health and human service assistance, compared to urban men.

METHOD

Sample

In this study, participants were recruited from frontier areas in two northwestern states in the United States using flyers and newspaper advertisements. Frontier was defined as a county of less than six persons per square mile. Inclusion criteria required that participants reside within a community with a population of fewer than 15,000 residents, and be a male caregiver who provided (or had provided) daily assistance with activities of daily living to a relative. Twelve non-Hispanic Caucasian men participated in this study. The men ranged in age from 45 to 87 years, with a mean of 58.9 years. Caregiving experience ranged from 1 to 28 years, with 8 of the 12 men providing care for 5 years or less. Nine of the men were caregivers for their wives and 3 of the men were caregivers for two family members each, resulting in a total of 15 care recipients for the 12 men. In addition to nine wives, care recipients included one adult daughter, one sister, three mothers, and one grandmother.

Ten of the men were lifelong residents of rural communities. The other two had lived in rural settings for 7 and 15 years, respectively. At the time of the study, two of the men lived on farms or ranches with the others living in towns with populations ranging from 150 to 12,228. Three of the men were retired; the others were working full- or part-time. All the men had careers in service and extractive industries. Generally, the men reported their health as good, with only two participants reporting chronic illnesses that impaired their ability to work in their chosen careers.

Family members receiving care from the study participants required assistance with activities of daily living and could not live independently without such care. Most of the care recipients suffered from musculoskeletal disorders, including three with spinal cord injuries. Five care recipients had dementia, three care recipients had experienced strokes, two had mental health disorders, one had amyotrophic lateral sclerosis, and one had cerebral palsy. All care recipients had primary care providers located within a few miles of their residences, and most required the care of a specialist on a semiannual basis requiring travel of 58 to 228 miles (one-way).

Data Collection Procedures and Analysis

Data were collected using in-depth interviews and observations consistent with constructivist grounded theory method (Charmaz, 2000, 2006). This method was deemed most appropriate since it is congruent with the study aims and assumptions that gender and culture are socially constructed phenomena. The method embraced the knowledge and experiences of participant and researcher as cocreators of a study's findings. Phenomena were deconstructed in order to explore hidden meanings, assumptions, and power relationships followed by construction of findings from data using inductive and generative processes. The method yielded an account of the meanings and actions of a social process rather than a simple explanation of a social process typical with other forms of grounded theory.

Participants contributed 18 interviews conducted both face-to-face and via telephone. Each interview lasted 45–120 minutes in length. A semistructured interview approach was used in order to accommodate conversation and optimal exploration. Latter interviews also included specific questions designed to explore emerging data categories, consistent with grounded theory methodology (Charmaz, 2000, 2006). Interviews were audio taped and transcribed by the author.

Data analysis began following the first interview with line-by-line open coding. Repetition of many of the codes was evident after four interviews. After eight interviews, 285 codes had been identified. These codes were collapsed into 21 broader focused codes. A situational map was used to help discern relationships among the focused codes. Subsequent interviews clarified emerging relationships and meanings in the data. From this process, four categories were constructed from the data: rurality, rural masculinity, caregiver challenges, and negotiating gender.

Findings were then compared to the extant literature for further clarification and refinement. Ultimately, a theoretical model was developed in which the core category, gender negotiation, was constructed as the chief explanatory and action category to account for the differences in experiences and perspectives among the participants.

FINDINGS

Rurality

The division between rurality and rural masculinity is obscure since both gender and culture are socially constructed phenomena and are intertwined in derivation and manifestation. Nevertheless, participants described attributes of rurality as applicable to most long-term residents of rural communities; whereas, attributes of rural masculinity were described as more prevalent or manifested more intensely in rural men than in rural women.

Geographic isolation was the most commonly discussed rural attribute. Although most participants lived within 50 miles of a health care provider, few lived close to health care specialists and comprehensive durable medical equipment providers. For example, one participant's wife had a subcutaneous pump that delivered pain medication continuously. The pump needed to be filled with medication every month, which required a 450-mile round trip to the medical office. All of the participants noted that driving long distances placed great financial, comfort, and time burdens on them and their care recipients. Two participants depleted their savings to purchase vans to transport their care recipients to medical appointments. One participant reported that he had become a member of a newly created ambulance service, in which an annual fee is paid to have a helicopter land in his community to transport his wife to an urban hospital when needed. Some participants emphasized that urban dwellers and health providers had little understanding or appreciation of such geographical challenges.

The participants described several social attributes of rurality. One attribute is a value for self-reliance and the hard work needed to maintain self-reliance. In discussing this value, participants did not use a vocal tone of admiration but rather a tone of matter-of-factness. One participant noted that his family and his wife's family were "Oregon Trail people," which fostered not only self-reliance but also ruggedness and independence. Related to self-reliance was a value of caring for one's own. Several participants commented that rural family values dictate that one care for one's family members when needed. Caregiving was not couched in negative terms of obligation or duty, but rather as a cultural norm that was so engrained that the adoption of the caregiver role did not foster much reflection. In answering a question about caregiver roles for spouses, one participant stated, "She'd be doing exactly what I'm doing because we both believe in the same things, the same kind of principles." Later, this participant commented about how someone had approached him at an urban restaurant and complimented him while he was helping his wife to eat. He was perplexed by the compliment and stated,

> [T]he way I take care of her and the attention I give her, I figure that's part of it, that's what I'm supposed to do. I told her [his wife] a long time ago that that's why she hired me on forty years ago.

Other participants noted that this value may be generational and worried that younger rural dwellers may be less likely to assume a caregiving role.

Seemingly paradoxical to self-reliance is the rural attribute of community support. Participants described rural community support as offers for assistance for tasks that would exceed the capacity of any normally self-reliant individual. They also noted that these offers were expected of others as a normative behavior of rural neighbors. An example was the offers of cutting and baling hay for a participant. Community support was described as "good neighborliness" and was viewed as a pervasive and beneficial characteristic typical of rural, but not urban, communities. In emphasizing the rural/urban difference in community support, one participant commented,

> I'll give you an idea. I had car troubles at 11:30 at night. I opened my hood, and right away some guy from the Forest Service and a retired mechanic comes over. One sheriff guy comes over. Then one other person. I have no idea who he was, but he comes over. . . . I mean everybody sticks up their finger in the air when they wave to you and drive along, your index finger goes up like a peace sign or whatever. In [urban home town], it's the MIDDLE finger that goes up!

However, community support may be predicated on having an insider status. Two participants who had not lived in their communities for many years commented on having an outsider status and perceived themselves as lacking common histories with local residents and fewer interdependent relationships. Although an outsider status did not impair their ability to receive desired services, being an outsider led to a perception that increased time was needed to establish community connectedness.

Faith communities were an important source of community support. In noting the difference between general community support and faith community support, one participant noted, "I guess [work colleagues] were more analytical, or 'What can we do to help?' Church people were there not only to help with physical things, but spiritual." The importance of faith community support was acknowledged even by those who did not attend a specific church. One participant commented,

> It kind of elevates you. . . . You depend upon prayer chains from denominations in this community. That's a really nice thing about being in a small town, is you know, you're not known in just your faith community. You're known in many groups. And, so, I'd meet folks in the grocery store who'd say, 'I'm praying for you, your wife and you.' Which, you know, is humbling, uplifting, and it's sustainable.

Another participant noted that rural communities have two kinds of tight-knit families: the "church family" and the "bar [tavern] family," with both families having regular members who spend time together and look out for each other. Each of these smaller communities may provide caregivers focused and ongoing support as opposed to the general support and encouragement provided by the community at large.

Participants identified faith as another rural attribute. Faith was less about church attendance and more about belief in a higher power and spirituality. Participants believed that God provided rural dwellers hardiness to endure life's challenges. For example, "God plants us the seeds to be strong and get us through tough times." In addition, participants articulated a somewhat fatalistic perspective when those challenges were beyond human intervention. For these challenges, rural dwellers accepted God's will. One participant commented, "We said that we married for better or for worse. We just happened to draw the worse card. You [have to] take life as it comes."

Rural Masculinity

The participants described rural masculinity in very personal and visceral language. Participants discussed attributes that not only described themselves but also the perspectives they had of other rural men. No rural masculinity attribute was discussed as much as self-reliance. Participants indicated that self-reliance was a keystone characteristic of rural masculinity. In addition, the participants described self-reliance in more detail as it related to masculinity than they did for rurality.

Participants described masculine self-reliance as a deep sense of independence with a strong unwillingness to ask others for assistance. This unwillingness did not stop at physical assistance with tasks, but included advice or feedback on their plans and actions as well. An unwillingness to ask for assistance is what separated the self-reliance of rural men from the self-reliance of rural women, whom these men perceived to be more willing to seek advice from peers. Self-reliance influenced how men approached work and challenges in all aspects of their lives and how they viewed themselves as men. Self-reliance was also described as including a "can-do" attitude which promoted ingenuity and a "hands-on" and pragmatic approach to problems. For example, although having access to durable medical equipment and physical therapy services for his injured wife, one participant felt not only an unwillingness to ask for these services but also felt that such services would not be needed because he could provide the services himself. He noted,

> I started manufacturing different things to get her up and walk, and even had her in the shop . . . used an engine hoist to get her up in the walker. Yeah, we had all different kinds of things. And when she goes to the potty, why I got an overhead wench that I run on a rail that I transfer her into the bathroom and the shower.

Participants noted that an unwillingness to ask for assistance was present even if it became apparent to the participant that he needed assistance with caregiving. The participants explained this unwillingness as a general resistance to relinquish control of a situation. According to the participants, relinquishing control by having others come in to provide caregiving was a frank admission that they, as men, were unable to complete the work and somehow had failed as caregivers. This belief was most common in terms of the personal and intimate aspects of caregiving, and less prevalent in asking for help with large and highly visible tasks such as farm work.

Discussion of independence, or possibly aversion to dependence, was common in the participants' descriptions of self-reliance. One participant commented on how important it was for him for his wife to become as independent as possible, not as a way to avoid work for himself, but as a way for her to improve self-esteem. One way he fostered independence in his wife was to intentionally fumble at caregiver tasks. He stated,

> And it gives her more incentive to do more for herself. And I'm a firm believer in that 'cause that's just the way it seems. If you do everything for them . . . she gets in the habit of it, but if you drag your feet, well, she'll figure out a way of doing it. I used to dress her up until about four or five months ago, and now she says, 'I'll do it myself!' And, thank God, she does a pretty good job of dressing herself.

Self-reliance also meant doing all work necessary, regardless of previous or stereotypical gendered divisions of labor. The participants were explicit that they did not see housework as feminine, but rather as work that had to be done, as is all work on a farm or ranch. If their wives could no longer perform housework, they pitched in and did it themselves. A typical comment was that "You gotta do what you gotta do." One participant stated that this "just do it" perspective was modeled to most rural men by their fathers and other men in their communities. One participant commented,

> [My father] was just a doer, you know, washing dishes, making dinner and everything. All my life he was like that. If mom worked at the hospital . . . how many Thanksgiving dinners did this man make? You know, I mean changing the kids' diapers, he was just a hands-on kind of guy, and at the same time he'd be underneath the car pulling the transmission. . . . I could take lessons from this guy.

The attribute of focusing on outcomes was also described. Regardless of the specific task, work was simply a process that yielded results. When asked about the increased amount of work they were doing as caregivers, participants paused and stammered to provide a response. The question was nonsensical to them. Participants commented that they did not think much about the work itself. However, participants described in great detail the sense of pride they felt when they completed tasks or met some other work objective.

Another attribute described by several participants was a reluctance to meet their emotional needs. Although somewhat variable among the participants, if any assistance was sought, for most of the participants it was for caregiving tasks and not for coping with stress. When asked if he shares his feelings with friends during visits, one participant replied, "I don't bring up anything like that . . . I don't give them any hard luck stories, because it wouldn't do any good." Three of the participants described themselves as stoic loners, who responded to stress with solitude. They described actions such as leaving the home to go for a walk or drive, distracting themselves with chores, or going for a drink when feeling stressed or overwhelmed. Although many people employ some solitude strategies when stressed, these three men employed these strategies exclusively. Sometimes these actions were beneficial. These men discussed how they used self-talk when alone to help them reframe their problems and motivate themselves for caregiving. However, they also described situations in which they left their care recipients in questionable safety so that they could be alone to "cool off."

Similar to the reluctance to meet emotional needs was the reluctance participants had in meeting their own physical health needs. Although most of the participants described themselves as healthy, several participants reported chronic illnesses that required ongoing medical attention. These participants reported that they only sought medical attention when illness symptoms got in the way of their ability to work for a day or two. Some participants reported new health changes caused by caregiving (e.g., insomnia, back pain), yet did not self-treat or seek medical attention for these new problems.

Participants also commented that rural men value common sense. Several participants provided numerous accounts of how health and human service providers lack common sense by adhering to bureaucratic procedures that impaired efficient delivery of services. These actions caused great frustration among the participants. For example, one participant's wife needed hospitalization for an acute respiratory illness. The participant knew that the local rural hospital would not admit her and would transfer her to a distant urban hospital. When he tried to convince the rural emergency room staff of this, they insisted on a full medical evaluation prior to transfer. This evaluation was then duplicated at the urban hospital when she arrived, thus creating duplicate billing to Medicare and a delay of treatment. Common sense was also described in terms of their own learning of how to be a caregiver. None of the men reported receiving formal instructions from hospital and clinic nurses or home health personnel on how to complete caregiving tasks, such as transferring, medication administration, and personal hygiene. The men stated that they learned these skills by asking other family members, observation, and by common sense. One participant stated,

> When I first started taking care of her, I got a little bit of information from my stepdaughter. And myself, I got a lot of common sense. I figure myself pretty smart. I've watched other people, picked up a few things here and there. And I'm the type you show me something today, I'll remember ten years from now. I do what is necessary, and most of it is common sense.

The participants expressed pride in their common sense. Common sense served as a foundation for their ingenuity and enabled them to remain self-reliant.

Another attribute of rural masculinity offered by the participants was that of the importance of fulfilling the provider role for one's family. Being a provider meant more than completing immediate caregiving tasks; it also required advocating for an optimal caregiving environment. Some men had to battle agencies in order to meet the needs of their care recipients, or battle employers to allow for more flexible scheduling to allow for caregiving. Two participants had to contest local zoning ordinances in order to build additions to their homes to better accommodate caring for sick family members.

Caregiver Challenges

The participants described a myriad of challenges related to caregiving, including hard physical labor, emotional/behavioral problems of care recipients, fatigue, lack of time, poor sleep, disrupted intimate and emotional relationships with their wives, disruptions at work, financial hardship, and detriments to their personal health. These challenges led to a pervasive stress that most of the men recognized, but that most simply chose to endure. The participants described this stress in very few, but very powerful words. One participant commented, "It [the stress] gets pretty tough. (Long pause) It can be real tough."

Gender Negotiation

Negotiation, or a redefining of one's gender role, is the core category constructed from the data and best accounts for how these men responded to caregiver stress. Caregiving required that the men confront situations, adopt behaviors, and complete tasks to which they were unaccustomed. For one participant, these changes produced no reported stress. For the rest of the men, some new behaviors and tasks conflicted with their individually constructed gender roles. These men underwent a process, which varied over time, in which various attributes of rural masculinity had to be rectified with caregiving responsibilities. This process was not always completed in a self-reflective manner; indeed, for most of the men, this process occurred in a reflex-like manner to sudden care recipient changes, to periods of markedly increased caregiver stress, or to both. However, for others the rectification process became quite overt and adopted a more negotiation-like process that allowed them to reduce any dissonance between caregiving responsibilities and their individual perspectives on their gender roles. Three general patterns of addressing gender role conflict were noted: gender compromise, gender conflict preservation, and gender reconstruction.

Gender Compromise: Accommodation

Some men implemented a compromise between necessary caregiving work and one or more attributes of their rural masculinity. Compromise allowed for tolerance of the conflict, made possible by recognizing that compromise would allow for completion of caregiver tasks. These men perceived themselves as "getting by" or "making do" with the challenges presented to them, resulting in a stage of accommodation with any perceived gender conflict. Any discomfort with conflict was balanced by the personal satisfaction of meeting a challenge and producing an end product, namely effective caregiving. Sometimes, compromise meant reaching out for help from others, but seeking help only occurred in a transient fashion. Such a pattern is analogous to the farmer, who ordinarily is independent in farm work, but seeks assistance only at harvest time. These men did not seek help for purposes of respite or self-growth. One participant stated,

> The advice I would give anyone taking care of someone is to evaluate the amount of care, then decide, if you are able to do the job. Sometimes the care required can be more than one person can give.

The men expressed very pragmatic perspectives. Managing conflicts between caregiving and gender was not an internal, self-reflexive process but rather a visibly external and outcome-focused process.

Gender Conflict Preservation: Edge of Crisis

Another group of men stubbornly clung to attributes of their rural masculinity, particularly the attributes of what might be considered an excessive self-reliance, a need for total control of the caregiver context, and neglect of their own physical and psychosocial health needs. These men resisted all assistance offered by others, even to the detriment of the care recipient, accepting help only when it was forced upon them by others. One participant complained bitterly about being forced to go to a nursing home after his own cardiac surgery, which required him to find someone else to take care of his wife during his absence. Another acquiesced to home health services only after his wife (his care recipient) refused to continue with the poor care she was receiving from him. These men reported anger, bitterness, and high levels of stress. Unlike the other men in the study, these men adopted routine patterns of disengagement from others, including their care recipients, when feeling overwhelmed. These men described themselves as loners. Frequently, they would leave the house for drives, walks, or "alone time" in a workshop during periods of stress. Occasionally, this disengagement involved drinking alcohol in their solitude. These men used disengagement as their primary stress reduction measure. None of these men seemed aware that their behavior had negative consequences to themselves and to their care recipients. The men were unable to quantify the length of time of disengagement periods, stating that they returned to the caregiver environment when they had "cooled off." It is noteworthy that care recipients were left unattended during periods of disengagement. One participant admitted that his care recipient wife complained frequently about being left on the commode for as long as an hour while he left the house to "clear his mind." Frequent disengagement often accelerated the caregiving context toward crisis, a situation in which the quality of caregiving becomes so poor that disruptions in the care recipient's health could require institutionalization or human service intervention.

Gender Reconstruction: Resiliency

This transformational process represents the third pattern of gender negotiation among the men. Men in this group had experienced caregiver trajectories in which the intensity of caregiver challenges had eventually overwhelmed them, overloading any gender compromise that may have been in place. Unlike men who employed a gender compromise pattern, men using gender reconstruction sent out more frequent, less task-specific calls for help. These men sought assistance from all sources including friends, neighbors, faith communities, as well as assistance from professional service organizations. The diversity of support addressed a plethora of needs, not just immediate or transient caregiver tasks. As support was utilized, these men reported that they had time to reflect upon recent changes in the caregiver dynamic, how they felt about caregiving, and how caregiving was affecting them as men.

These men described individual epiphanies of awareness of the benefits of assistance-seeking and assistance-accepting in enhancing the quality of the caregiving work, the improvement in their emotional health, and ultimately their abilities as caregivers. They acknowledged that the value they had placed in being independent, self-reliant, and in control was excessive to the point of making them ineffective as caregivers. They realized that letting go of control and asking for help was essential to avoid crisis. Importantly, these men identified these specific rural masculinity attributes as something their peers had in common, not as things that were uniquely characteristic of themselves. One participant commented,

> You know, I'm macho, and I'm a guy, and I figured I could do it all. So, in retrospect, I could have had hospice in here two or three months sooner . . . it would have been nice.

Continuing with his advice to other men, this participant shared,

> Don't be afraid to ask for help. Just know that there are resources out there . . . don't be as fussy as I was. . . . There is always somebody, and you don't know who that is. It might be somebody you don't expect.

These men reported that they had become much more adept at identifying personal emotional and instrumental needs and at locating appropriate resources to meet their needs. Importantly, these men did not seek help to remove themselves from the primary caregiver role. Instead, these men remained active in the day-to-day hands-on care of the care recipient and described their new roles as caregiver team leaders. These men also described a newly found resiliency to stress stemming from caregiver challenges. This resiliency was not a result of experience, but rather as a result of changed self-perceptions and changed behaviors. The men employing the gender reconstruction pattern did not describe their individual transformations as an emasculating experience. Instead, these men described a reprioritization of rural masculinity attributes. They described how they learned to de-emphasize the importance of self-reliance and emphasize the importance of being a good provider to loved ones. Being a good provider meant that they had to seek and accept assistance.

Gender-Cultural Model of Caregiving: Rural Male Caregivers

A preliminary model was constructed to illustrate the process of gender negotiation (see Figure 12.1) constructed from the data. The model depicts the rural male caregiver imbedded in overlapping cultural and gender contexts. Attributes of caregiving, rural masculinity, and rurality serve as challenges and resources for caregivers. The interplay between challenges and resources moves the caregiver between episodes of high stress and caregiver crisis and episodes of low stress and caregiver success. At individualized points on a caregiver's trajectory, a stress point is reached in which he must respond to noncongruence between constructed gender and caregiver work. This response, gender negotiation, can take one of three pathways: gender conflict preservation resulting in an approach to crisis, gender compromise resulting in a state of accommodation, and gender reconstruction resulting in the development of resiliency.

DISCUSSION

Several attributes of rurality were evident in the study data, all of which are consistent with the extant literature. Pervasively, participants described geographic isolation consistent with rural areas (Bigbee, 1991; Wagenfeld, 2003). This isolation permeates the other rural attributes identified, both historically and influentially. In terms of caregiving services, although most of the men lived relatively close to emergency care services, other routine and specialty services were miles away. Travel to these services placed great emotional, financial, and physical stress on both caregivers and care recipients, a hardship common among rural dwellers (Bales, 2006; Findholt, 2006; Henson, Sadler, & Walton, 1998). Geographic isolation has perhaps made self-reliance necessary among rural dwellers. Self-reliance, according to the men, was valued among

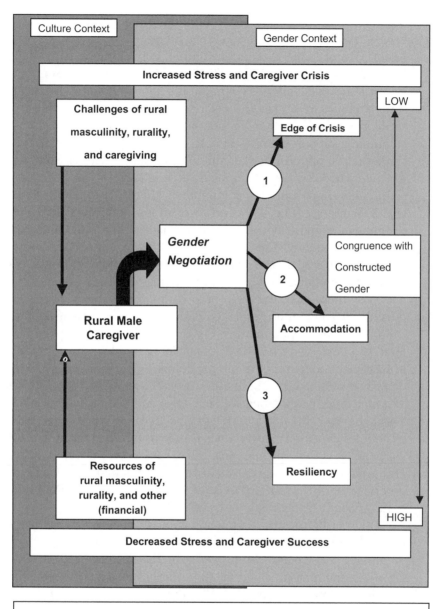

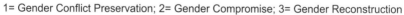

1= Gender Conflict Preservation; 2= Gender Compromise; 3= Gender Reconstruction

Figure 12.1. Gender-cultural model of caregiving: Rural male caregivers.

both men and women, and incorporated a strong sense of hardiness and hard work and is well supported in the literature (Bigbee; Koehler, 1998; Lee & Winters, 2004; Leipert & Reutter, 2005; Long & Weinert, 1989; Wirtz, Lee, & Running, 1998). The attribute of community support suggests the interdependence common in rural communities. Community support comes from a variety of sources, from individuals as well as from social groups such as faith communities. Although potential sources of community support are present in all communities, the pervasiveness of community support in rural communities is noteworthy as described by the men who had moved to rural areas from urban areas. High levels of community support in rural communities are described in the literature (Bales, Winters, & Lee, 2006); however, in some instances, access to this community support may depend upon having an insider status within the rural community. A few of the men who were new to their communities described a "clannish" aspect to their rural neighbors and perceived challenges in obtaining desired support. This perspective was not mentioned by those who resided in their communities for many years. It is possible that long-time residents were unaware of their insider status within their own communities. On the other hand, it is possible that men who perceived themselves as outsiders simply were not socialized in local behaviors and customs for help-seeking, since one newcomer described selfless offers of assistance from friends and strangers alike. The men described a strong faith in God as central to rural communities. This faith was evident in fatalistic perspectives, acknowledging that God sometimes sends challenges that cannot be overturned by hardworking people. As such, people must trust that God will see them through. Faith and prayer were central to these communities and have been described by others (Arcury, Quandt, McDonald, & Bell, 2000; Bennett & Lengacher, 1999; Gaskins & Lyons, 2000; Koehler).

As a socially constructed phenomenon, it is not surprising that attributes of rural masculinity identified in this study overlap with attributes of rurality. Most pervasive in overlap is the attribute of self-reliance. However, the men provided detailed clarifications of how self-reliance is different for rural men than for rural women. The men described self-reliance solely in positive terms for rural residents in general, namely hardworking, hardy, and independent. In relation to rural men, the men described additional characteristics of self-reliance that were both positive and negative. The participants believe that rural men are more likely to add a strong work orientation to self-reliance, incorporating a strong can-do attitude and doing anything and everything to accomplish desired work outcomes. These characteristics of self-reliance were described in very glowing terms and were a source of great pride among the men. On the other hand, with the exception of those men using a gender conflict preservation pattern of gender negotiation, the men noted that rural men took the independence aspect of self-reliance to the extreme, describing rural men as characteristically too independent, resistant to relinquishing control of their home caregiving context, and likely to display an excessive unwillingness to seek help. Awareness of this negative side of self-reliance appears to be an essential step to adopting a gender reconstruction pattern of gender negotiation. Other attributes of rural masculinity (see Table 12.1) were common, and served as either sources of challenges or resources within the caregiving context.

The academic literature is extraordinarily sparse on the topic of rural masculinity, particularly in terms of rural western masculinity. In theory, masculinity ideology among rural men is likely different than that

Table 12.1

ATTRIBUTES OF RURAL MASCULINITY

ATTRIBUTES AND SUB-ATTRIBUTES	SOURCE OF CHALLENGE	SOURCE OF RESOURCE
1. Self-reliance: Overly independent		
a. Resists relinquishing control	X	
b. Unwilling to seek help	X	
2. Self-reliance: Work-action orientation		
a. Can-do attitude		X
b. Focus on outcomes		X
c. Will do all work necessary		X
3. Reluctance to address emotional needs		
a. Loner perspective	X	
b. Isolation from male peers caregivers	X	
4. Neglects personal health	X	
5. Values outdoors/engages in hobbies		X
6. Values common sense/ingenuity		X
7. Values provider role		X

of nonrural men (Beynon, 2002; Courtenay, 2000; Good, Robertson, O'Neil, et al., 1995; Levant & Habben, 2003; Levant, Hirsch, Cozza, et al., 1992; O'Neil, Good, & Holmes, 1995; Pleck, 1995; West & Zimmerman, 1987). However, few scholars have provided clear descriptions of these differences, other than rural men are more likely to adopt traditional masculinity ideology (Levant & Habben). Perhaps due to the topics and directions of the interviews, the men did not provide evidence of support for the traditional masculinity ideology characteristics of homophobia and objectification of sexuality, but support was provided for the characteristics of toughness, self-reliance, restricted emotionality, and an importance on accomplishments and work.

The dearth of academic references of rural masculinity supports the examination of the popular media for support of the study's findings. There is no shortage of presentations of rural western men in print, film, and song. Often these presentations are stereotypes or caricatures of rural men; however, topical themes are evident within these media. The popular media tends to portray rural men consistent with traditional masculinity, with possibly the additional characterizations that rural men are unrefined, poorly educated, and cling to common sense as the primary source for personal knowledge. A couple of examples are illustrative.

In music, Michael Martin Murphy sings about rural masculinity in his song *Cowboy Logic* (Cook & Rains, 1990). The lyrics describe how cowboys solve problems, namely through common sense, a focus on outcomes, hard work, and simplicity.

> When the times are hard and the chips are down, he knows just what to do. Now the cowboy's got a set of rules that he lives by day to day, and if you ask him for his advice, he'll more than likely say . . .

Murphy then proceeds with a set of maxims.

> If it's a fence, mend it. If it's a dollar bill, spend it. . . . If it's a load, truck it. If it's a punch, duck it. If she's a lady, treat her like a queen. If it's a job, do it. Put your back into it, 'cause a little bit of dirt's gonna wash off in the rain. If it's a horse, ride it. If it hurts, hide it. Dust yourself off and get back on again. (Cook & Rains, 1990)

These maxims highlight values of hard work, toughness, and simple functionality. These values were expressed at length by the men in the study as well. Murphy then sings how these maxims are well-known to the point of universality.

> That's the cowboy logic. Every cowboy's got it. It's in the way he lives his life and the songs he sings. . . . He's got a simple solution to just about anything.

In literature many fictional accounts present an overly dramatic and inaccurate characterization of rural men. An historical and notable exception are the stories of Charles ("Charlie") Russell, who was identified by field placement community members as the best source for understanding both rural men and rural western culture. Although C. Russell lived nearly a century ago, his stories of rural men adapting to the changes of the twentieth century mimic the experiences of today's rural men adapting to increased technology and changing economic realities (Cristy, 2004). Challenges of role and work adaptation were expressed by a number of men in this study.

In C. Russell's stories (1927), the similarities in the thinking and actions of his characters to the cowboy logic noted earlier are seen. The basic plot of many of C. Russell's stories centers on a rugged and self-reliant man who is ranching, cowboying, hunting, or doing some other work endeavor. While working, the character comes across a surprising, and often dangerous, problem which requires swift and creative thinking. The character relies upon a response seemingly based on common sense, but the response does not quite solve the problem. Some calamity or unexpected series of events results, informing the reader that the character did not really have the common sense he thought he had. C. Russell twists this plot with humor to help drive home his point. This story line provides a helpful allegory for the collective experiences for the men in this study. These caregivers experienced new and unforeseen challenges. Approaches to these challenges were generally based on common sense and hard work (and perhaps a bit of luck). A focus on task outcomes made the hard work palatable, at times even enjoyable, and led to a great sense of pride when outcomes were met. However, these approaches were variably successful, often falling short of meeting outcomes if challenges were particularly intense or frequent. Calamity and near calamity were evident in the caregiver trajectories of some of the participants. Similar to C. Russell who informs the reader how expanded perspective might avert calamity, the men undergoing gender reconstruction developed insight that transformed their experiences.

In terms of caregiver challenges, the men in the study recounted burdens typical of those described at length in the literature. However, there was great variability in the interpretation of how these burdens affected them as individuals and how these interpretations changed over time. This variation lends support to the criticism made of the numerous quantitative caregiver studies which have examined phenomenon using cross-sectional designs (Coe & Neufeld, 1999; Harris, 1993; Kramer, 2000). In terms of caregiver rewards, rewards were most often described in terms of work accomplishment. These rewards served to strengthen or validate preexisting rurality and rural masculinity. Of notable exception were the men who used the gender reconstruction pattern of gender negotiation. These men described additional rewards much more characteristic of personal growth, such as a strengthening of faith, a new and more balanced perspective on life, or a deeper discernment of one's personal strengths and limitations.

Nothing was located in the literature that described a process of negotiating gender as a means to rectify conflicts between one's *constructed* gender and subsequent behaviors in the context of caregiving. Although informative, other qualitative studies examining male caregivers are generally thematic in nature and do not present processes men adopt to respond to conflicts with constructed gender (Archer & MacLean, 1993; Coe & Neufeld, 1999; Harris, 1993; Hilton, Crawford, & Tarko, 2001; Mays & Lund, 1999; Neufeld & Harrison, 1998; Parsons, 1997; R. Russell, 2004, 2007). However, most of the themes identified in these studies are supported by the focused codes constructed in the present study.

LIMITATIONS

The small sample size and exploratory nature of this study present significant limitations to the generalizability of findings. The constructed findings are representative of a homogenous subsample of rural male caregivers. The model constructed from the findings provides a very preliminary framework for understanding how men might negotiate conflicts between gender and caregiving. In this study, men negotiated gender but not rurality. It is likely that in other ethnic and racial groups, negotiation of both gender and culture might occur. Also, the study did not provide findings that adequately explain possible shifts in gender negotiation patterns as one journeys along a caregiver trajectory. Further research is needed to investigate possible pattern shifts and factors that facilitate pattern shifts in order to more fully develop the model. Further research is also needed in other subgroups of caregivers in order to more fully understand gender attributes and their effect on caregiver and care recipient health and quality of life.

IMPLICATIONS FOR PRACTICE

R. Russell (2007) noted the importance of constructed gender in our understanding of caregiving. Such understanding is essential in developing strategies that will enhance men's ability to experience and provide caregiving with greater satisfaction and quality. Although individual participants variably adopted identified rural masculinity attributes, findings from this study suggests possible attributes of masculinity that may differ from those of other subgroups of men. In terms of a caregiving context, attributes of overly independent self-reliance (characterized by a strong resistance to seek help and an unwillingness to relinquish perceived control of the caregiving context) and reluctance to meet emotional needs (characterized by lonerism and escapism) promoted negative caregiving experiences and outcomes which may result in poor caregiver and care recipient health. Men who became aware of the potential harm caused by these gender attributes and who reconstructed their perspectives on these attributes were able to adopt new behaviors that provided improved caregiving quality and satisfaction. However, this awareness and behavior change occurred after enduring much stress.

Health and human service providers could potentially identify men who cling strongly to attributes associated with negative caregiver experiences and assist them to develop awareness and behavior change before reaching caregiver crisis. Identification might occur through questioning men on how they (a) feel about asking for and accepting help from others, (b) access sources of support, (c) manage their stress, and (d) take care of their own health and emotional needs. Such questioning can serve as an initial exploration for caregiver and provider alike and determine baseline perspectives and strategies caregivers possess as they progress through their caregiver trajectories. It is important to note that gaining awareness of one's perspectives on gender roles and adopting new behaviors are not easy tasks, and for these participants, occurred only as they approached a perceived crisis. Crisis can be averted, however, if providers work cooperatively with caregivers early in their caregiver trajectories.

Providers must not use an approach that negates a caregiver's baseline constructed gender. Simply pointing out attributes held by the caregiver that are problematic in a caregiving context will only result in an emasculating tone that will possibly be rejected by the caregiver. Therefore, providers should offer information and assistance that emphasize attributes of rural masculinity and rurality associated with positive experiences that might already fall within an individual's constructed gender and culture. Such attributes include a self-reliance that is outcome-focused and celebratory of hard work, a value for caring for one's own family, a value of a common sense approach to work, a recognition and acceptance of available community support, and a value on being a good provider. Helping caregivers elevate these attributes may serve as a deterrent to less helpful attributes held by the caregiver. For example, for the participants in this study who adopted a gender reconstruction pattern, the value of being a good provider deterred their preponderance to resist asking for help. Providers might focus a discussion on how reaching out for help yields better outcomes and is not a sign of personal failure, similar to the need to seek assistance at harvest time. Services that respect the caregiver's desire to provide caregiving, as well as privacy and dominance in the home setting may also be beneficial. These services might include in-home services in which the caregiver is taught necessary caregiving skills and is mentored to adopt a team leader role. It is troubling that none of the participants in this study received any instruction from health and human service providers on how to provide caregiving. Home health workers who come into a home and only provide assistance to the care recipient fosters caregiver escapism, denounces caregiver personhood, and is perceived as highly intrusive. By refocusing the caregiving context on positive attributes, providers will help reduce the stress of caregiving and allow the caregiver the respite needed to facilitate gender reconstruction and personal growth.

Routine family assessment and service intake procedures may need to be examined to accommodate the exploration of the constructed genders of clients. Many providers may need continuing education on established theoretical foundations of gender and may require mentoring on how to conduct gender assessments in a sensitive and respectful manner. In addition, educators in health and human service academic programs need to instruct students on the importance of gender and the clinical complexities resulting from variable and competing gendered attributes.

Most likely, such content is rare in academic programs. However, educators may find using current academic content on culture to be an effective conduit for gender content, since culture also includes variable and competing constructed attributes that affect health and wellness. Use of this type of conduit can provide students an appropriate scaffold from relatively familiar to unfamiliar content.

CONCLUSIONS

This study provides initial insight into the processes used by a group of male rural caregivers. Using qualitative methods and a constructivist approach, the findings suggest that these men experienced conflict with personal gender roles as they adopted necessary caregiver work. This conflict produced variable levels of stress. These men managed their stress in one of three patterns: gender conflict preservation, in which men avoided conflict resolution by employing actions of detachment; gender compromise, in which men accepted conflict by doing what was necessary to get the caregiving work completed; and gender reconstruction, in which men reframed their perspectives on gender so that caregiving work no longer provided conflict with personal gender. Men using the gender reconstruction pattern reported greater caregiver success and personal growth. Implications of this study for health and human service providers include the need to explore the constructed genders of male caregivers in order to optimize caregiver success and health.

ACKNOWLEDGMENTS

Acknowledgments to Deborah Messecar, PhD, RN, and Judy Kendall, PhD, RN, from the School of Nursing, Oregon Health & Science University, and to Helen Lee, PhD, RN, who served as dissertation committee members for this study, for their guidance and their support.

REFERENCES

Acton, G. J., & Winter, M. A. (2002). Interventions for family members caring for an elder with dementia. *Annual Review of Nursing Research, 20,* 149–179.

Archbold, P. G., Stewart, B. J., Greenlick, M., & Harvath, T. A. (1992). The clinical assessment of mutuality and preparedness in family caregivers to frail older people.

In S. Funk, E. Tornquist, M. Champagne, & R. Wiese (Eds.), *Key aspects of elder care: Managing falls, incontinence, and cognitive impairment* (pp. 328–339). New York: Springer.

Archer, C., & MacLean, M. (1993). Husbands and sons as caregivers of chronically ill elderly women. *Journal of Gerontological Social Work, 21* (11/2), 5–23.

Arcury, T. A., Quandt, S. A., McDonald, J., & Bell, R. A. (2000). Faith and health self-management of rural older adults. *Journal of Cross Cultural Gerontology, 15* (1), 55–74.

Arno, P. S. (2006). *Economic Value of Informal Caregiving*, presented at the Care Coordination and the Caregiving Forum, Dept. of Veterans Affairs, NIH, Bethesda, MD, January 25–27, 2006.

Bailey, M. C. (1998). Outsider. In H. J. Lee (Ed.), *Conceptual basis for rural nursing* (pp. 139–148). New York: Springer.

Baillie, V., Norbeck, J. S., & Barnes, L. E. (1988). Stress, social support, and psychological distress of family caregivers of the elderly. *Nursing Research, 37* (4), 217–222.

Bales, R. L. (2006). Health perceptions, needs, and behaviors of remote rural women of childbearing and childrearing age. In H. J. Lee & C. A. Winters (Eds.), *Rural nursing: Concepts, theory, and practice* (2nd ed., pp. 66–78). New York: Springer.

Bales, R. L., Winters, C. A., & Lee, H. J. (2006). Health needs and perceptions of rural persons. In H. J. Lee & C. A. Winters (Eds.), *Rural nursing: Concepts, theory, and practice* (2nd ed., pp. 53–65). New York: Springer.

Ballantyne, J., & Buehler, J. (1998). Experiences of HIV-infected men with rural health care. In H. Lee (Ed.), *Conceptual basis for rural nursing* (pp. 366–377). New York: Springer.

Bennett, M., & Lengacher, C. (1999). Use of complementary therapies in a rural cancer population. *Oncology Nursing Forum, 26* (8), 1287–1294.

Beynon, J. (2002). What is masculinity? In J. Beynon (Ed.), *Masculinities and culture* (pp. 1–25). Philadelphia: Open University Press.

Bigbee, J. L. (1991). The concept of hardiness as applied to rural nursing. In A. Bushy (Ed.), *Rural nursing* (Vol. 1, pp. 39–58). Thousand Oaks, CA: Sage.

Bigbee, J. L. (1993). The uniqueness of rural nursing. *Nursing Clinics of North America, 28* (1), 131–144.

Bookwala, J., Newman, J., & Schulz, R. (2002). Methodological issues in research on men caregivers. In B. J. Kramer & E. Thompson (Eds.), *Men as caregivers: theory, research, and service implications* (pp. 69–98). New York: Springer.

Buehler, J., Malone, M., & Majerus, J. (1998). Patterns of responses to symptoms in rural residents: The symptom-action-time-line process. In H. Lee (Ed.), *Conceptual basis for rural nursing* (pp. 318–328). New York: Springer.

Bull, C. N., Krout, J. A., Rathbone-McCuan, E., & Shreffler, M. J. (2001). Access and issues of equity in remote/rural areas. *Journal of Rural Health, 17* (4), 356–359.

Carpenter, E. H., & Miller, B. H. (2002). Psychological challenges and rewards experienced by caregiving men: A review of the literature. In B. J. Kramer & E. H. Thompson (Eds.), *Men as caregivers: Theory, research, and service implications* (pp. 99–126). New York: Springer.

Center on an Aging Society. (2003, January). Data profile: Rural and urban health. *Challenges for the 21st century: Chronic and disabling conditions*, 1–6.

Charmaz, K. (2000). Grounded theory: Objectivist and constructivist methods. In N. K. Denzin & Y. S. Lincoln (Eds.), *Handbook of qualitative research* (2nd ed., pp. 509–536). Thousand Oaks, CA: Sage.

Charmaz, K. (2006). *Constructing grounded theory: A practical guide through qualitative analysis.* Thousand Oaks, CA: Sage.

Coe, M., & Neufeld, A. (1999). Male caregivers' use of formal support. *Western Journal of Nursing Research, 21* (4), 568–588.

Cook, D., & Rains, C. (1990). *Cowboy Logic* [Recorded by M. M. Murphy] [Music]. New York: Warner Bros. Records.

Courtenay, W. H. (2000). Constructions of masculinity and their influence on men's well-being: A theory of gender and health. *Social Science and Medicine, 50* (10), 1385–1401.

Cristy, R. J. (2004). *Charles M. Russell: The storyteller's art.* Albuquerque: University of New Mexico Press.

Dybbro, J. A. (1998). Ethnocentrism. In H. J. Lee (Ed.), *Conceptual basis for rural nursing* (pp. 287–296). New York: Springer.

Eberhardt, M., Ingram, D., & Makuc, D. (2001). *Urban and Rural Health Chartbook, Health, United States, 2001* (No. 76-641496). Hyattsville, MD: National Center for Health Statistics.

Findholt, N. (2006). The culture of rural communities: An examination of rural nursing concepts at the community level. In H. J. Lee & C. A. Winters (Eds.), *Rural nursing: Concepts, theory, and practice* (2nd ed., pp. 301–312). New York: Springer.

Gaskins, S., & Lyons, M. A. (2000). Self-care practices of rural people with HIV disease. *Online Journal of Rural Nursing and Health Care, 1* (1).

Gitlin, L. N., Belle, S. H., Burgio, L. D., Czaja, S. J., Mahoney, D., Gallagher-Thompson, D., et al. (2003). Effect of multicomponent interventions on caregiver burden and depression: The REACH multisite initiative at 6-month follow-up. *Psychology & Aging, 18* (3), 361–374.

Goins, R. T., & Mitchell, J. (1999). Health-related quality of life: Does rurality matter? *Journal of Rural Health, 15* (2), 147–156.

Good, G. E., Robertson, J. M., O'Neil, J. M., Fitzgerald, L. F., Stevens, M., DeBord, K. A., et al. (1995). Male gender role conflict: Psychometric issues and relations to psychological distress. *Journal of Counseling Psychology, 42* (1), 3–10.

Gwyther, L. (1992). Research on gender and family caregiving: Implications for clinical practice. In J. Dwyer & R. Coward (Eds.), *Gender, families and elder care.* Newbury Park, CA: Sage.

Harris, P. B. (1993). The misunderstood caregiver? A qualitative study of the male caregiver of Alzheimer's disease victims. *Gerontologist, 33* (4), 551–556.

Harris, P. B. (2002). The voices of husbands and sons caring for a family member with dementia. In B. J. Kramer & E. Thompson (Eds.), *Men as caregivers: Theory, research, and service implications* (pp. 213–233). New York: Springer.

Henson, D., Sadler, T., & Walton, S. (1998). Distance. In H. J. Lee (Ed.), *Conceptual basis for rural nursing* (pp. 51–60). New York: Springer.

Hewitt, M. (1992). Defining 'rural' areas: Impact on health care policy and research. In W. Gesler & T. Ricketts (Eds.), *Health in rural North America: The geography of health care services delivery* (pp. 25–54). New Brunswick, NJ: Rutgers University Press.

Hilton, B., Crawford, J., & Tarko, M. (2001). Men's experiences of coping with their wives' breast cancer involved focusing on the cancer and treatment and focusing on family to keep going. *Evidence-Based Nursing, 4* (1), 31.

Houde, S. C. (2002). Methodological issues in male caregiver research: An integrative review of the literature. *Journal of Advanced Nursing, 40* (6), 626–640.

Koehler, V. (1998). The substantive theory of protecting independence. In H. J. Lee (Ed.), *Conceptual basis for rural nursing* (pp. 236–256). New York: Springer.

Kramer, B. J. (1997). Differential predictors of strain and gain among husbands caring for wives with dementia. *Gerontologist, 37* (2), 239–249.

Kramer, B. J. (2000). Husbands caring for wives with dementia: A longitudinal study of continuity and change. *Health and Social Work, 25* (2), 97–107.

Kramer, B. J. (2002). Men caregivers: An overview. In B. J. Kramer & E. Thompson (Eds.), *Men as caregivers: Theory, research, and service implications* (pp. 3–19). New York: Springer.

Kumar, V., Acanfora, M., Hennessy, C. H., & Kalache, A. (2001). Health status of the rural elderly. *Journal of Rural Health, 17* (4), 328–331.

Ladner, C., & Cuellar, N. (2002). Depression in rural hospice family caregivers. *Online Journal of Rural Nursing and Health Care, 31* (1).

Lawton, M. P., Kleban, M. H., Moss, M., Rovine, M., & Glicksman, A. (1989). Measuring caregiver appraisal. *Journal of Gerontology, 44* (3), P61–P71.

Lee, H. J. (1998a). Concept comparison: Old-timer/newcomer/insider/outsider. In H. J. Lee (Ed.), *Conceptual basis for rural nursing* (pp. 149–155). New York: Springer.

Lee, H. J. (1998b). Lack of anonymity. In H. J. Lee (Ed.), *Conceptual basis for rural nursing* (pp. 76–88). New York: Springer.

Lee, H. J., & Winters, C. A. (2004). Testing rural nursing theory: Perceptions and needs of service providers. *Online Journal of Rural Nursing and Health Care, 4* (1). Retrieved September 6, 2006, from http://www.rno.org

Leipert, B. D., & Reutter, L. (2005). Developing resilience: How women maintain their health in northern geographic isolated settings. *Qualitative Health Research, 15* (1), 49–65.

Levant, R. F., & Habben, C. (2003). The new psychology of men: Application to rural men. In B. Stamm (Ed.), *Rural behavioral health care: An interdisciplinary guide* (pp. 171–180). Washington, DC: American Psychological Association.

Levant, R. F., Hirsch, L. S., Cozza, T. M., Hill, S., MacEachern, M., Marty, N., et al. (1992). The male role: An investigation of contemporary norms. *Journal of Mental Health Counseling, 14* (3), 325–337.

Lishner, D. M., Richardson, M., Levine, P., & Patrick, D. (1996). Access to primary health care among persons with disabilities in rural areas: A summary of the literature. *Journal of Rural Health, 12* (1), 45–53.

Long, K., & Weinert, C. (1989). Rural nursing: Developing the theory base. *Scholarly Inquiry for Nursing Practice: An International Journal, 3*, 113-127. New York: Springer.

Marks, N. (1996). Caregiving across the lifespan: National prevalence and predictors. *Family Relations, 45*, 27–36.

Mays, G. D., & Lund, C. H. (1999). Male caregivers of mentally ill relatives. *Perspectives in Psychiatric Care, 35* (2), 19–28.

Miller, B., & Cafasso, L. (1992). Gender differences in caregiving: Fact or artifact? *Gerontologist, 32* (4), 498–507.

Morgan, D. G., Semchuk, K. M., Stewart, N. J., & D'Arcy, C. (2002). Rural families caring for a relative with dementia: Barriers to use of formal services. *Social Science and Medicine, 55* (7), 1129–1142.

National Alliance for Caregiving and American Association of Retired Persons [NAC & AARP]. (1997). *Family caregiving in the U.S.: Findings from a national survey* (Report). Washington, DC.

National Alliance for Caregiving and American Association of Retired Persons [NAC & AARP]. (2004). *Caregiving in the U.S.* (Report). Washington, DC: National Alliance for Caregiving.

National Institute of Nursing Research [NINR]. (1994). *Family caregiving.* Retrieved April 8, 2003, from http://www.nih.gov/ninr/research/vol3/FamCare.htm

National Institute of Nursing Research [NINR]. (1995). *Chapter 2: Rural America: Challenges and opportunities.* Retrieved April 9, 2003.

National Rural Health Association [NRHA]. (2007). *What's different about rural health care?* Retrieved December 21, 2008, from http://www.ruralhealthweb.org/go/left/about-rural-health/what-s-different-about-rural-health-care

Neufeld, A., & Harrison, M. J. (1998). Men as caregivers: Reciprocal relationships or obligation? *Journal of Advanced Nursing, 28* (5), 959–968.

O'Lynn, C. (2006). The symptom-action time line: A literature review and recommendations for revision. In H. J. Lee & C. A. Winters (Eds.), *Rural nursing: Concepts, theory, and practice* (2nd ed., pp. 138–152). New York: Springer.

O'Neil, J. M., Good, G. E., & Holmes, S. (1995). Fifteen years of theory and research on men's gender role conflict: New paradigms for empirical research. In R. F. Levant & W. S. Pollack (Eds.), *A new psychology of men* (pp. 164–206). New York: Basic Books.

Opinion Research Corporation (ORC). (2005). *Attitudes and beliefs about caregiving in the U.S.: Findings of a national opinion survey.* Opinion Research Corporation.

Parsons, K. (1997). Male experience of caregiving for a family member with Alzheimer's Disease. *Qualitative Health Research, 7*, 391–407.

Pearlin, L. I., & Schooler, C. (1978). The structure of coping. *Journal of Health and Social Behavior, 19*, 2–21.

Pinquart, M., & Sorensen, S. (2006). Gender differences in caregiver stressors, social resources, and health: An updated meta-analysis. *Journals of Gerontology. Series B: Psychological Sciences and Social Sciences, 61B* (1), P33–P45.

Pleck, J. H. (1995). The gender role strain paradigm: An update. In R. F. Levant & W. S. Pollack (Eds.), *A new psychology of men* (pp. 11–32). New York: Basic Books.

Robinson, B. C. (1983). Validation of a caregiver strain index. *Journal of Gerontology, 38* (3), 344–348.

Russell, C. M. (1927). *Trails plowed under.* Lincoln: University of Nebraska Press.

Russell, R. (2004). Social networks among elderly men caregivers. *The Journal of Men's Studies, 13* (1), 121–142.

Russell, R. (2007). Men doing "women's work": Elderly men caregivers and the gendered construction of care work. *Journal of Men's Studies, 15* (1), 1–19.

Ryan-Nicholls, K. (2004). Health and sustainability of rural communities. *Rural and Remote Health, 4* (242), 1–11.

Schulz, R., Beach, S. R., Lind, B., Martire, L. M., Zdaniuk, B., Hirsch, C. (2001). Involvement in caregiving and adjustment to death of a spouse: Findings from the caregiver health effects study. *Jama, 285* (24), 3123–3129.

Stoller, E. (2002). Theoretical perspectives on caregiving men. In B. J. Kramer & E. Thompson (Eds.), *Men as caregivers: Theory, research, and service implications* (pp. 51–68). New York: Springer.

Thompson, E. H. (2002). What's unique about men's caregiving? In B. J. Kramer & E. H. Thompson (Eds.), *Men as caregivers: Theory, research, and service implications* (pp. 20–50). New York: Springer.

U.S. Census Bureau. (2002). *U.S. summary: 2000* (Census profile No. C2KPROF/00-US). Washington, DC: U.S. Department of Commerce.

U.S. Census Bureau. (2004). *U.S. interim projections by age, sex, race, and Hispanic origin.* Retrieved February 27, 2007, from http://www.census.gov/ipc/www/usinterim-proj/

Vitaliano, P. P., Zhang, J., & Scanlan, J. M. (2003). Is caregiving "hazardous to one's physical health"? A meta-analysis. *Psychological Bulletin, 129,* 946–997.

Wagenfeld, M. O. (2000). Delivering mental health services to the persistently and seriously mentally ill in frontier areas. *Journal of Rural Health, 16* (1), 91–96.

Wagenfeld, M. O. (2003). A snapshot of rural and frontier America. In B. Stamm (Ed.), *Rural behavioral health care: An interdisciplinary guide* (pp. 33–41). Washington, DC: American Psychological Association.

West, C., & Zimmerman, D. H. (1987). Doing gender. *Gender and Society, 1* (2), 125–151.

Wirtz, E., Lee, H., & Running, A. (1998). The lived experience of hardiness in rural men and women. In H. Lee (Ed.), *Conceptual basis for rural nursing* (pp. 257–274). New York: Springer.

Yee, J. L., & Schulz, R. (2000). Gender differences in psychiatric morbidity among family caregivers: A review and analysis. *The Gerontologist, 40,* 147–164.

Young, R. F., & Kahana, E. (1989). Specifying caregiver outcomes: Gender and relationship aspects of caregiving strain. *Gerontologist, 29* (5), 660–666.

Zarit, S., Reever, K. E., & Bach-Peterson, J. (1980). Relatives of the impaired elderly: Correlates of feelings of burden. *The Gerontologist, 20* (6), 649–655.

13

Complementary Therapy and Health Literacy in Rural Dwellers

JEAN SHREFFLER-GRANT, ELIZABETH NICHOLS,
CLARANN WEINERT, and BETTE IDE

Adequate health literacy is necessary in today's health care market place so that consumers are able to understand and evaluate information regarding conventional or allopathic health care (Institute of Medicine [IOM], 2004). Health literacy is defined in *Healthy People 2010* as "the degree to which individuals have the capacity to obtain, process, and understand basic health information and services needed to make appropriate health decisions" (U.S. Department of Health and Human Services, 2000, Section 11-2).

Health literacy is even more important for evaluating complementary and alternative medicine (CAM). Health care consumers usually have some assistance from providers to interpret information about allopathic care and often receive instructions and advice to guide health care decision making and action taking. This is less likely with CAM. These therapies are often self-prescribed or self-directed in nature and are less regulated or controlled by governmental agencies or allopathic providers. Further, studies have found that often there is limited communication between consumers and allopathic providers about consumers' use or potential use of CAM (Eisenberg, Kessler, Foster, et al., 1993; Eisenberg, Davis, Ettner, et al., 1998; Vallerand, Fouladbakhsh, & Templin, 2003).

During the past several decades, the use of CAM in the United States has grown significantly (Barnes, Bloom, & Nahin, 2008; Eisenberg et al., 1993; Eisenberg et al., 1998; IOM, 2005). CAM has become an important component of the U.S. health care system as consumers, including those living in rural areas, increasingly use CAM as an adjunct to or substitute for conventional health care (Arcury, Preisser, Gesler, & Sherman, 2004; Astin, 1998; Eisenberg et al., 1998; Harron, & Glasser, 2003; McFarland, Bigelow, Zani, Newson, & Kaplin, 2002). In addition, the recent downturn in the economy has fueled an increase in the use of CAM products in place of allopathic treatments because of the lower cost of CAM (Associated Press, 2009). The National Center for Complementary and Alternative Medicine (NCCAM; 2006) defines CAM as a group of diverse health care systems, practices, and products that are not presently considered a part of allopathic health care. The CAM therapies and products are not considered part of allopathic care in large part because there is insufficient evidence that they are safe and effective (NCCAM, 2008). Types of CAM range from therapies provided by practitioners, such as naturopathic physicians and acupuncturists, to self-care practices, such as herbs and magnets.

In 2007, approximately 40% of adults in the United States used some form of CAM in the past 12 months (Barnes, Bloom, & Nahin, 2008) which is slightly more than the 36% use rate found in a comparable national study conducted in 2003 (Barnes, Pewell-Griner, McFann, & Nahin, 2004). In addition, the results of the Barnes et al. study demonstrated that approximately one in nine (11.8%) children used CAM in the past 12 months. Not surprisingly, use among children whose parents used CAM was significantly higher (23.9%) than among children whose parents did not use CAM (5.1%). In 2007, when cost concerns caused a delay in seeking allopathic care, CAM was more likely to be used by both adults and children than when cost was not a concern (Barnes et al.). Despite the widespread use and acceptance of CAM in the general population, consumers are reluctant to inform allopathic providers that they used CAM (Eisenberg et al., 1993; Eisenberg et al., 1998).

Based on the literature, the demographics of those in the general United States population who use CAM vary; but in general, CAM is used more often for chronic than acute health conditions and use is more common among women than men, younger adults than older, those with higher incomes and more education, and those living in the west than in other parts of the country (Astin, 1998; Astin, Pelletier, Marie, & Haskell, 2000; Cherniack, Senzel, & Pan, 2001; Eisenberg, et al., 1998). Studies have found that individuals with chronic illness have a variety of reasons for using CAM, including (a) symptom relief, (b) ineffectiveness of allopathic treatments, (c) side effects of allopathic treatments, (d) dissatisfaction with allopathic care, (e) concerns about adverse effects of allopathic care, (f) desire for control, and (g) the ready availability of CAM (Johnson, 1999; Montbraind & Laing, 1991; Rao, Mihaliak, Kroenke, et al., 1999; Vincent & Furnham, 1996).

Despite extensive searches, no empirical studies have been located in the literature specifically on health literacy about CAM. There is also very limited evidence in general about how much CAM users know about the products and treatments they use, what sources of information they use, or how they evaluate and use the information they have or acquire (IOM, 2005). Evidence is also lacking about how consumers in the United States decide when and how to use CAM and whether or not they comply with instructions from CAM providers or product labels. One study found that while 80% of older study participants reported using two or more CAM therapies, their self-rated knowledge about most of the therapies was very low (King & Pettigrew, 2004). The IOM cited three primary sources of information that consumers use about CAM: word of mouth, the Internet, and health food stores. The few studies evaluating the quality of information available from these sources suggested that quality may be a concern.

The purpose of this chapter is to present a summary of a series of research studies conducted by a team of investigators at the Colleges of Nursing at Montana State University-Bozeman and the University of North Dakota on the use of CAM by older rural dwellers. The results of these projects have raised a number of researchable questions regarding the health literacy levels about CAM among older rural adults, particularly rural adults with chronic illnesses.

HEALTH CARE CHOICES: A STUDY OF COMPLEMENTARY THERAPY USE AMONG OLDER RURAL DWELLERS

At the time this study was conducted, a number of well-known studies had demonstrated that use of CAM was growing among the general population in the United States, but little was known about use of these therapies among rural residents. Most of the national studies did not report where study participants lived and some used only urban participants. To address this gap in the literature, the Health Care Choices study was conducted with older adults living in sparsely populated rural areas in Montana and North Dakota (Shreffler-Grant, Weinert, Nichols, & Ide, 2005). The purpose of the study was to explore the use, cost of,

and satisfaction with the quality and effectiveness of CAM from the perspectives of the older rural adult participants. The study was conducted
during 2000–2003 and funded by NCCAM (1R15AT09501). A descriptive survey design was used to generate data from a random sample of
older adults in 19 rural communities in Montana and North Dakota. An
interview instrument was developed to elicit data addressing the specific
aims and was piloted prior to use. Telephone interviews were conducted
with 325 older adults. Participants ranged in age from 60 to 98 years
($m = 71.7$). Most of the participants (67.7%, $n = 202$) reported having
one or more chronic illnesses. Only 17.5% ($n = 57$) reported using CAM
providers, while 35.7% ($n = 116$) used self-prescribed CAM practices.
When these two categories of use were combined, a total of 45.2% of
the participants used some form of CAM, or used CAM providers, self-
prescribed CAM practices, or both. This finding demonstrated that these
older rural residents were using as much or more CAM than participants
in national studies (36%–40%) that included all adult age groups.

Relevant to the issue of health literacy about CAM, the participants
in this study most often learned about the CAM therapies by word of
mouth from relatives or friends, consumer marketing, or reading, rather
than health care professionals (Shreffler-Grant et al., 2005). Much of
the CAM used by participants of this study was self-prescribed, raising
questions about whether the participants had sufficient knowledge and
information for safe and effective use of the CAM products. In addition,
a majority (64.6%, $n = 210$) of the participants reported that they had at
least one significant acute or chronic health problem and 32.3% ($n = 105$)
had two or more significant health problems. The research team wondered about the potential for adverse drug-herb or drug-vitamin interactions with this population of vulnerable older adults who likely were
taking multiple prescription medications and had aging, impaired physi-
ological responses, or both.

HEALTH CARE CHOICES: OLDER RURAL WOMEN

Additional analyses were conducted on a portion of the data set generated in the first Health Care Choices study to answer the following
research question: What factors predict use of CAM among older rural
women (Shreffler-Grant, Hill, Weinert, Nichols, & Ide, 2007). Men
were excluded from this analysis because too few men in the larger
data set used CAM, which is consistent with the literature about CAM

use. Potential predictors were selected from the literature and observations from practice and included education, age, rurality, marital status, income, spirituality, number of chronic illnesses, and health status. Logistic regression analysis was used to examine factors associated with use of CAM by the rural women participants (n = 156). A total of 25.6% of the women had used CAM recently and most of the therapies they used were self-prescribed. Women most likely to use CAM were those who were fairly well educated, not currently married, and in their early older years (60–69 years of age). They had one or more significant chronic illnesses and lower health related quality of life due to emotional concerns such as depression or stress.

Although this analysis did not yield additional information about health literacy about CAM per se, the results reinforced and expanded the findings of the main study discussed above. The women who reported use of CAM in this analysis used primarily self-prescribed CAM, which again raises concern about their level of knowledge about CAM. Women with one or more chronic illnesses were more likely to use CAM than those without chronic illness. Specifically, for each additional chronic illness reported, the odds of CAM use increased by 46%. By identifying characteristics of older rural women who are more or less likely to use CAM, the results can be used to tailor educational interventions to improve health literacy about CAM.

HEALTH CARE CHOICES: CHRONIC ILLNESS

The purpose of this study was to provide a better understanding of older rural adults' use of CAM, their perceptions of efficacy of the CAM they used, and the sources of information they used about CAM (Nichols, Sullivan, Ide, Shreffler-Grant, & Weinert, 2005). The study was conducted during 2003–2004 and funded by the Center for Research on Chronic Health Conditions in Rural Dwellers (CRCHC) at Montana State University–Bozeman College of Nursing (NIH/NINR IP20NR07790-01). Ten participants between 60 and 80 years of age who reported using CAM in the original Health Care Choices study and who had two or more chronic illnesses were interviewed by telephone. Qualitative analysis was used to organize content and identify themes. Participants primarily used self-prescribed CAM therapies such as dietary supplements and herbs, taken to compensate for perceived dietary deficiencies. Participants were generally satisfied with the results they attributed to the CAM. With regard to health literacy about CAM, the participants attempted to use reputable sources of information about the CAM products they used, but it was clear that some used the products in an inconsistent manner and did not understand what the products did. Some individuals reported seeking information about CAM from sources other than their allopathic providers due to a perception that the providers were too busy to answer their questions about CAM.

HEALTH CARE CHOICES: CAM PROVIDERS IN RURAL LOCATIONS

This study was motivated by the results of the first Health Care Choices study in which the older rural adults reported limited use of CAM providers, in contrast to self-prescribed CAM. The study's purpose was to determine the availability of CAM resources in 20 small rural towns in Montana and North Dakota and to explore the contribution of one type of CAM provider, naturopathic physicians, to rural health care (Nichols, Weinert, Shreffler-Grant, & Ide, 2006). The study was conducted during 2004–2005 and funded by the Center for Research on Chronic Health Conditions (CRCHC) in Rural Dwellers at Montana State University-Bozeman College of Nursing (NIH/NINR IP20NR07790-01). CAM resource data were collected by Internet and telephone directory searches and an online survey of naturopaths in Montana. Seventy-three CAM providers were identified in the 20 towns. Most naturopaths were located in population centers but some offered outreach clinics to rural communities. Based on the results, the team concluded that local availability is not the critical factor in use of CAM providers by older rural adults. Although there were likely fewer choices of CAM providers in these small rural towns than in larger towns or cities, there were CAM providers available if the rural residents chose to use them. Rural residents are also known to travel outside their local communities to see health care providers who are acceptable to them (Shreffler-Grant, 2006.)

HEALTH CARE CHOICES: CAM HEALTH LITERACY

Due to the questions concerning CAM health literacy identified in the results of the studies discussed above, the research team designed and is seeking funding for the next Health Care Choices project on CAM health literacy. The purpose of the proposed study is to develop a psychometrically sound instrument to measure CAM health literacy. A new instrument is needed due to the limitations of currently available measures of health literacy. The health literacy instruments available essentially evaluate basic reading and math skills in a health care context (IOM, 2004) and not the more complex aspects needed to make reasoned decisions about the use of CAM.

The proposed study will contribute to a fuller understanding of health literacy as it relates to CAM. Data from this study, together with results of the team's prior work will contribute to the development of an educational intervention with older rural adults with chronic health conditions. It is anticipated that this instrument can be adapted to assess health literacy in other self-care decision-making situations with individuals with chronic health conditions.

The research team completed preliminary work on this project with funding from an Intramural Block Grant (2008–2009) from Montana State University-Bozeman College of Nursing. A conceptual model was developed to guide item construction for the new instrument. The model was reviewed and critiqued by a panel of CAM and health literacy experts and revised based on their input. In addition, potential items for the new instrument have been developed and will be reviewed and critiqued by a nationally known expert on scale development. Once funding is obtained for the larger Measuring CAM Health Literacy study, work will commence to finish development of the new instrument and conduct psychometric evaluation of the instrument.

DISCUSSION

Over the past decade, this research team conducted the series of studies discussed above on use of CAM among older rural adults. This work has led us to ask compelling questions about the level of health literacy about CAM among this population, particularly those with chronic illnesses. Health care consumers in any location, particularly those with chronic illnesses, make numerous decisions about health care and use a wide variety of self-care health products and therapies; decisions often made independent of allopathic providers. This is particularly true of older rural adults who are known to be more independent, engage in more self-care, and have less access to allopathic care than those living in urban areas (Shreffler-Grant et al., 2007). Those with chronic illnesses are also more likely to use CAM therapies (Astin, 1998; Astin et al., 2000; Barnes et al., 2004; Eisenberg et al., 1998; Shreffler-Grant et al., 2007).

Making informed decisions about the use of CAM requires a sophisticated level of health literacy on the part of the consumer. Without adequate CAM health literacy, older rural consumers may not know of all the appropriate health care choices that may benefit them, may fall victim to scams or unscrupulous sales practices, or may ingest potentially harmful substances. Informed use of CAM can increase health and illness management options and support well-reasoned decision making regarding self-care for older rural adults living with chronic illnesses.

ACKNOWLEDGMENTS

These research studies were funded in part by grants from the NCCAM (1R15AT09501), the CRCHC at Montana State University-Bozeman College of Nursing (NIH/NINR IP20NR07790-01), and an Intramural Block Grant (2008–2009) from Montana State University–Bozeman College of Nursing.

REFERENCES

Arcury, T. A., Preisser, J. S., Gesler, W. M., & Sherman, J. E. (2004). Complementary and alternative medicine use among rural residents in western North Carolina. *Complementary Health Practice Review, 9* (2), 93–102.

Associated Press. (January 13, 2009). With economy sour, consumers sweet on herbal medicines. Washingtonpost.com

Astin, J. (1998). Why patients use alternative medicine: Results of a national study. *Journal of the American Medical Association, 279* (19), 1548–1553.

Astin, J., Pelletier, K., Marie, A., & Haskell, W. (2000). Complementary and alternative medicine use among elderly persons: One-year analysis of a blue shield Medicare supplement. *Journal of Gerontology, 55A*, M4–9.

Barnes, P. M., Bloom, B., & Nahin, R. L. (2008). Complementary and alternative medicine use among adults and children: United States, 2007. *National health statistics reports, No. 12.* Hyattsville, MD: National Center for Health Statistics.

Barnes, P. M., Pewell-Griner, E., McFann, K., & Nahin, R. L. (2004). Complementary and alternative medicine use among adults: United States, 2002. *National health statistics reports, No. 343.* Hyattsville, MD: National Center for Health Statistics.

Cherniack, E. P., Senzel, R. S., & Pan, C. X. (2001). Correlates of use of alternative medicine by the elderly in an urban population. *Journal of Alternative and Complementary Medicine, 7*, 277–280.

Eisenberg, D., Davis, R., Ettner, S., Appel, S., Wilkey, S., Van Rompay, M., & Kessler, R. (1998). Trends in alternative medicine use in the United States, 1990–1997: Results of a follow-up national survey. *Journal of the American Medical Association, 280* (18), 1569–1575.

Eisenberg, D., Kessler, R., Foster, C., Norlock, F., Calkins, D., & Delbanco, T. (1993). Unconventional medicine in the United States. *The New England Journal of Medicine, 246–252.*

Harron, M., & Glasser, M. (2003).Use of and attitudes toward complementary and alternative medicine among family practice patients in small rural Illinois communities. *The Journal of Rural Health, 19* (3), 279–284.

Institute of Medicine (IOM; 2004). *Health literacy: A prescription to end confusion.* Washington, DC: The National Academies Press.

Institute of Medicine (IOM; 2005). *Complementary and alternative medicine in the United States.* Washington, DC: The National Academies Press.

Johnson, J. (1999). Older rural women and the use of complementary therapies. *Journal of Community Health Nursing, 16* (4), 223–232.

King, M. O., & Pettigrew, A. C. (2004). Complementary and alternative therapy use by older adults in three ethnically diverse populations: A pilot study. *Geriatric Nursing, 25* (1), 30–37.

McFarland, B., Bigelow, D., Zani, B., Newsom, J., & Kaplan, M. (2002). Complementary and alternative medicine use in Canada and the United States. *American Journal of Public Health, 92,* 1616–1618.

Montbraind, M., & Laing, G. (1991). Alternative health care as a control strategy. *Journal of Advanced Nursing, 16,* 325–332.

National Center for Complementary and Alternative Medicine (NCCAM; 2006). *What is complementary and alternative medicine (CAM)?* Retrieved June 10, 2006, from http://nccam.nih.gov/health/whatiscam/

National Center for Complementary and Alternative Medicine (NCCAM; 2008). *Expanding horizons of health care: Strategic plan 2005–2009.* Retrieved March 17, 2009, from http://nccam.nih.gov/about/plans/2005

Nichols, E., Sullivan, T., Ide, B., Shreffler-Grant, J., & Weinert, C. (2005). Health care choices: Complementary therapy, chronic illness, and older rural dwellers. *Journal of Holistic Nursing, 23* (4), 381–394.

Nichols, E., Weinert, C., Shreffler-Grant, J., & Ide, B. (2006). Complementary and alternative providers in rural locations. *Online Journal of Rural Nursing and Health Care, 6* (1). Retrieved July 14, 2005, from http://www.rno.org

Rao, J., Mihaliak, K., Kroenke, K., Bradley, J., Tierney, W., & Weinberger, M. (1999). Use of complementary therapies for arthritis among patients of rheumatologists. *Annals of Internal Medicine, 131,* 409–416.

Shreffler-Grant, J. (2006). Acceptability: One component in choice of health care provider. In H. J. Lee & C. A. Winters (Eds.), *Rural nursing, concepts, theory, and practice* (2nd ed., pp. 166–176). New York: Springer.

Shreffler-Grant, J., Hill, W., Weinert, C., Nichols, E., & Ide, B. (2007). Complementary therapy and older rural women: Who uses and who does not? *Nursing Research, 56* (1), 28–33.

Shreffler-Grant, J., Weinert, C., Nichols, E., & Ide, B. (2005). Complementary therapy use among older rural adults. *Public Health Nursing, 22* (4), 323–331.

U.S. Department of Health and Human Services (2000). *Healthy People 2010, Section 11-2: Health Communication Objective.* Retrieved July 14, 2005, from www .healthypeople.gov

Vallerand, A. H., Fouladbakhsh, J. M., & Templin, T. (2003). The use of complementary/ alternative medicine for self-treatment of pain among residents or urban, suburban, and rural communities. *American Journal of Public Health, 93,* 923–925.

Vincent, C., & Furnham, A. (1996). Why do patients turn to complementary medicine? An empirical study. *British Journal of Clinical Psychology, 35,* 37–48.

Acceptability: One Component in Choice of Health Care Provider

14

JEAN SHREFFLER-GRANT

Since the early 1980s, access to health care has deteriorated in many rural areas in the United States as a result of the closure of rural hospitals and the associated loss of local providers and services that often accompany hospital closure. Historically, much of the blame for closures has been attributed to factors external to rural communities, such as limited Medicare reimbursement, the declining rural economy, and provider shortages. In contrast, a substantial volume of evidence now indicates that the closures may, in part, be due to influences closer to home. Some rural hospitals are underutilized by local residents who bypass them to seek care in larger towns and cities (Amundson, 1993; Bauer, 1992; DeFriese, Wilson, Ricketts, & Whitener, 1992; Liu, Bellamy, & McCormick, 2007; Radcliff, Brasure, Moscovice, & Stensland, 2003; Reinert, 1991).

Since the early 1990s, variations of Critical Access Hospitals (CAHs) have been implemented as alternatives to hospitals that are at risk for closure. CAHs must be located in remote rural areas, are limited to short-stay lower-acuity services and are allowed more flexibility in staffing and other licensure requirements. They are also reimbursed by Medicare on the basis of reasonable cost instead of prospective payment as compared with traditional rural hospitals. Cost-based Medicare reimbursement is considered advantageous for small hospitals that often serve a high proportion of older patients and are less likely to be able to average risk across large numbers of admissions as may be necessary under prospective payment (Christianson, Moscovice, Wellever, & Wingert, 1990). Following implementation of the Rural Hospital Flexibility Program, passed into law in 1997, CAHs became a national model and have gained broad support in rural areas across the nation (Shreffler, Capalbo, Flaherty, & Heggam, 1999). By 2006, less than a decade after the CAH model was passed into law, a large majority (80%) of small rural hospitals and more than 60% of all rural hospitals had converted to CAHs (Pink, Holmes, Thompson, & Slifkin, 2007). As of September 2008, there were 1,294 certified CAHs nationwide (Rural Assistance Center, 2008). Whether these new CAH models will be any more viable than traditional rural hospitals will likely be tied to how they are viewed and used by the rural residents they are intended to serve.

Improving equity in access to care has been an ongoing concern throughout most of the past half-century (Aday, Bagley, Lairson, & Slater, 1993; Patrick & Erickson, 1993), and rural access to care has been a particularly persistent problem (Gamm & Hutchison, 2003). Although equitable access to health care in and of itself may be intuitively desirable, it is through presumed links between access to quality health services, appropriate use, and resulting positive health outcomes that access becomes important (Millman, 1993). I conducted a study (1996) to examine rural residents' perspectives on access to health care in six communities in Montana with CAHs. The concept of "acceptability" is one dimension of access to care that can be used to explain why people do or do not use local rural health care services. As part of the larger study, a scale to measure acceptability was developed and validated. In this chapter, I will focus on the Acceptability Scale (see Table 14.1).

CONCEPTUAL FRAMEWORK

Access to care was the conceptual framework guiding this study. I conceptualized access to care as having two dimensions. *Potential access to care* includes properties of the population and health care system that affect opportunities to enter into the health care system. *Actual or realized access to care* includes utilization and willingness to use the health care system and satisfaction with the care received (Aday & Andersen, 1975; Andersen, McCutcheon, Aday, Chiu, & Bell, 1993).

Table 14.1

INDIVIDUAL ITEMS INCLUDED IN THE "ACCEPTABILITY SCALE"

1. How would you rate [*facility name*] in each of the following categories?

	CIRCLE ONE ANSWER FOR EACH CATEGORY					
	EXCELLENT	GOOD	AVERAGE	FAIR	POOR	
a. Overall quality of care	5	4	3	2	1	Don't know
b. Medical care	5	4	3	2	1	Don't know
c. Nursing care	5	4	3	2	1	Don't know
d. Staff concern/compassion	5	4	3	2	1	Don't know
e. "Personal" aspects of care	5	4	3	2	1	Don't know
f. Building cleanliness and condition	5	4	3	2	1	Don't know
g. Acceptability as source of care	5	4	3	2	1	Don't know

2. How would you rate each of the following aspects of overall medical care provided in your community? (Care provided by physicians, nurse practitioners, physician assistants, or other primary care providers at their office or local hospital.)

	CIRCLE ONE ANSWER FOR EACH CATEGORY					
	EXCELLENT	GOOD	AVERAGE	FAIR	POOR	
a. Competence of primary care providers	5	4	3	2	1	Don't know
b. Concern/compassion for patient	5	4	3	2	1	Don't know
c. "Personal" aspects of care	5	4	3	2	1	Don't know
d. Competence of support staff	5	4	3	2	1	Don't know
e. Acceptability of provider as source of care	5	4	3	2	1	Don't know

In several studies published in the 1980s on the relationship between access to care and utilization of care, Penchansky and Thomas (1981; Thomas & Penchansky, 1984) defined access as the fit between clients and the health care system—an adequate degree of fit was measured by objective utilization and subjective satisfaction. They identified five components of potential access that are referred to as "the 5 As":

1. Availability—an adequate supply of providers and services relative to clients' needs;
2. Accessibility—where services are located relative to where clients are;
3. Accommodation—how services are organized to accept clients;
4. Affordability—costs of services relative to resources of clients; and finally,
5. Acceptability—the clients' attitudes and opinions about the characteristics of providers and services.

Discriminant validity of Penchansky and Thomas' (1981; Thomas & Penchansky, 1984) components of access to care was supported in their studies, and subsets of clients were found to differ significantly in utilization of health care based on how satisfied they were with the components that were salient for them. Although these investigators measured acceptability chiefly by consumers' attitudes and opinions about the physical environment in which care was delivered, they proposed that attitudes about personal and technical practice characteristics of providers and services were also relevant.

METHODS

In the larger study to examine rural residents' perspectives on access to health care (Shreffler, 1996), I employed a descriptive survey design. I sent surveys to a random sample of 100 households in each of six communities with CAHs, and I interviewed a subset of respondents by telephone. I obtained a 63.5% response rate on the mail survey ($n = 381$).

My principal aims in this study were to identify the predictors of use and willingness to use local health care and satisfaction with care. In interpreting the term *predictors*, it should be noted that I sought significant statistical relationships rather than cause and effect relationships. It was not possible to determine from the data whether people used local health care because they thought it was acceptable or whether they thought it was acceptable because they had used it.

There were four dependent variables in the analyses to address actual access to care. They were (a) use of the local CAH, (b) use of the local primary care provider, (c) willingness to use the local CAH, and (d) willingness to use the local provider. These *use* variables were dichotomous *yes* or *no* indicators of whether or not the respondents reported actual use of the CAH and the local provider in the recent past. The *willingness to use* variables were dichotomous *yes* or *no* indicators constructed from responses to a question about where respondents would first seek care for a variety of future health concerns. The future health concerns counted as *yes, willing to use* were concerns for which the local CAH and provider(s) offered health care services rather than other services included in the question that were not available locally and for which patients would need to be referred elsewhere.

The major independent variables, or potential predictors, included potential access to care factors. All were measured by respondents' self-report and from their perspectives (versus from the perspectives of the hospitals or providers). These included characteristics of the population (e.g., age, income, health insurance, and health status) and characteristics of the health care system that I operationalized according to "the 5 As" from Penchansky and Thomas' work (1981; Thomas & Penchansky, 1984) (i.e., availability, accessibility, accommodation, affordability, and acceptability).

The Acceptability Scale comprised the summed values of responses to twelve 5-point Likert-type rating questions related to the concept of acceptability included on the mail survey. I based my selection of the questions for inclusion in the scale on Penchansky and Thomas' work (1981; Thomas & Penchansky, 1984). I then validated the questions in telephone interviews from responses to the question: "When you and your household members choose a medical care provider and a hospital to use, can you tell me what factors are important to you?" Responses were related to the technical quality of care, the "art" of care, and the appearance of the facility or office.

The Acceptability Scale items were components of two questions that asked respondents to rate a wide variety of aspects of health care in their local communities (see Table 14.1). Response options included *excellent, good, average, fair, poor,* and *don't know.* The scale had a possible point range of 12–60. The reliability coefficients for the Acceptability Scale were Cronbach's alpha = 0.97 and the Standardized item alpha = 0.97; the inter-item correlations analysis ranged from 0.54 to 0.88.

To identify the predictors of use and willingness to use local health care, I built four separate multivariate logistic regression models (one for each dependent variable) in which I first regressed the dependent variable on a set of six community (dummy) variables to control for confounding by community. Then I added independent variables to the model together as a group (not stepwise). Next, I calculated odds ratios and 95% confidence intervals for the independent variables with $p \leq .05$.

I analyzed qualitative comments on several short answer questions on the mail survey and open-ended questions from the telephone interview regarding access to care by using content analysis methods. I read all qualitative data multiple times and sorted them into similar categories based on the words used in the comments (manifest content) and the apparent meaning of the words (latent content; Catanzaro, 1988). I sought patterns and categories that might add to the understanding of rural residents' views on access to health care in their local communities. I then summarized these themes and categories and identified relevant themes using the actual phrases of the respondents.

RESULTS

Table 14.2 shows the descriptive results of the use of and willingness to use the dependent variables I examined. As can be seen on the table, relatively few respondents ($n = 37$, 9.7%) reported that anyone in their household had used the local CAH for inpatient care in the prior 2 years, whereas roughly two-thirds of the respondents ($n = 260$, 68%) reported use of the local provider in the past year. Less than half of the respondents indicated willingness to use the CAH ($n = 162$, 43%) and local providers ($n = 182$, 48%) for future health concerns.

I computed Acceptability Scale scores for 261 of the total 381 households; I excluded the remaining because of missing values or *don't know*

Table 14.2

FREQUENCIES OF DEPENDENT VARIABLES "USE OF" AND "WILLINGNESS TO USE" LOCAL HEALTH CARE ($n = 381$)

VARIABLE	n	%
"Used the CAHs" for inpatient care in prior 2 years	37	9.7
"Used local provider(s)" in the past year	260	68.0
"Willing to use the CAH" in the future	162	43.0
"Willing to use the local provider(s)" in the future	182	48.0

Note: CAHs = critical access hospitals.

Table 14.3

RESULTS OF MULTIVARIATE LOGISTIC REGRESSION MODELS TO IDENTIFY PREDICTORS OF USE OF AND WILLINGNESS TO USE LOCAL HEALTH CARE

	β	SE	OR	95% CI
Use of CAHs and				
• Knowledge of local health care	.836	.400	2.308	(5.05, 1.06)
• Respondent age	.035*	.017	1.036	(1.07, 1.01)
• Household income	−.533*	.221	.587	(0.61, 0.56)
Use of local provider and				
• Acceptability scale score	.096**	.024	1.100	(1.15, 1.05)
Willing to use CAHs and				
• Acceptability scale score	.065**	.021	1.067	(1.11, 1.02)
• Use local provider	.936*	.452	2.549	(6.18, 1.05)
Willing to use local provider and				
• Acceptability scale score	.088**	.023	1.092	(1.14, 1.04)
• Used provider in the past	1.879**	.504	6.546	(17.58, 2.44)
• Community affiliation	1.540**	.549	4.664	(13.69, 1.59)

Note: SE = standard error; OR = odds ratio; 95% CI = 95% confidence interval of the odds ratio. Data include significant independent variables only.
*$p <$ or $= .05$
**$p <$ or $= .01$

answers. The mean Acceptability Scale score was 46.48 (SD = 9.87; Range = 18–60 points [possible range = 12–60 points]).

Based on the logistic regression analysis (summarized in Table 14.3), respondents for households most likely to use the CAH for inpatient care were those who rated their knowledge of local health care highly, were older in age, and reported lower incomes. The odds ratio indicates the factor by which the odds of use or willing to use change when the corresponding variable is changed by one unit. Because in this chapter I focus on the Acceptability Scale, I do not discuss the other results at length, but just as illustration, for every unit increase in the knowledge rating category with an odds ratio of 2.308, the odds of use of the CAH increased by 130%. An odds ratio of 1 is equal odds, so anything significantly over or under 1 is considered. The Acceptability Scale as well as other variables in this model (distance from CAH, use of local provider, ease of transportation, and community affiliation) were not significant predictors of use of the CAH. I anticipated that few if any covariates would be significant in this model, with only 37 households who had reported use of the CAH.

Households most likely to use the local provider(s) were those that had higher Acceptability Scale scores. For each additional point on the scale, the odds of use of the provider increased by 10%. Other variables in this model (knowledge of local health care, distance from CAH, respondent age, income, transportation, and community affiliation) were not significant predictors of use of the local provider.

Households most likely to be willing to use the CAH for future health problems were those with higher Acceptability Scale scores and those that used the local provider(s) in the past year. Based on the odds ratios, for each additional point on the Acceptability Scale, the odds of indicating willingness to use the CAH increased by 7%. Other variables in this model (knowledge, distance from CAH, age, income, transportation, and community affiliation) were not significant predictors of willingness to use the CAH.

Residents most likely to be willing to use the local provider(s) in the future were also those with higher acceptability scores, who used the local provider(s) in the past year, and reported that they were affiliated with the local community. Each point on the Acceptability Scale increased the odds of willingness to use the provider by 9%. Other variables in this model (knowledge, distance from CAH, age, income, and transportation) were not significant predictors of willingness to use the local provider.

Among those who used local health care, the Acceptability Scale score was also a significant predictor of satisfaction with care. Because I included only those households that had used both the CAH and local provider(s) in the recent past ($n = 36$) in this analysis, I used Mantel-Haenszel chi-square tests to examine relationships between satisfaction and selected covariates. There was insufficient power to analyze this relationship using multivariate logistic regression models. The Acceptability Scale score was significantly associated with satisfaction with the local CAH, emergency care, local primary care provider(s), and the availability of night or weekend care ($p \leq .01$). Other variables examined were not significantly associated with satisfaction with care.

In the qualitative comments, the rural respondents offered many perspectives related to the relationship between acceptability and use of local health care. "He knows what he's doing. He knows my son and my son knows him and that's comforting." "He's a country type doctor. I like that." "The way a hospital is equipped. I want a doctor who is top of the line." "For the doctor—that you have rapport with him, that he gives you accurate information, that you're comfortable that he knows what he's doing." "For the hospital—the nursing care, cleanliness. The doctor—personality. I go to see him the first time—did the medicines help, did the care help the problem?" "They don't have the services, the doctor's not as good, and it's not as good a hospital."

DISCUSSION AND CONCLUSIONS

In this study, the Acceptability Scale was the most consistent predictor of use and willingness to use local rural health care as well as satisfaction with care. Acceptability is that component of access to care that reflects potential clients' attitudes and opinions about the characteristics of providers and services. Unlike other aspects of access, acceptability reflects opinion, judgment, and personal preferences on the part of consumers. The current rural reality for obtaining most goods and services including health care is that with access to vehicles, modern highways, and health insurance, rural residents are not as affected by distance in choosing health care as they once were. And this study suggests that those who do not find local health care acceptable go elsewhere.

It is interesting to note that a large majority (95%) of the respondents in this study indicated that having local health care was very or somewhat important to their household members and "keeping" or maintaining the health services and providers they had was the predominant theme in the qualitative comments—yet only 9.7% of the households had a family member hospitalized in the CAH in the prior 2 years, and only 68.2% had used the local provider(s) in the prior year. A clarification of this discrepancy may be found by considering a second theme that emerged from the data—"just in case." "You always have certain people who are doubters . . . but they still want emergency care available in case they need it, even though they don't support it for everyday things." "I know that it's not paying its way in taxes but we need it. It's like having an insurance policy. Insurance policies don't pay for themselves either but you need it just in case." Clearly there was support in these six communities for keeping their local health care, but acceptability was associated with use of local health care whereas support or indicating its importance were not.

By improving researchers' understanding of what rural consumers deem acceptable in terms of services and providers, the Acceptability Scale can be used to improve health care access for rural residents. In the practice arena, attending to community residents' perceptions of competence, quality, the art of care, and appearance of facilities as well as developing strategies to strengthen and improve these perceptions may reduce out-migration for health care that is available locally. In the policy arena, as new models of care are developed or refined, paying substantial attention to features or characteristics that influence acceptability to consumers can make the difference between services that will be used and valued and services that will be bypassed by the residents they are intended to serve. When it comes to rural health care, Kinsella's (1982) old baseball adage, "If you build it, [they] will come" does not necessarily hold, unless what is built is acceptable to rural residents.

ACKNOWLEDGMENTS

This research was funded by Health Care Financing Administration Dissertation Grant 30-P-90510/0-01, Hester McLaws Award, Sigma Theta Tau Zeta Upsilon Research Award, and Montana State University–Bozeman College of Nursing.

REFERENCES

Aday, L. A., & Andersen, R. (1975). A framework for the study of access to medical care. In L. A. Aday & R. Andersen, *Development of indices of access to medical care* (pp. 1–14). Ann Arbor, MI: Health Administration Press.

Aday, L. A., Bagley, C. E., Lairson, D. R., & Slater, C. H. (1993). *Evaluating the medical care system: Effectiveness, efficiency, and equity.* Ann Arbor, MI: Health Administration Press.

Amundson, B. (1993). Myth and reality in the rural health service crisis: Facing up to community responsibilities. *The Journal of Rural Health, 9,* 176–187.

Andersen, R. M., McCutcheon, A., Aday, L. A., Chiu, G. Y., & Bell, R. (1993). Exploring dimensions of access to medical care. *Health Services Research, 18* (1), 49–74.

Bauer, J. C. (1992). The primary care hospital: More and better health care without closure. In L. A. Straub & N. Walzer (Eds.), *Rural health care: Innovation in a changing environment* (pp. 65–74). Westport, CT: Praeger.

Catanzaro, M. (1988). Using qualitative analytical techniques. In N. F. Woods & M. Catanzaro, *Nursing research: Theory and practice* (pp. 437–456). St. Louis: C. V. Mosby Co.

Christianson, J. B., Moscovice, I. S., Wellever, A. L., & Wingert, T. D. (1990). Institutional alternatives to the rural hospital. *Health Care Financing Review, 11* (3), 87–97.

DeFriese, G. H., Wilson, G., Ricketts, T. C., & Whitener, L. (1992). Consumer choice and the national rural hospital crisis. In W. M. Gesler & T. C. Ricketts (Eds.), *Health in rural North America* (pp. 206–225). New Brunswick, NJ: Rutgers University Press.

Gamm, L., & Hutchison, L. (2003). Rural health priorities in America: Where you stand depends on where you sit. *The Journal of Rural Health, 19* (3), 209–213.

Kinsella, W. P. (1982). *Shoeless Joe Jackson comes to Iowa.* New York: Ballantine Books.

Liu, J., Bellamy, G. R., & McCormick, M. (2007). Patient bypass behavior and Critical Access Hospitals: Implications for patient retention. *The Journal of Rural Health, 23* (1), 17–24.

Millman, M. (Ed.). (1993). *Access to care in America.* Washington, DC: National Academy Press.

Patrick, D. L., & Erickson, P. (1993). *Health status and health policy: Quality of life in health evaluation and resource allocation.* New York: Oxford University Press.

Penchansky, R., & Thomas, J. W. (1981). The concept of access: Definition and relationship to consumer satisfaction. *Medical Care, 19,* 127–140.

Pink, G. H., Holmes, G. M., Thompson, R. E., & Slifkin, R. T. (2007). Variations in financial performance among peer groups of Critical Access Hospitals. *The Journal of Rural Health, 23* (4), 299–305.

Radcliff, T. A., Brasure, M., Moscovice, I. S., & Stensland, J. T. (2003), Understanding rural hospital bypass behavior, *The Journal of Rural Health, 19* (3), 252–259.

Reinert, B. R. (1991). The impact of hospital closures on rural Texas residents: A nursing perspective. *Dissertation Abstracts International, 52,* 1958. (No. 9128345)

Rural Assistance Center. (2008). CAH frequently asked questions. Retrieved December 26, 2008, from http://www.raconline.org/info_guides/hospitals/cahfaq.php

Shreffler, M. J. (1996). Rural residents views on access to care in frontier communities with medical assistance facilities. *Dissertation Abstracts International, 57,* 3131. (No. 9630109)

Shreffler, M. J., Capalbo, S. M., Flaherty, R. J., & Heggam, C. (1999). Community decision-making about Critical Access Hospitals: Lessons learned from Montana's Medical Assistance Facility program. *The Journal of Rural Health, 15,* 180–188.

Thomas, J. W., & Penchansky, R. (1984). Relating satisfaction with access and utilization of services. *Medical Care, 22,* 553–568.

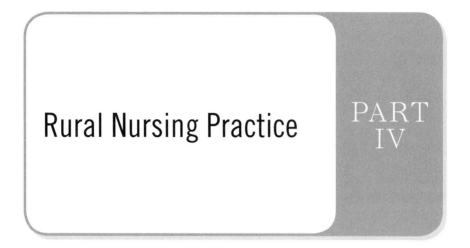

Rural Nursing Practice

PART
IV

15

The Distinctive Nature and Scope of Rural Nursing Practice: Philosophical Bases

JANE ELLIS SCHARFF

LOOKING BACK

Plenty and little have changed in 10 years. Rural nursing practice seemed a dichotomous set of the routine and the extraordinary to me back then, as it does now. I was an insider, if not an old-timer, and my findings, although remarkable to some, seemed simply confirmatory to me. Already a budding pragmatist and not yet fully a scientist, I thought, at the time, it was enough to have empiric validation for the practice that I had known and in which my former workplace colleagues continued. For that reason and so many others, I did not publish the findings of my master's thesis in 1987. Subsequently, I have been cited frequently, misrepresented occasionally, and poached a time or two when it comes to references about the world of rural nursing. It is time to uphold my responsibility to nursing science and to set the record straight. The nature and scope of rural nursing *is* distinctive. I am now willing to be quoted on that. Furthermore, rural nursing can now be given a definition based on that distinctiveness.

Rural nursing practice, be it hospital practice, private practice, or community health practice, is distinctive in its nature and scope from the practice of nursing in urban settings. It is distinctive in its boundaries, intersections, dimensions, and even in its core. Ten years ago I was loath to claim distinctiveness within rural nursing's core. It seemed too bold to proclaim that at the very level of essence, and not attributable to setting alone, rural nursing could be so different. Today, I am determined to claim it: The core of all nursing is care, and care is the substance of the relationship between nurse and patient; consequently, what happens at the core of rural nursing is something apart from what happens at the core of nursing anywhere else.

Still a pragmatist, my job is to get readers as close to the experience as I can. Thankfully, my growth as a scientist makes the job easier than it was some years back. Although no longer in the practice, I understand rural nursing better today than I did then. The importance of rural nursing has not decreased as my worldview has expanded. On the contrary, the more I dissect and reconstruct my thoughts about life and truth and nursing science, the more clearly I see the beauty emanating from the nature and scope of rural nursing, and the more clearly I appreciate its relevance to all of nursing science.

From an ontological viewpoint, I will share some information about what it means to "be" a rural nurse, and from an epistemological viewpoint, I will express a little of what it means to "know" rural nursing practice. What came as primary expression to me, because I lived it, breathed it, and studied it, is secondary expression as I write it; and I will do my best to translate the experience through common language. However, the story I tell will require imagination to transcend time and space and to gain a sense of the reality of rural nursing practice. The information for this chapter comes from my ethnographic study of rural hospital nurses in the Inland Northwest completed in 1987, from dialogue with key informants before then and up until today, and from my personal experiences within rural health care systems over the past 20 years.

In the last 10 or 15 years, I have made some presentations about portions of this work to nurse clinicians, nurse researchers, and non-nurse health care audiences. Inevitably, following such presentations, I was approached by one or two individuals who had been rural nurses who wanted to tell me that the presentation struck a chord. I understood their need, that which stemmed from the human desire to be recognized and understood. It stems from the frequent, albeit unintended, distortion of truth about rural nursing communicated by those who do not fully understand what it means to walk a mile in a rural nurse's duty shoes. I may not be able to change that, but I offer my perspective nonetheless.

CONCEPTUALIZING RURAL NURSING PRACTICE

Being Rural

There was a wonderful line in the 1984 science fiction film *The Adventures of Buckaroo Banzai: Across the Eighth Dimension* (Rausch). The line was delivered by the main character, Buckaroo, a multi-skilled neurosurgeon, particle physicist, rock musician, and Zen warrior who, in the midst of chaos matter-of-factly declared, "No matter where you go, there you are." If this sounds simple, I would caution that it is hardly simple. Buckaroo was talking about being in the moment, so imagine for a moment what it means to have *gone* rural. What of rural nursing identity? While the imagery may seem silly or surreal, the truth is real, authentic, important, credible, respectable, and as serious as any nursing practice anywhere. However, as indicated earlier, rural nursing practice is also distinctive from nursing anywhere else. Although I use the analogy of Buckaroo Banzai hoping it will bring a smile, rural nurses will recognize the script of playing a cool and noble professional, simultaneously enacting multiple roles, and managing the continual transition from one part to another with the frankness of Buckaroo.

Being rural means being a long way from anywhere and pretty close to nowhere. Being rural means being independent or perhaps just being alone. Being a rural nurse means that when a nurse saves a life, everyone in town recognizes that she or he was there; and when a nurse loses a life, everyone in town recognizes that she or he was there. Being rural means turning inward for answers, because there may be nobody to turn to outward. Being rural means that when a nurse walks into the emergency room, it may be her or his spouse or child who needs a nurse, and at that moment, being a nurse takes priority over being anyone else. Being a rural nurse means being able to deal with what she or he has got, where she or he is, and being able to live with the consequences.

Knowing Rural

Certainly every reader has heard that a little knowledge can be a dangerous thing. The adage was probably modified from what Alexander Pope (1711) said in the seventeenth century: "A little learning is a dangerous thing." I dispute it now and say that a little knowledge can be a lifesaving thing. The demarcation between danger and safety is the difference between *having* knowledge and *using* knowledge. From time to time, I have had conversations with academic colleagues about dangerous nurses. In these conversations, we have agreed that dangerous nurses are not those who know they do not know what they are doing—although there is certainly an element of danger in that scenario, which ultimately must be addressed. The greater danger, however, emerges with those nurses who think they do know, but actually do not know, what they are doing. Although I have no statistics on the prevalence of such nurses, it is my belief that they hide more easily in urban settings than they do in rural settings.

Knowing rural means knowing that what one knows may be all one has. Knowing rural means personally knowing everyone with whom one works and having knowledge about nearly everyone for whom one cares. As a rural nurse, knowing means sharing knowledge in an informal, yet crucially important, exchange with other professionals, where the addition of one mind can mean expanding the knowledge base by 100%. Although *whom* one knows can be important in any setting, the distinction between rural and urban dynamics of whom one knows is that in the urban setting whom one knows is more likely to be related to competitive advantage, whereas in the rural setting whom one knows is more likely to be related to cooperative advantage. Knowing rural means that knowledge can mean the difference between perishing, surviving, and thriving; and, therefore, knowing is inextricably connected to *being* when one is rural.

THE NATURE AND SCOPE OF NURSING

For practicality, a framework for the study of the nature and scope of rural nursing practice was sought to identify and describe the distinctive characteristics of practice in rural settings. The American Nurses' Association (ANA) Social Policy Statement (1980) provided the framework for a logical sequence of investigation into details of rural nursing practice. The policy statement includes an organized and systematic approach to studying nursing nature and scope.

1. *Nursing's Nature.* Within the policy statement, the nature of nursing is characterized as a relationship between the nursing profession and society that is mutually beneficial, and nursing itself is deemed an essential outgrowth of the society that it serves.

Nursing is described as existing in response to society's needs. From that standpoint, my study of rural nursing was based on assumptions that rural nursing emerges from and is essential to rural society, and distinctions of rural nursing are due, in part, to distinctive interests and needs of rural society.

2. *Nursing's Scope.* The scope of nursing includes four definitive characteristics that are intersections, dimensions, core, and boundary (ANA, 1980). These four characteristics became conceptual foundation blocks for my study of rural nursing.

   a. *Intersections.* Nursing intersects with other professions involved in health care. These intersections are points at which nursing meets and interfaces with other professions as well as expands its practice into the domain of other professions as necessary.

   b. *Dimensions.* Characteristics such as philosophy, ethics, roles, responsibilities, skills, and authority are examples of nursing dimensions. These are qualities that add depth to nursing practice. They are characteristics underscored and influenced by interpersonal relationships and intimacy as well as the intrapersonal quality of nursing.

   c. *Core.* The concept of the core of nursing is complex and somewhat more difficult to discuss than are the other concepts. It is oversimplification to say that the needs of people are the core of nursing, although such is true. Nursing exists to deal with human response to health issues, and human response can be equated to human need with respect to health. The patients' *needs* and their *responses* are outgrowths of who they are as human *beings*. The nursing care we provide is an outgrowth of who we are as human *beings*. The core of nursing is the dynamic of nursing care juxtaposed with human response.

   d. *Boundaries.* Nursing's boundaries change and expand in direct reflection of the intersections, dimensions, and core of practice. Boundaries are nebulous, unseen, intangible lines of demarcation between what is clearly within the nature and scope of nursing and what is questionably within nursing's scope. Unlike physical boundaries, nursing's boundaries are metaphysical, are relationally and contextually based, and sometimes have origins outside the control of nursing.

METHODS

In an effort to describe the nature and scope of rural nursing, it was determined that an ethnographic method, using participant observation and interviewing techniques, would yield the most pertinent data for analysis. Data were gathered throughout several stages of conceptualization concerning rural nursing phenomena. Field notations, printed news media, and taped interviews were employed. The study of rural hospital nurses included an exploratory phase in which eight rural nurses from northwest Montana were interviewed. These interviews were audio taped, and from initial open-ended questions, a more refined interview guide was developed that contained both closed and open-ended questions. Twenty-six rural hospital nurses in one of four rural towns in eastern Washington, northern Idaho, or western Montana were interviewed. All interviews were audio taped and then transcribed verbatim. The findings reported in this chapter are related to many aspects of rural nursing practice and are based on the responses of all 34 rural nurses, as well as several other key rural informants and my own observations. All samples were convenience, and all informants elected to be included in the studies.

FINDINGS

Informant Demographics

All of the informants were women ranging in age from 25–61 years with an average age of 40 years. The number of years actively employed as a registered nurse (RN) was 3–35 years. The mean number of years spent working in rural hospitals was eight years and, for most informants, was roughly half the total active nursing years. Most informants were originally diploma-prepared, seven were baccalaureate graduates, and four were associate graduates. Two informants had achieved a master's degree in nursing. Although informants were not asked about marital or parental status, nearly all said during the interview that they were married and were parents.

Most of the informants worked full-time, and those who worked part-time averaged 23 hours per week. In addition, many were placed "on call" if they were not working. On call status could be attributed to low census, high census, operating room call, cardiac care call, or emergency department call. Most informants reported one or two days of overtime per month. In almost every case, informants indicated a need to be flexible about their working schedules with regard to the events of the rural practice setting. Turnover rates were low at all facilities, and the most senior nurses had been on staff from 16–25 years.

Hospital Demographics

Information about the hospitals was obtained through interviews with nursing, fiscal, administrative, or other personnel, as well as from public records and the participant observation process. The hospital organizations were between 20 and 60 years in existence, the present structures were between 3 and 35 years old, and all had undergone some renovation over time. Ownership of the hospitals was stated as nonproprietary, public district, or community. Each hospital was governed by a board of directors of 3–10 individuals who held fiduciary and decision-making authorities, and to whom the administration was accountable. Board membership was either self-perpetuating or community elected. One facility was accredited by what was then the Joint Commission on Accreditation of Hospitals (JCAH). Administrative personnel said that there was little to be gained by small rural hospitals having JCAH accreditation, especially in light of what the JCAH charged for the process.

The hospitals had licensure ranging from 20–44 acute care beds, 0–3 intensive or cardiac beds, 5–7 newborn bassinets, and 3–5 swing beds for extended care. In every case, occupancy was at a fraction of licensure, and occupancy figures averaged to be about 20%–40% for acute care beds. There was some variability in the use of the other services at each facility. Two had fairly active use of the cardiac or intensive care beds. Two had fairly active obstetrical departments. Three had active surgical departments. Emergency cases at these hospitals ranged from 3–13 per 24-hour day during the previous fiscal year. One relied on the constant occupancy of swing beds to maintain financial solvency. The number of physicians on medical staff ranged from 3–17. Typically, physicians who held admitting privilege at a given facility did not necessarily live within the community. Undoubtedly, the variety of medical practitioners on staff impacted the occupancy of each facility. Usually, nurses were expected to be able to float from medical–surgical areas to emergency, obstetrical, and intensive care areas, but not to the operating room, which seemed to be the one sacrosanct specialty area.

The Rural Communities

At the time of the study, I spent several weeks traveling to and about four separate communities in western Montana, northern Idaho, and eastern Washington to gather information regarding the nature and scope of rural nursing. Each of these towns fit the operational definition of being geographically isolated and of having less than 5,000 residents. Upon arrival in each community, time was taken to drive about, observe the local terrain, look for indicators of economy, walk around town to observe the pace and lifestyle, note the casual conversations taking place in public areas, and read each community's local weekly newspaper.

There were many similarities and few differences between the communities in terms of how they appeared to the outsider. Each town was located near railroad tracks, all of which were currently used. Three of the towns were on a river in forested mountain terrain and were logging or lumber mill towns. The fourth town was on an expansive plain and was an agricultural community. Each town was inhabited mostly by Caucasian people, and each was laid out in typical western fashion with one main street and several auxiliary streets at which the center of the business district was found. Each town boasted the typical hardware stores, grocery stores, restaurants, farm or logging machinery shops, tool shops, post office, drug store, employment office, beauty shops, ice cream stands, feed stores, junk shops, small motels, bars, and churches. Each town had a well-kept appearance, although each had a few empty buildings or storefronts in the business district.

Residents in these communities were friendly and helpful. They recognized me as an outsider, and, although willing to answer my questions, were curious and wanted to know the purpose of my presence in their town. When I explained myself, the residents registered sincere interest and pleasure that their community had been targeted for this study. They acted like they felt privileged and eagerly conveyed their high regard for nurses in general and *their* nurses specifically. Never did these residents express animosity toward the community of nurses. Most of them had a story to tell about how a friend or relative's life was saved at the local hospital.

Rural Hospital Nurses

The rural nurses I observed and interviewed were a dynamic group of women who could certainly be called *expert generalists*. They moved quickly, and for the most part easily, from one role to another as circumstances required. They explained that most rural nurses have a great deal of knowledge regarding a variety of nursing practice areas. When beginning work in a rural hospital, many nurses suffer reality shock due to the variety of demands placed on them. One seasoned nurse told me, "Although you might start out and you don't have that wide knowledge, you better get it quickly." A relative newcomer nurse expressed admiration about the knowledge level of her rural colleagues, calling them "impressive." The nurses I interviewed routinely worked in three or four different specialty areas of nursing practice every week, and sometimes every day. When talking with one respondent about this phenomenon and how easy certain nurses made it look, she said, "The ones who are experienced in rural nursing seem to be very comfortable in switching back and forth between specialties."

Nursing Staff Tenure and Group Acceptance

At all facilities nurses were heard to use the terms *new* or *newcomer* and *old* or *old-timer* in reference to a given nurse's tenure on the staff. There was no particular time limit identified when a nurse makes the transition from new to old, nor how one arrives at a level of acceptance. However, tenure of less than 2 years was apparently definitely considered new, and tenure of 3–5 years in combination with competence generally constituted acceptance. Tenure beyond 10 years was considered seasoned, and in special cases of achieving high proficiency or social acceptance, one of these nurses might be called an old-timer, but usually this term was reserved for someone who had been around for 20 or more years. What I discerned was some gray area depending on a nurse's tenure, level of proficiency, and sociability related to group fit. It seemed that a nurse who was very skillful, flexible, and likeable might reach old-timer status sooner than a nurse who was lacking one of those characteristics.

Although I cannot pinpoint a "typical" rural nurse, certain characteristics were confirmed as traits of distinctive advantage for a rural nurse's success. For example, good common sense, good judgment ability, the ability to set priorities, good physical assessment skills, and physical and emotional strengths were considered of survival significance to these nurses, due, in part, to the aloneness of their practices. They made comments such as, "You have to make all your own decisions. There's no one to do that for you." "You have to be able to be autonomous." "You can't go to somebody for concurrence with decision making." "At any time during your shift, your assignment may change drastically." "You can make the difference between life or death—the judgment calls are yours." All informants were adamant that the prevalent feeling of aloneness and serious responsibility were distinctive to the rural setting. None would concede that the feeling was anything like that experienced in an urban setting. These nurses expressed a very real and pervasive sense of responsibility that rural nurses bear for their patients. The nurses who do not have the ability consistently to carry the burden of such decisional responsibility are the ones who do not survive as rural nurses. Old-timers claimed they could often tell right away, or within a few weeks, if a newcomer was going to catch on or not. Old-timers based such predictions on their assessments of a newcomer's characteristics as mentioned above, combined with evidence of adaptation to the new environment.

Education and Professional Development

The burden for self-responsibility of education is greater in the rural setting than in the urban setting, and most rural nurses accept this burden in stride. There are a wide variety of sources from which rural nurses receive their continuing education, such as out-of-town workshops or conferences, in-service education, journals, textbooks, practice sessions, physicians, and other nurses. The greatest educational needs voiced were in cardiac, trauma, maternal/child, and complex medical nursing.

Informants indicated a thirst for knowledge in accredited professional continuing education. Several respondents reported attending more than ten continuing education events in a year. Most attended between three and ten events annually. These events were developed and held locally, developed elsewhere but held locally, or developed and held in urban settings. Although expenses were a factor, they were not the central factor in respondents' attending continuing education events.

Nearly all informants also relied on journals for new information, read journals regularly, and reported the most popular journals to be *Nursing, American Journal of Nursing, RN, Journal of Nursing Administration,* and *Nursing Management,* in that order. Current journals were visible in each facility, and notations were seen hanging on bulletin boards in nursing report rooms or locker rooms with a suggestion from one nurse to others that everyone review a given recent journal article germane to a given current case.

Rural nurses, in fact, identify one another as their most important single source of information and education. This was often explained as information being imparted from a peer when it was needed most, so that learning occurred while doing, which tended to heighten the memory. Comments that supported these phenomena included, "We try to share everything we can with each other." "New nurses sometimes come in with great new information or real current ideas. It helps a lot." "Sometimes the new girls expect you to know things, and I don't, and it can be embarrassing. So we look it up together." "When you've been around for awhile, you develop a camaraderie. We know what we can expect from each other."

Out-of-town workshops were identified as the next most important source of continuing education to rural nurses. Informants qualified this by stressing that the topic or presentation needed to be relevant to the rural environment. One informant said, "It's got to be meaningful. You know, you go up to the city and they tell you how to do something, and they don't realize how different the setup is."

Interpersonal Relationships and Nursing Practice

Rural nurses know everyone who works at the hospital, all of the physicians, and most of their patients. Rural nurses say that the interpersonal closeness of knowing everyone with whom they work and for whom they care generally has a positive influence on their practice. The intensity of this interpersonal dynamic is unique to the rural setting. Although it is likely that nurses in any setting develop close relationships, rural nurses are in a distinctive situation of being personally acquainted with all of those around them, so that the depth of interaction is potentially greater, and the accountability for interpersonal exchange is a constant that is simply not present in other settings. An informant explained the bond she felt with coworkers by saying, "It's nice to know the people you're working with. You work more together, you try harder, and you work closer." Another nurse shared that among many rewarding qualities of rural nursing, "The cooperation of the other nurses and the cohesiveness of the group is probably the biggest."

An old-timer at one hospital said, "I don't have to explain when I say something. They believe me, and they do it without wasting time." It was easy to verify this through observation. Certain old-timers could communicate a virtual reassignment of responsibilities through the tone of their voices as they disappeared momentarily to deal with arisen crises, such as the admission of trauma victims in the emergency room. On occasions it was like watching a dance, the motions of which were so well understood; each dancer so valued and respected, that without missing a step, workers would change places based on available expertise and would back each other up without visible cues. Even physicians were seen deferring to old-timer nurses at such times. Yet, the choreography depended heavily on the direction of the one in charge; and on other occasions, with an inexperienced newcomer directing, the dance was frantic and the flow chaotic.

Practicing Medicine

Rural nurses are understandably reluctant to admit that they practice medicine, but they know their boundaries are sometimes stretched by circumstance. "You take it upon yourself and do what has to be done to make sure the patient's stable before you can call the doctor," said one nurse to me. When patient crises occur, calling the physician is considered important, but it simply does not rank at the top of the list. The nurses I interviewed and watched used a standard A-B-C (airway, breathing, circulation) order of setting priorities to respond to patient needs. Thus, they often began written or unwritten medical protocols while the aide would be sent to summon the physician. Physician response times varied from 5–30 minutes at the rural hospitals, resulting in nurses being responsible for considerable decision making during the time lapse. At each site, I heard or saw variations on the themes of nurses stabilizing cardiac or trauma victims and nurses managing precipitous births without benefit of physicians present. In interviews, nurses were adamant that they had a responsibility to the patients to do whatever was required during an emergency, and although it sometimes felt uncomfortable, inaction would have constituted neglect. The words of one nurse summarize the collective opinion, "We do it because we have to, because it would be wrong if we didn't."

There were also circumstances of newcomer physicians relying on seasoned nurses for insight into or even direction regarding a given patient case. Per physician request, the nurse would literally advise what medications and treatments to order in cases where the doctor did not have the familiarity with a patient's history that the nurse did. This was especially true in after-hours situations of physicians covering for another's patients. My assessment of these circumstances is that each party acted within unseen lines of mutual trust and understanding with the dynamic of trust specific to a given relationship.

Another observation I made at these facilities, which struck me then and which I have informally reconfirmed on multiple occasions since, is that rural physicians seem more likely to read and respond to nurses' notes about patients than do urban physicians. Doubtless there is great individual variability, yet it is tempting to hypothesize that rural professionals have a better grasp than do their urban counterparts of pertinent information that is necessary to communicate to the health care team. Certainly, further study would be required to confirm the probability.

Rural Expertise: Aces and Pinch Hitters

Rural nurses generally believe that no one can be an expert in every area of rural nursing practice. However, a few nurses are extremely proficient in all clinical areas, and these nurses become role models and mentors to the other nurses with whom they work. At two study sites many informants identified a colleague or two who fit this category. Interestingly, those who were identified by others as *aces* did not identify themselves as such. Each nurse was very modest about her own capability, but the pride toward aces among the staff was obvious. I was aware that talking to or watching these aces in action was as much an honor for the locals as it was for me as an investigating outsider.

All rural nurses interviewed agreed that they must be competent in more than one clinical area to be considered an acceptable staff member. The top four clinical areas deemed to be most important for competency were emergency nursing, obstetrical nursing, intensive or coronary nursing, and medical-surgical nursing. A supervisory nurse told me, "There's a difference between competent and expert. I think everybody who works in this hospital should be able to walk into any specialty area and function." But there was an expectation held by all informants that they be clinically strong, if not expert, in at least two of the above-named areas and be able to float to any other department and still function well in a pinch.

With regard to functioning in a pinch, in the early 1980s two rural Montana nurse executives who are admitted baseball fans coined the *Pinch Hitter Theory of Rural Nursing*. One of those persons, Jean Shreffler, now an academic, is author of other chapters in this text. The second person, Maura Fields, was then and remains today the nurse executive at a rural hospital in Montana and is arguably one of the most innovative and masterful nurse leaders I have ever had the good fortune to know. Her rendition of the theory went like this:

> In rural nursing, you have to be like a pinch hitter. You may not perform a task or procedure or work on a very specialized case but once a year. But when you go to do it, you have to do it like you do it every day. In baseball, a batting average of 300 is good. But the pinch hitter, well, you want them to be better than that, really, you want them to bat a thousand. That's what it's like for a rural nurse, when they go to work, you want them to bat a thousand. (Personal conversation, Maura Fields, 1983)

For those readers who are doubting that there can be that many instances in which the above theory becomes important, rest assured that it happens all the time. Industrial and recreational traumas are frequent in these communities. Rural citizens experience their share of severe burns, drug overdoses, cardiac arrests, head injuries, freak accidents, and critical illness. Although transfer to larger medical centers is sometimes preferred, stabilization is first necessary, and transfer is sometimes not possible. One hospital in this study is 90 road miles from the nearest medical center of any size and 150 road miles from a trauma center. Rotary blade or fixed wing aircraft are often used to transport cases that require more care than can be delivered locally, but northwest mountain weather conditions can be a significant factor in keeping aircraft grounded.

Although rural nurses do not expect an easy routine, frustration is common surrounding the conflict of trying to achieve expertise in such a complex practice. Boredom is rare as they face the constant variety of demands. One informant related the example of the prior day's evening shift. The informant was one of two RNs on duty at the time, assisted by one aide. The scenario she described began after change of shift report and went like this:

> Just yesterday evening there were seven patients in the house with nothing going on. Within an hour, there was one admitted with a depression state, an OB came in, and there were four or five cases in the ER, one being a child with rectal bleeding, which makes you wonder about child abuse.

Although two nurses and an aide would have no difficulty caring for seven stable medical surgical patients, the admission of the depressed patient was a wrench in the works. Mental health diagnoses are among those which rural nurses feel least appropriately prepared for, and they lack confidence in rural physicians' ability to treat mental health patients appropriately, as well. The depressed patient required suicide precautions for a period of time which meant that the aide was assigned to remain with the patient at all times. The pediatric patient in the emergency room required careful documentation, delicate interaction, and a social services consultation. The obstetrical patient admission required nurse assessment and individual care until it was determined that the patient was in early labor. One nurse moved back and forth between the emergency room and the general care unit; the other moved back and forth between the labor room, the depressed patient, and the general care unit.

Here is an account from another informant about another evening shift where three RNs were on duty but without assistance from an aide:

> Not long ago we had an OB with a bad baby, small for gestational age; and at the same time we got two ambulances five minutes apart, and they were both cardiacs with chest pain. While that was happening, there was surgery going on, and there was somebody in the unit. I don't know if God is watching you or what, but, for the most part, things seem to come out okay in the end.

In this case, one nurse was already assigned to the intensive care unit, and one was required to remain with the obstetrical patient to do monitoring and other procedures. When the first ambulance arrived, the third nurse was dispatched to the emergency room. Fortunately, some ambulance crew members were emergency medical technicians and could help with continued patient monitoring and calling in the physician, laboratory, and respiratory personnel. Also fortunately, the physician arrived within 10 minutes and was designated to care for both patients. The final good fortune is that nothing went wrong on the general care unit while hell was breaking loose elsewhere.

Knowing Patients Personally

Most rural nurses subscribe to the belief that when they know patients personally, they can give better care. The possibility of experiencing fear when caring for family members or best friends notwithstanding, the rewards are considered rich. A gradual loss of anonymity occurs to rural nurses as they become immersed in and assimilated into rural society, making anonymity nonexistent for old-timers. "I can be more support-ive emotionally when I know them," one said, and another elaborated, "Let's say in the ER, with chronic lungers, you know them, and they feel secure because they know we remember them." I saw instances of rural nurses informally calling to check on patients after discharge. As far as I know, patients were always glad to have these calls. The loss of anonymity is generally considered reassuring for those professionals who are comfortable with rural life, but it can be constricting as well. It should not be assumed, however, that negative aspects of anonymity loss are necessarily related to poor patient outcomes. On the contrary, one informant told me,

> I know of several situations where knowing my OB patients who had poor outcomes made a difference to them, where I was really able to help them get through the experience. It's a real emotional drain, but you're ahead of the game because the trust is there.

The argument could be made that patients perceive their care to be better based on the close personal contact that is often made in the rural setting. A nurse who believes that her relationship to a patient made a difference in the patient's outcome said,

> I recovered my little neighbor girl after her surgery. Most little kids are scared when they wake up, but when she woke up she knew me and wasn't afraid and recovered really fast. Because fear generates pain, but she wasn't afraid, she recovered faster than usual.

It is a cultural expectation of many rural people to be taken care of by someone they know. This differs from the expectation in urban set-tings. For the most part, informants agreed that rural people do expect to have their medical needs met, even though they live far from a major medical center. However, one informant said that rural patients often wait until they are "half dead" before they seek intervention and are "grateful for what they get." Another nurse said, "People have told me they were glad I was on when they were here, that if I said it was going to be okay, then it was going to be okay."

Nearly all rural nurses could confirm that sometimes they had patients from out of town who had previously experienced urban hospi-tal admissions. These patients, whether vacationing in the rural setting or passing through the rural area, ended up in rural hospitals for reasons not important to this story. Their comments about the care they received in rural hospitals are important. The nurses were told by these patients that the care was of better quality, that they felt more cared for, that the rural nurses took more time to listen, that care was accomplished more quickly and smoothly, and that they felt more like people and less like numbers in the rural hospital than they did in any urban hospital. The outsider patients often expressed surprise at the high level of competence they encountered in the rural setting.

DISCUSSION

Rural Nursing's Distinctive Nature and Scope

Analyses of the reports of rural nurses show that the nature and scope of rural nursing are clearly distinctive. Using a framework to focus the discussion, the distinctions can apparently be categorized as those pertaining to rural nursing's nature, as well as the four components of rural nursing's scope, those being intersections, dimensions, core, and boundary.

The Nature of Rural Nursing

Most rural nurses have difficulty defining their practice, although they can describe it. Their descriptions are a variety of rich, thoughtful, colorful, and articulate responses. Rural nursing is generalist nursing, not to be mistaken for mundane, and includes an intensity of purpose which makes it distinctive. Rural nurses may feel misunderstood and poorly recognized by the larger nursing community, but they are nonetheless a proud lot.

The Scope of Rural Nursing

The intersections of rural nursing are distinctively marked and fluid. Rural nurses consistently and necessarily practice well within the realm of other health care disciplines, the most notable being respiratory therapy, pharmacy, and medicine. The intersection between nursing and medicine has the most extensive implications. It is a gray area that hinges on circumstances and relationships, and the most complex intersections occur during emergent situations; "until the doctor gets there." Some rural nurses embrace this intersection more willingly than others, but none do it casually. Reflective concern is apparent in comments related to this intersection. One informant said, "It means putting your neck out there on the line, but you have to make the judgment and go on." Another told me, "It sometimes feels uncomfortable, but it's part of my responsibility to the patient."

It is evident that the practice of rural nursing is dimensionally distinctive. Rural nurses embrace an ethic of openness and honesty that is pervasive. The dimension of interpersonal knowing is viewed as a positive feature of rural practice, and it exists between nurses and patients as well as among coworkers. A nurse administrator shared with me that, "in terms of practice outcomes, your accountability is right in front of your face." Rural nurses talked about being able to accomplish goals more quickly with their patients and said that guidance, teaching, and counseling behaviors are automatic to their practice in the rural environment. Communication patterns in the rural setting are more direct and suffer less obfuscation than do those in urban settings. There are fewer barriers to go through when imparting messages from one to another. As a result, there are probably fewer errors of omission and commission related to practice in the rural setting than there are in the urban setting. Confronting and managing conflict is more common in the rural setting, avoidance being an unacceptable dynamic for group cohesiveness that stems from mutual concern and regard for one another. Independent decision making is a given in rural practice, but rural nurses are aware of their limitations. One said, "You have to know when you don't know, and you have to know where to go to find out." Rural nurses are mindful, if not fully informed, about the legal dimensions of their practice. However, with respect to questions of patient safety and survival, rural nurses sometimes decide their ethical obligation to do what is right for their patients carries more weight than their legal responsibility to uphold the law. These cases generally become lessons of learning, are scrutinized and discussed by the group, and are entered into memory for future reference.

Human responses, which nurses diagnose and treat, are the core of nursing. Some sources have suggested, and informants in this study agreed, that rural dwellers are known to delay health seeking and tend to define health as the ability to get out of bed and go to work. Thinking in terms of nursing diagnosis, one might call this behavior "dysfunctional perceptual orientation to health" which requires distinctive intervention at nursing's core. Rural nurses are faced with determining an appropriate line of demarcation between a rural dweller's rugged individualism and stubborn disregard for health. Inextricable from rural nursing's core are the relational issues of what it means to be rural. As introduced earlier in this chapter, from an ontological standpoint, rural nursing is distinctive at its very core.

Boundary being dependent on the intersections, dimensions, and core of nursing, there can be no question as to rural nursing's distinctive boundary. Rural nursing is constantly changing in response to complex intersections and dimensional intricacies distinctive to rural society. The boundary is, therefore, neither smooth nor even static. When nurses come to a rural setting from an urban setting they are very aware that the boundary of their practice changes. The transitional period for these nurses is not always easy, and boundary expansion can be accompanied by ambivalence, anxiety, and frustration. Newcomers must become adjusted to the rural culture to function effectively, and not all survive. Rural experts can play a key role in the success of newcomer transition, and those aces who invest themselves in the orientation and mentoring of newcomers know the importance of the payoff.

Defining Rural Nursing

Rural nursing is a special variety of nursing in which the nurse must have a wide range of advanced knowledge and ability, in combination with commitment, to practice proficiently in multiple clinical areas simultaneously along the career trajectory. The practice requires constant and continual personal and professional adaptation in developing identity. A rural nurse has both an ontological sense of being and an epistemological sense of knowing that connect the nurse with the surrounding community, and through which the rural nurse creates a reality of rural professional nursing practice. In no other setting is a nurse's practice so thoroughly and integrally a constant factor in a nurse's life. In a society where separating one's private life from one's professional life is considered obligatory, rural nurses are singularly challenged, stripped of their own anonymity while simultaneously charged with protecting their patients' privacy.

CLOSING THOUGHT

The newcomer practices nursing in a rural setting, unlike the old-timer, who practices *rural nursing*. Somewhere between these spectral extremes lies the transitional period of events and conditions through which each nurse passes at her or his own pace. It is within this temporal zone that nurses experience rural reality and move toward becoming professionals who understand that having gone rural they are not less than they were, but rather they are more than they expected to be. Some may be conscious of the transition and others may not, but in the end a few will say, "I am a rural nurse."

REFERENCES

American Nurses' Association (ANA). (1980). *Nursing: A social policy statement* (Publication No. NP-63 20M 9/82R). Kansas City, MO: Author.

Pope, Alexander. (1711). Essay on criticism. Cited in B. Evans (Ed.), *Dictionary on quotations* (1978). New York: Avenel Books, Delecort Press.

Rausch, E. M. (Screenplay Author). (1984). *The adventures of Buckaroo Banzai: Across the eighth dimension*. [Film]. (Available through Vestron Video.)

16 The Rural Nursing Generalist in the Acute Care Setting: Flowing Like a River

KATHRYN (KAY) AYRES ROSENTHAL

Nurses working in rural hospitals are characterized as expert generalists, often caring during single shifts for a diverse group of patients who would have been admitted to a specialty unit had the care occurred in an urban setting. As a generalist, however, the nurse is held to the same standards of care established by specialty nursing (e.g., operating room [OR], intensive care unit [ICU], obstetrics [OB], and postanesthesia care unit [PACU]). This can create struggles, opportunities, and threats to generalist nurses specific to the practice of rural nursing. In this chapter, I illuminate the issues and concerns and rewards and challenges faced by rural nurses by presenting an overview of my research (Rosenthal, 1996). I present subthemes, themes and the metatheme, as well as one example of a story cocreated by me on the basis of the data I obtained. I describe implications for nursing practice, administration, education, and research.

DESIGN

I chose exploratory descriptive as the design for the study. I encouraged nurses to tell stories of their experiences working in a rural acute care hospital to illustrate the lived experience of the rural nurse generalist.

The assumptions of the design include (a) the topic has not previously been studied or explored or has not been studied from the point of view of the participant or informant, and (b) the participants had personal experience in, or knowledge about, the topic (Brink & Wood, 1989, p. 145).

I use narrative to present the findings. Polkinghorne (1988) defined *narrative* as the equivalent of story, the primary form by which human experience is understood and made meaningful. Narrative processes organize human experiences into meaningful episodes providing a means of increased understanding of life's events and a mechanism to verbalize unspoken aspects of life.

Research Question

What are the stories told of the lived experience of rural generalist nurses who work in an acute care hospital with fewer than 25 beds located in a mountain setting?

Agency Access and Setting

Two rural hospitals with fewer than 25 beds were the settings for this study. These hospitals were located in western mountain communities in the United States. Hospital A was approximately 90 minutes and Hospital B was approximately 3 hours from urban hospitals. Neither hospital selected for this study provided high technological care (e.g., cardiac catheterization, angioplasty, neurosurgery). Hospital A had computer axial taxonomy (CAT or CT) scanning capabilities. Hospital B had magnetic resonance imagery (MRI) and CT scanning.

Referrals to larger hospitals were made when technological support services were needed. Patients were sent to larger hospitals for continued treatment, transported by personal car in non-acute situations, by ambulance when ground transport was appropriate, or by helicopter when time was critical. Helicopter transports took less than 30 minutes from Hospital A to reach metropolitan hospitals north or south of its location. Hospital B had fixed-wing transportation that arrived in a metropolitan area within 40 minutes. Transferring patients within the "golden hour" of emergency medicine—the hour that predicts mortality and morbidity, success or failure—was easily met in normal weather situations. In typical mountain weather conditions (e.g., lightening storms in May and June, low cloud covering common in the winter and spring months, and intermittent wind storms throughout the year), the uncertainty of helicopter support was an ever-present issue at Hospital A. Hospital B was less affected by weather because of fixed-wing navigational capabilities.

Sample

The Director of Nursing (DON) at each hospital obtained facility permission to conduct the study, identified generalist nurses who worked in multiple subspecialties within the hospital (e.g., OR, emergency department [ED], OB, medical-surgical, and gastrointestinal lab [GI]), and scheduled interviews with them. The study sample comprised seven registered nurses (RN) and one licensed practical nurse (LPN) who agreed to participate in the study (see Table 16.1). Three nurses worked entirely in a rural setting; the other five nurses in the study had multiple years of experience in rural and urban settings. One of the eight nurses had rural nursing practicum as part of her

Table 16.1

DEMOGRAPHICS

	HOSPITAL A NURSES				HOSPITAL B NURSES			
Characteristic	1	2	3	4	5	6	7	8
Age	44	66	52	39	44	51	36	56
Gender	F	F	F	F	F	F	M	F
Ethnic	C	C	C	C	C	C	C	C
Education	DIPL	DIPL	ASSOC	LPN	BSN	DIPL	ASSOC	DIPL
Rural/Clinical	N/N	N/N	N/N	Y/Y	N/N	N/N	N/N	N/N
Work status	FT	FT	FT	FT	FT	FT	FT	FT
Total years in nursing	23	40	4.5	19	22	26	3	34
Rural nursing, years	20	28	4.5	19	18	20	2	34
Career in rural nursing, %	86	70	100	100	81	86	66	100

Note: F = Female, M = Male; C = Caucasian; ASSOC = Associate Degree, BSN = Baccalaureate, DIPL = Diploma, LPN = Licensed Practical Nurse; FT = Full Time; Rural/Clinical = Rural nursing clinical offered in nursing program/Participated in rural clinical; N = No, Y = Yes.

nursing education. Ethical approval was obtained for the study from the University of Colorado, Denver, Review Board.

Interviews

Interviews were conversational in style and manner. Each interview began with an introduction to the lens under which I conducted the study, the research question, and a list of probing questions, which facilitated but did not prescribe the interview direction. I conducted interviews after assuring the nurses that I would maintain their confidentiality and anonymity. In these interviews, I encouraged the nurses to share their stories. I audio taped and transcribed the interviews. I disguised specifics in the story that would aid the reader in identifying the person or place. For example, a motorcycle accident became a car accident; I changed the nurses' name to a pseudonym, and omitted the highway number. I verified interviews in writing with each nurse. I collected stories until redundancy occurred and no new themes emerged.

Data Analysis

According to Brink and Wood (1989), the analysis of data for an exploratory study "requires a fluid, flexible, somewhat intuitive interaction" between the data and researcher (p. 151). Living with the data, explained as reading and rereading the transcripts, looking for what is present, absent, what fits, and what does not fit, is recommended. Data analysis for the present study had two distinct aspects. One was the identification of themes with supporting subthemes and exemplar transcripts. I sent transcripts, themes, subthemes, and stories to the participants as well as faculty members for confirmation. The second aspect of data analysis was the creation of narratives, stories rewritten by me on the basis of the interviews with rural generalist nurses.

FINDINGS

Four themes emerged from the data: (a) *Going with the Flow: Fluid Role*; (b) *Fish Out of Water: Expert to Novice*; (c) *Still Waters Run Deep: Self-Reliance*; and (d) *Life in a Fishbowl: Contextual Knowledge of Patients*. I explicate briefly each of the themes here. See Rosenthal (1996) for a full description of the themes and subthemes with supporting transcript excerpts.

Going with the Flow: Fluid Role

The first theme, *Fluid Role*, emerged from several subthemes: (a) *Flexibility* was needed by the rural nurse as the workload and type of nursing care to be delivered varied based on the patients' ages and diagnoses; (b) *Shifting Priorities* occurred throughout the rural nurse's day (e.g., the nurse in the middle of one procedure may be required to move immediately to another more urgent priority); (c) *Continuity of Care* was demonstrated by nurses caring for patients from ED to OR and PACU all in the same shift; (d) the *Lack of 24–Hour Ancillary Support* forced the rural nurses to fill these roles (e.g., cook, dispatcher, phone operator, laboratory, and x-ray personnel) on the off-shifts and weekends; (e) the *Anticipatory Generosity with Regard to Limited Availability of Nursing Staff* was described as off-duty RNs hearing sirens and coming to the hospital to see if help was needed; and (f) the feelings of *Team Support*, *Interdisciplinary Rapport*, the *Give and Take of the Team*, and *Implicit Trust* were illuminated; instances of Role Transcendence were described in which nurses may act in the role of physician until the physician arrived and the physician acted as RN in the absence of another nurse.

Fish Out of Water: Expert to Novice

The second theme, *Expert to Novice*, represented the dualism within the nurse's knowledge base. Although rural nurses could be experts in surgical nursing, they were concomitantly novices in other areas of nursing. Many nursing skills were transferable from one specialty to another, but some skills were specific to a certain branch of nursing. Nurses came to the rural nursing setting feeling confident of their previous knowledge base. Their confidence is challenged almost immediately because of the breadth of knowledge needed in the rural setting. The theme *Expert to Novice* was a compilation of the subthemes discussed by the nurses in their interviews. The rural nurses who were former urban nurses described how *Urban Nurses Are In for a Big Surprise* when they decide to "go rural." The nurses felt they *Never Have Enough Knowledge* and sometimes had to learn in the midst of actions, which they termed *Trial by Fire*. They frequently were alone in situations where they realized they were the *Most Qualified*; in situations where they were caught not knowing a particular skill or theory, they would *Know That Next Time*. Rural nurses sought out continuing education opportunities as *Their Confidence Increased through Certification*.

Still Waters Run Deep: Self-Reliance

The third theme, *Self-Reliance*, emerged from subthemes of the rural nurse's ability to *Thrive on Variety*. One nurse commented, "I stay sane by changing my job within the facility, clinically too. I learned OB, ED, then ICU . . ." instead of being threatened by it. The nurse's ability to Stay Calm in the middle of chaotic situations was described by one nurse who stated, "And I can stay very calm . . . I do get flustered by things but they happen inside." *Self-Reliance* addresses the rural nurses' realization that *One Is Alone; You're It* in many situations, when one would like to have had another professional's guidance or support, as well as *Humor and Confidence* while dealing with one's own humanness. One nurse described having been taught to start intravenous lines (IVs), but not having done any. When a patient needed an IV, the DON said, "Go in and start it," and she did.

Life in a Fishbowl: Contextual Knowledge of Patients

The final theme, *Contextual Knowledge of Patients*, illustrated the unique position of the rural nurses in that the majority of the patients would be personally connected to themselves, their family, or friends in the context of the community. In the urban setting, nurses working across town would rarely care for patients that they knew personally. In the rural setting, all employees were known; if they or their children came to the hospital for service, the rural nurses provided the care. Because the community was small, the odds of caring for an acquaintance or family member were greatly increased. That can be terrifying for rural nurses. Even the tourists could be connected to the rural nurse because they were often visitors of friends of the nurse.

Subthemes of *Contextual Knowledge* include (a) *Caring for a Known Person*, (b) the *Discomfort of Caring for a Friend*, (c) the *Positive Aspects of Knowing the Patient*, and (d) how knowing the patient *Touches Your Heart and Soul*. One nurse described dealing with rape cases and how upsetting that was. "Almost everything that goes on in a rural hospital this size, it touches one's heart and soul really, because you know everybody or almost everybody."

Metatheme

The metatheme, *Flowing Like a River*, emerged from reviewing the transcripts, the four themes, and their subthemes. The metatheme is an image that united all the findings of the study and provided an overall impression of the lived experience of rural nurses.

STORIES OF RURAL NURSING

The creative outcomes of the interviews of rural nurses were a compilation of six stories explicating the lived experience of rural nurses. I wrote the stories in the first person so that emotions could be expressed. They were based on the data but certain aspects of the interviews were fictionalized (i.e., names of participants, date, time, and place). However, the substance of the stories' situations and events were true to the transcribed interviews. "Injured? Dying? This Can't be Happening!" reflected the nurses' stories of caring for patients who are family members or acquaintances. "Man, Am I a Good Metro Nurse! I'll Show Those Rural Nurses a Thing or Two" reflected interview content from former urban nurses who moved to rural areas thinking it would be easy because they know more than their rural colleagues, but find they have a lot to learn. "Code Blue Boots" reflected the training scenarios practiced to help prepare staff for "what-if" situations that will eventually occur while they were on duty. "We're All In This Together" reflected the community collegiality between the school and the hospital in the rural setting. "Orientation. You Call This Orientation?" described how despite orientation, or lack thereof, rural nurses became oriented to the variety of roles. I present here excerpts from one story, "Western Slant."

> It was Labor Day. The town was hosting multiple events. The parade of horses, antique cars, motorcycles always left us short staffed. We had three nurses scheduled and a fourth on call for the ED. The day started out quiet enough. Then we heard a vehicle in the ambulance bay.

It was Rancher Bob, former board member of the hospital, very prominent businessman in the community, director of the city planning committee. He had his horse trailer blocking the ambulance bay and wanted our help. Of all things, he wanted his horse's leg x-rayed. Bring out the portable x-ray machines, work quickly we need to keep the bay open for "real" emergencies! I couldn't believe my eyes and ears. I've worked in the rural setting for three years now and knew the local vet sometimes borrowed OR lights, some drugs from the pharmacy but this really caught me off guard. As we were finishing up, the ambulance pagers blared.

"Multiple motor vehicle accident (MVA) on the pass, two vans with multiple passengers involved in a head on." Primary and secondary crews were being dispatched. They asked, "Could we please coordinate the staffing of the third vehicle?"

"No." I respond. "They are staffing the parade in the event of injuries." A flurry of thoughts enter my head. We need to get that horse out of the ambulance bay. Start calling the disaster roster list. As I think of staffing, it hits me what a mess this is going to be. We'll need help and most of the employees are either at the parade, at work already or out of town for the holiday. Well, just start calling.

Admitting tells us that there is a husband and wife in the lobby, the wife has an ankle injury. "Tell them we are setting up the ED for a major car accident and they are going to have to wait." Tossing her an ice pack and pillow, I add, "Here, put an ice pack on the ankle, take this pillow to elevate her leg." Calling out after her I ask her to, "Ask how much discomfort or pain she is in and let me know if it's a lot. We'll come out and check her as soon as we can." I say somewhat tersely.

"Is that horse out of the ambulance bay?" I speak into the room. "Yes," comes a reply. Hearing Cindy in the corner of the room and seeing her setting things up I delegate: "Cindy, can you go look at this ankle in the lobby . . . ? I'll finish opening the trauma tray and I'll pull the chest tube trays while you're gone. . . ."

Report is called in, one Black (Dead on Arrival, DOA), one Red (Critical), permission to chopper from the site received. Six Yellow (Unstable), and two Green (Stable, "Walking Wounded"). Two nurses from Home Health Care have arrived. I assign one to the morgue. I assign the other to the two patients triaged as "greens" telling her, "Take them to the . . . chemotherapy room, that way if you need to lay them down, the chemo chairs stretch out."

A nursing home aide comes to command center, how can she help? "Go to the Med-Surg floor and ask for a census and status report from one of the nurses." I recognize I am not using please or thank you, I'm just barking out commands. . . . OK. I've got six nurses in the ED. Next person that comes in can cover the floor or switch places with one of the floor nurses in the ED. Patients one and two arrive. Ten minutes later patient three arrives. We're starting IVs, hanging blood and IV fluid, inserting chest tubes, foleys, nasogastric tubes, recording assessments, doing EKGs, x-rays, running labs.

The patient in the lobby is what?! Complaining about the what?! The wait! Tell them we're sorry but we have to take care of the critical patients in this accident first and they are just going to have to wait.

Patients four and five arrive. Another nurse, who just happened to hear the ambulance sirens by her house, came in to see what was going on. Great!

"Go assess the patients on the floor and see where they are at with meds, treatments, are they doing OK? There's an aide there that can help you."

"Wait," one of the floor nurses says, "You start this IV, I can't get it and I'll go check the patients on the floor, I know them already."

"Good idea. Let's go." Patient six arrives and is no longer a yellow, he is retriaged a red and we need a chopper now.

There are no more carts, I thought maintenance was bringing one from the basement? Where is it?

The x-ray technologist asks, "Are we done with all the x-rays? Can we do the lady in the lobby? Hey, who are all those people in the lobby anyway?"

"What do you mean?" I go to the lobby and there are at least twenty people there. I quietly tell the admitting clerk "Let's get some traffic control here. . . ."

Seeing a housekeeper walk in, I send him to command center and tell them to assign him as Security.

Finally the chopper arrives and after assessing the patient themselves, listening to report, they are out of the building. One down, five to go.

"Let's see if we can transport the two patients in room four in the same ambulance. Patient #4–1 needs to be transported to Metro OR and patient #4–2 needs to get a CT scan," I say. . . .

"I'll go see them (the greens in chemo) when we get the yellow's taken care of," says ED doc number two.

The ambulance bay doors open and it's one of the local family practitioners walking in, "Need any help? I was at the parade and heard a lot of commotion, what's going on?"

"Here," Jane calls out, "we've had a major MVA [motor vehicle accident], go see the patient in five, possible head injury and rib fracture." She tells him, "x-rays have been done and are in the room. Let us know if they need to go to Metro for a CT or MRI."

He comes out after assessing the patient and announces calmly, "Let's admit to our hospital and just watch closely."

"OK," I say, "But you're taxing my staffing. Almost everyone is here right now and nights will only have three nurses on. How close are we going to have to watch him?" We decide if he's the only "yellow" that we keep we'll have adequate staffing.

"Come see the patient in bay one, he might have abdominal injuries from his seat belt," calls Cindy. We decide to send him to Metro Trauma ED for abdominal CT and surgical consult. We'll send bay three with him for a surgical consult unless Orthopedics can come up and do surgery here. Then we reconsider, a C-arm (specialized x-ray equipment) will probably be needed so we better send him down.

"Let's send the two kids to Children's Metro, their injuries aren't too bad but they can watch them closer," ED doc one yells to the unit secretary.

She starts dialing Children's Metro. "ER or ICU?" she clarifies. "ER, and pull some antidumping law (COBRA) forms and start copying the chart as soon as you can. Did anyone fax those labs to Metro OR when they came back?" No one knows. Lab is paged to fax the results and copy the charts of the kids so they can go down by ambulance. It's interesting how all departmental lines, minimal as they are, disappear in an emergency; x-ray is copying charts, getting maps for friends in the lobby so they can meet them at Children's Metro, cleaning the cart when bay two leaves by chopper. The paramedics and EMTs are all helping with vitals, writing the nurses' notes as dictated by the RN's assessment; helping hold legs while foleys are inserted, and helping cut off clothes so we can really see the extent of injuries.

Now, back to deal with the greens, ED doc number one goes to evaluate and hopefully discharge to home. ED doc number two is debriefing with the ED staff.

"Hey," I call out, "let's do this later, get this ankle out of the lobby before the prima donna or her husband strokes from waiting, her x-rays are over there."

Finally, the ED is cleaned out but the husband of the woman with the hurt ankle has come unglued. We've called the police department back in to remove him from the ED. The officer approaches the doctor and the husband who are yelling at each other at the top of their lungs. The doctor pulls the officer's pistol, aims it at the husband and says, "You can just get out of my ER." We all stand there flabbergasted! In Metro ED it's the patients or visitors who draw the guns, here it's the doc!

"CALM DOWN EVERYONE," yells the police officer. He takes his gun from the doctor and secures it in his holster. I grab the arm of the ED doc and kind of push/pull him into room five, closing the door behind us and tell him to "Stay." By now I'm visibly shaking. It's been enough to deal with the accident to now have to deal with this. The police officer has taken the husband outside and has threatened to take him to jail if he doesn't calm down.

Cindy has called the debriefing team, but since it's a holiday she had to leave a message, they'll get back to us Tuesday. ED doc number one has discharged the greens downstairs and has agreed to put a splint on the lady with the broken ankle and discharge her.

In the meanwhile, we are cleaning the ED and getting ready for the next round just in case. Happy Holiday! NOT. The safety director/Certified Registered Nurse Anesthetist (CRNA) says, "Let's write this one up so we don't have to have a fake disaster drill." We all agree! This one was enough for the whole year.

"But YOU write it up," calls ED doc number two from room five. He is shaking his head and says he's "off to the showers." He's cooled off and embarrassed, we nickname him "Quick Draw McGraw" . . . behind his back and all start laughing when he is out of hearing range. We hope he was out of hearing range!

DISCUSSION

In the story, "Western Slant," written with actual interview data, I incorporate the reality of rural nursing on a holiday shift. In the story I demonstrated several of the themes and components of the metatheme. *Going with the Flow: Fluid Role* was evidenced by the nurses' flexibility, changing priorities, limited staff, and the team support during the emergency. *Fish Out of Water: Expert to Novice* was demonstrated by the nurse on the floor, possibly an expert in OB, coming to ED to help where she may be a novice. *Still Waters Run Deep: Self-Reliance* is demonstrated by the variety of the situation, the need to stay calm during the emergency, and the sense of humor exhibited by the staff to survive the stress of the situation. *Life in a Fishbowl: Contextual Knowledge of Patients* was not clearly illuminated in this story as victims were not identified as family members or visitors of any of the employees.

Implications for Nursing Practice

The nurses described characteristics of successful rural nurses during the interviews. These characteristics included "flexibility," "emotional strength," and "being able to ask for help from a coworker or knowing when advice is needed from a Metro ED, ICU, or burn unit." The successful rural nurse "cannot be afraid to ask questions." The rural nurse needs personal accountability to "learn from the situation because there are times when she must go ahead and do something, carry out a new procedure, or administer a medication for the first time, when there is no one else to ask or to help." The nurse who "looks up the information before or after the situation" will be prepared for the next time. The rural nurse who is able to "recognize skills and knowledge of others" and "tap into their strengths without feeling that she is less proficient or less of a nurse for not knowing" will be more successful in the rural setting. Furthermore, the nurse who is determined to succeed in the setting and "desires to live in a rural community" will have a greater rate of success. Nurses are bound to be "self-critical" and constantly assess their work. The nurse should be "confident but not overly so."

Rural nurses need to love the challenge of learning, the thrill of doing it all, and being a "jack-of-all-trades." Nurses who "thrive on variety" and do not like the comfort and security of established routines may excel in rural nursing. Rural nurses need to know how to get along with people because the ability to build relationships and establish community rapport is crucial. Tact and assertiveness and being a team player are skills needed by rural nurses. Being able to read instructions and policies and procedures in front of patients during a crisis may be required. Rural nurses must be practical, "have common sense," "know how to triage, set priorities, delegate, and use good judgment." Having the ability to implement theory and be able to turn knowledge into action even if they have never done the procedure before will enhance the nurses' confidence.

Nurses may act as physicians in the absence of physicians—starting the resuscitation procedures, administering medications per Advanced Cardiac Life Support protocol, and determining what IV solution to hang before the physician arrives. Nurses may begin appropriate diagnostic tests, laboratory and x-ray, so that when physicians arrive they will have the information needed to immediately begin treating the patient.

The nurses spoke of rewards and benefits of rural nursing. One reward identified was "having time to do the little things for patients. To be able to sit with the patient and talk about what is really going on in [his or her] life. To give back rubs and offer foot soaks." Because there is less hierarchy in the rural setting, nurses' voices are more easily heard. Nurses can make a difference and feel ownership of the rural hospital. Although there are few positions for promotion, nurses who want to learn will identify many opportunities for lateral promotion into different clinical and nonclinical opportunities.

Implications for Nursing Administration

Cross training rural nurses so they feel prepared for any situation is a critical aspect of nursing administration. Financial support for training as well as providing multiple support systems are essential. The nurses recommended support systems that enable the rural nurse to function with limited resources. Systems were also recommended to relieve nurses during traumatic events when the situation involves a family member. A system to cover extreme fluctuations in census during popular community events (e.g., a rodeo) or sick calls and holidays is needed. With no ability to "divert" the patient to a different unit, to a different floor, or to a different hospital within town, systems are needed to support the nurses on duty.

The stories (Rosenthal, 1996) can be used as orientation scenarios to help decrease fear of "what if"—who might come in the ED doors or be admitted to the floor. New nurses will need assistance with planning, identifying personnel to be called in, appropriate supplies to be pulled for use in an emergency, and determining division of tasks. These scenarios will assist to prepare rural nurses for multiple possibilities and to preplan what their responses could be.

The nurses in this study identified a need for assertiveness training and conflict resolution skills so they could confront coworkers and physicians while maintaining a collegial relationship. Professional and practice organizations (e.g., the Emergency Nurses' Association, the state's nurses' association, American Association of Critical Care Nurses, and Sigma Theta Tau International) can link rural nurses with other nurses for information exchange and support (Long & Weinert, 1989).

Implications for Nursing Education

Several implications for nursing education arose from this study. They include increasing faculty and students' sensitivity to the unique and challenging aspects of rural nursing and providing insight into the lives of rural nurses, particularly the diversity, ambiguity, and uncertainty of rural practice. Further implications for nursing education encompass exchange programs between rural and urban hospitals and universities. For example, university faculty could provide in-services to rural nurses and urban nursing students could be assigned to rural clinical rotations. Urban nurses might provide educational outreach (e.g., trauma courses offered on site at the rural setting). Contracts between urban and rural facilities enable rural nurses to practice in specialized urban settings to strengthen skills.

The stories (Rosenthal, 1996) composed by me from the interviews can be used by nursing faculty to ask nursing students how they would respond to the situations. Or the stories could be used as exemplar cases in ethics discussions. Benner (1991) calls for an increase in storytelling in both practice and ethical discussions. There are no right or wrong answers to be determined from the stories, only multiple possibilities, multiple realities, and multiple choices that could be discussed between faculty and students.

Implication for Nursing Research

Implications of this study for future research include further narrative inquiries and expansion of the stories to develop rural nursing theory. Gadow (1990) suggested, "The cultivation of personal knowing as a form of inquiry may be the most important contribution of nursing to the human sciences" (p.167). Perhaps this study will encourage others to expand their inquiry into personal knowing and further ask, "What is it like?" regarding other aspects of nursing.

Future research may focus on what sociologists would call deviant case analysis. Strauss and Corbin (1990) discussed negative cases and stated, "The negative or alternative cases tell us that something about this instance is different. Following through on these differences adds density and variation to our theory" (p.109). Research questions might include: What are the stories of unsuccessful rural generalist nurses? What are the stories of rural generalist nurses who remain in the setting but are not comfortable in the generalist role, who stay in the setting not by choice but because of family obligations? In this study, the DON recruited successful rural nurses. Altering the sample selection method may reveal totally different perceptions of the lived experience of rural nurses. Repeating this study with nurses from other rural settings would provide additional insight into the lived experience of the rural nurse generalist.

In future studies, another style of interview or research methodology could be used. I did not share my personal stories with the participants. It would be an interesting comparison to repeat the study with the researcher engaging in the interviews instead of staying passive. Being more openly empathic might encourage nurses to share more threatening stories, to further expand on stories, or offer insight into why treating a known patient was so difficult. Another possibility would be a focus group of rural nurses. This technique might reveal other stories that are stimulated by participation of other group members.

SUMMARY

Conducting this study generated a rich data source. It examined a setting rarely studied that encompasses a focus on patient care and nursing services. It adds to the knowledge base of rural nursing practice and of nursing administrators and sensitizes nursing educators and others to the needs of rural nursing staff and their leaders.

REFERENCES

Benner, P. (1991). The role of experience, narrative, and community in skilled ethical comportment. *ANS, 14* (2), 1–21.

Brink, P., & Wood, M. (1989). *Advanced design in nursing research.* Newbury Park, CA: Sage.

Gadow, S. (1990). Response to "Personal knowing: Evolving research and practice." *Scholarly Inquiry for Nursing Practice: An International Journal, 4,* 167–170.

Long, K. A., & Weinert, C. (1989). Rural nursing: Developing the theory base. *Scholarly Inquiry for Nursing Practice: An International Journal 3,* 113–127. New York: Springer.

Polkinghorne, D. (1988). *Narrative knowing and the human sciences.* Albany: State University of New York Press.

Rosenthal, K. (1996). *Rural nursing: An exploratory narrative description.* Unpublished doctoral dissertation, University of Colorado, Denver, CO.

Strauss, A., & Corbin, J. (1990). *Basics of qualitative research.* Newbury Park, CA: Sage.

C.

17

The Rural Nursing Generalist in Community Health

LINDA E. TROYER and HELEN J. LEE

Fewer nurses live and work in rural settings as compared with urban settings. According to Stratton, Dunkin, Juhl, and Geller, in 1995, the mean registered nurse (RN)-to-population ratio was twice as large in metropolitan areas compared with nonmetropolitan areas. And yet a higher percentage of rural nurses works in community-based nursing—11.8% compared with 7% of the overall RN population (Dunkin, Stratton, Movassaghi, & Kindig, 1994). Rural nurses are described as generalists (Bigbee, 1993; Scharff, 1987). Although literature on rural nursing has increased since the late 1980s, the majority of literature describing the characteristics of rural nurses is based on descriptions of hospital-based nurses. Our purpose in this chapter is to describe a study conducted by the first author (L. Troyer) to explore whether the concept of rural nurse generalist could be extended to the practice of community health nurses.

In my study, I used the four characteristics of the scope of nursing used by Scharff (1998) in a previous chapter: intersections, dimensions, core, and boundaries. The most distinctive finding of Scharff's study was that rural hospital nurses do not specialize but rather expand the scope of their practice.

METHODS

My study was qualitative descriptive in design; I collected data using interviews of a convenience sample of rural community-based nurses. *Rural* was defined as a nonmetropolitan county not having a city of 50,000 in population within its boundaries.

Sample

I recruited a convenience sample of seven rural community-based nurses in central and eastern Montana through networking with Montana State University–Bozeman community health faculty. Three participants were exclusively public health nurses (PHNs), three were home health nurses (HHNs), and one nurse was a tribal nurse with both PHN and HHN responsibilities. All participants were female, ranging in age from 27–56 years. Three nurses had a Bachelor of Science degree in nursing, whereas the remaining four held associate degrees in nursing. Reported nursing years of experience varied from 3–24 years, and experience in rural community-based nursing ranged from 2–14 years. The sample included nurses with and without previous urban work experience. Four nurses worked full-time; three were part-time, working 20–32 hours per week. Nurses who worked full-time were on call up to 20 nights of the month. All full-time nurses reported working overtime, varying from a few hours a month to 20 hours per week.

Procedures

Following approval by the Human Subjects Review Committee of the College of Nursing, Montana State University–Bozeman, I collected data using focused semistructured interviews. After I collected demographic information from the study participants, I asked broad general questions followed by prompts pertaining to the scope of their practice and experience. Examples of the questions included: "Tell me what you do," "Describe a typical work day," "Tell me about the people you care for," "To whom are you responsible?" and "If you had complete control of your job, what would you change?" The interview ended by quoting Scharff's (1998) definition of rural nursing: "a special variety of nursing in which the nurse must have a wide range of advanced knowledge and ability, in combination with commitment, to practice proficiently in multiple clinical areas simultaneously along the career trajectory" (p. 37).

I then asked the participants whether they saw themselves fitting the definition. I audio taped and transcribed interviews for analysis.

Data Analysis

I summarized and categorized demographic information by the community-based practice represented—home health, public health, and tribal nurse. I categorized and organized into tables the percentage of time spent and the job responsibilities verbalized by the participants. Then, I performed content analysis of the data (Mayring, 2000) in two stages. In the first stage, I coded all data systematically for emergent categories (inductive coding). I used open coding to find tentative categories and their properties. In the second stage (deductive coding), I used the codes (intersections, dimension, core, and boundary) derived by Scharff (1987) from the 1980 American Nurses Association (ANA) Social Policy Statement to categorize the data pertaining to the interviewed nurses' practice. As the deductive coding progressed, particularly for the dimension of nursing, the similarities and differences between the three categories of nursing represented in the sample became evident.

RESULTS

I present the study findings in three sections. First, I report the percentage of time nurses spent in general job responsibilities. Then, I describe community-based nursing using Scharff's (1998) scope of nursing codes derived from the 1980 ANA Social Policy Statement. That description includes a comparison of the community-based nursing responsibilities between and among the three types of community-based nurses represented in the sample. Finally, I present the continuum of autonomy, job variety, and job satisfaction that emerged from the inductive content analysis process.

Nursing Job Responsibilities

Table 17.1 shows the percentage of time spent in general nursing job responsibilities. The majority of the nurses' time was spent with client contact (range = 15%–50%) and paperwork (range = 8%–50%). The nurses, whether home health, tribal, or public health, had unique ways of dividing their time; no clear-cut differences in their use of time could be seen between the three categories of nurses. Driving took up a considerable amount of work time for most of the nurses in the sample (range = 2%–30%).

Table 17.1

PERCENTAGE OF TIME SPENT ON GENERAL JOB RESPONSIBILITIES

JOB RESPONSIBILITY	HHN#1	HHN#2	HHN#3	Tribal RN	PHN#1	PHN#2	PHN#3
Client contact	50	30	15	50	35	50	45
Paperwork	10–20	50	33	8	15	15	40
Driving	10–20	10	6	30	25	2	5
Meetings	<5	2	15	10	10	5	5
Phone calls	10	10	12	2	10	5	2
Computer	10	2	0	0	5	5	0
Other							
Public relations	5						
In-services, public relations				19			
Continuing nurse education							3

Note: HHN = home health nurse; PHN = public health nurse; RN = registered nurse.

Intersections

The intersections of nursing are points where nursing meets, interfaces, and extends its practice into other areas of other professions. The interview data revealed that rural community-based nursing practice intersects or subsumes the practice of several other professions. One nurse said, "You get so used to doing different things that you may do more in the scope of another discipline than you realize."

In home health nursing the greatest overlap was with mental health and the social work issues of finances and insurance coverage. In public health nursing the greatest overlap with other allied health areas was with nutrition and social work.

Dimensions

The dimensions of nursing are the roles, responsibilities, and skills that nurses use in practice. The dimensions of nursing provided further description of the scope of nursing. The nurses' philosophy, ethics, and authority influenced these dimensions.

The practice of the rural community-based nursing distinguished itself in terms of the wide variety of roles within each practice and between types of practice as shown in Table 17.2. Most of the listed nursing responsibilities are self-explanatory except for "gap-filling."

Table 17.2

RESPONSIBILITIES OF COMMUNITY-BASED NURSES

RESPONSIBILITIES	HHN ($n = 3$)	PHN ($n = 3$)	TRIBAL NURSE
Administration	3/3	3/3	yes
Allied health tasks	3/3	3/3	yes
Assessment	3/3	3/3	yes
Continuing education	3/3	3/3	yes
Coordination of care	3/3	3/3	yes
Family planning	0/3	2/3	yes
Gap-filling	0/3	3/3	yes
Head Start[a]	0/3	3/3	yes
Home visits	3/3	2/3	yes
Hospice	3/3	0/3	yes
Immunizations	0/3	3/3	yes
Maternal/child health	0/3	3/3	yes
On call	3/3	0/3	yes
Patient education	3/3	3/3	yes
Prison	0/3	1/3	yes
Reimbursement[b]	3/3	1/3	no
Satellite clinics	0/3	2/3	yes
School nursing	0/3	3/3	yes
Staff supervision	3/3	1/3	yes
Travel to > 1 county	3/3	3/3	no
Well-child care	0/3	3/3	no
WIC nutrition program	0/3	3/3	no

Note: HHN = home health nurse; PHN = public health nurse; WIC = Women-Infant-Children. Data for HHN and PHN represent ratio of nurses with responsibility to the total number of nurses.
[a]Head Start Developmental and Health Screening.
[b]Reimbursement responsibilities included (1) ensuring services and supplies were covered by insurance, and (2) grant paperwork.

Reported by the PHNs and the tribal nurse, gap-filling means adding services based on the needs of individuals and agencies in the community. For example, if the local hospital stopped teaching prenatal classes, the PHNs would start childbirth classes.

In analyzing the interview data, the similarities and differences between and among the study participants became evident. The following paragraphs describe the contrast.

Similarities Among HHNs

As the HHN served mostly older clients, all were concerned with cuts in Medicare reimbursement for home health care especially for clients who lived long driving distances from the home health office. They reported spending long hours completing Outcome and Assessment Information Set (OASIS) forms (Center for Health Services and Policy Research, 1998) and other paperwork.

Differences Among HHNs

Two HHNs were in combined administrative and staff positions. One HHN did not have a hospice program in the counties where she worked. She thought her cancer patients did not get the number of visits they required because of Medicare reimbursement issues. She reported making unpaid visits to these clients; she ultimately quit her home health job because of this issue.

Similarities Among PHNs

The three PHNs conducted similar mandated programs, such as the Women-Infant-Children Nutrition Program (WIC), well-child clinics, immunizations, maternal/child health programs, and Head Start developmental and health screening. They were responsible for the nursing administration tasks of their offices. They kept records of the services provided to justify funding of programs. Often the paperwork required to justify a program took more time than the actual program itself.

Differences Among PHNs

One PHN primarily provided school nursing for her county, did not deliver elder programs, and did very little maternal/child health. The other two PHNs completed home visits for clients who did not meet home health agency guidelines and traveled to satellite clinics. One PHN set up medications for the prison inmates in her county.

Tribal Nurse—Both a PHN and an HHN

The tribal nurse carried out PHN programs, such as immunizations and maternal/child health, but did not do well-child clinics or WIC. In addition, she undertook school nurse responsibilities for an outlying school on the reservation. In conjunction with the county home health office, the tribal nurse participated in home visits and hospice nursing.

Core

The core of nursing deals with human responses to health or illness issues. Based on the rural nursing theory work, nurses in the rural setting keep in mind that often the clients' view of health is the ability to work, to be productive, and to do usual tasks (Long & Weinert, 1989). HHNs reported that typically clients waited too long before getting hospice or home care, whereas, PHNs frequently encountered clients too proud to use public health services.

Boundary

The boundary of rural community-based nursing is a combination of the intersections, dimensions, and core of nursing. As with rural hospital nursing, rural community-based nurses' boundaries of practice changed continually as the nurses moved between nursing activities, as the following accounts from two different nurses portray.

> I walked in the office at 7 a.m. and the phone was ringing off the hook. My client 50 miles away pulled out his central intravenous line. The closest ambulance couldn't make it to his place because it was broken down. I called the ambulance here but I beat them out there and applied pressure until they got there. When I got back, a client 30 miles away in another direction was having cardiac problems. I went out there and had to call the ambulance because he was in third degree heart block. And cell phones don't work out here so I can't get things done while I'm driving.

> On my way to work, I was flagged down and informed that someone had been sick all night. I haven't got a telephone in the car because cell phones don't work out here. That client needed to go to the emergency room. I always follow up and go to the emergency room with a client. You're always breaking rules. So you have to have good common sense on when to break the rules. Then there was a sick baby somewhere where the child had a positive blood culture and they want me to find the baby so the parents can bring the child in. Then I got a report on children somebody was neglecting. I got an anonymous call to check on them because they were left alone. So I had to go out and check if they were left alone and then call social services. Our social service department is overwhelmed. If there is medical neglect, the public health nurses deal with that too. Then a school called to say that five kids have head lice. They're brought to my office and we treat the head lice and contact the parents and educate the parents on the treatment of head lice. Then the clinic called me to say there's a lady in

labor and she's 17 and she's scared, can you come over and give her a crash course on some breathing exercises? How can you say no? So you throw down all your paperwork and run over to the clinic and start demonstrating the blowing and puffing. It's just too wild sometimes. You have to be very flexible.

Fit of *Rural Nurse Generalist* Definition

When asked whether they fit the *rural nurse generalist* definition provided by Scharff (1998), these community health nurses all agreed they did. Two responses are shared below:

> Yes, I fit this definition but I don't consider myself to have advanced knowledge, I mean, I'm learning every day. But you have to know something of everything in order to work in a rural setting. Like peds, maternity, geriatrics, med-surg, orthopedics, dermatology. There's always something to learn.

> As a new graduate I am working towards this knowledge and ability but I have a long ways to go. I see that I need a wide range of knowledge in different areas. Being aware of other resources that are available to get the knowledge I need, I'm gradually getting to that point. I don't have all that knowledge in myself but I'm learning who I can go to. Like social work, physical therapy, occupational therapy, speech therapy. Knowing who your resources are and being aware that I don't have to be totally knowledgeable in all those areas, although it would be good to have a greater knowledge in those areas. Definitively a lot of the knowledge falls into nursing. But if someone is available with greater knowledge, I feel it is my job to refer to those people. Nursing is cool in that we have a little bit of knowledge in a lot of areas and we can do a lot of things. Sometimes a specialist can only work so many hours or only get reimbursed so much, so then it is our place to go back in and work with them and make sure they are getting followed up on adequately.

Summary

The content analysis of the interview data using Scharff's (1998) constructs demonstrated that the rural community-based nurses in the sample were generalists and did not specialize. The roles they included in their practice were flexible and expanded to meet the needs of their rural communities. Because the majority of their clients were older with acute health care needs, HHNs experienced the most similarity in tasks performed. The practice of HHNs was also more similar to rural hospital nurses than other community-based nurses. The practice of PHNs included more variety in the ages of clients served and the many different programs with which they were involved. While PHNs did home visits, HHNs reported that they were not responsible for public health programs. The tribal nurse experienced the greatest amount of variety in her practice as it included both home health and public health nursing.

CONTINUUM OF AUTONOMY AND JOB VARIETY AND SATISFACTION

The content analysis of the responsibilities of the community-based nurses and the comparison of the three differing levels of nurses resulted in a continuum based on (a) autonomy, (b) job variety, and (c) job satisfaction. *Autonomy* referred to being able to function alone and make independent decisions (Davis, 1991). *Variety* in the job was defined as the ability to be flexible in adapting to the needs of the individual and the community; not being tied to one area of nursing (Troyer, 2000, pp. 37, 47). *Job satisfaction* referred to being happy while fulfilling the job requirements (Mish, 1989, p. 646).

The seven nurses were placed on the continuum starting from left to right, from less to more job autonomy, job variety, and job satisfaction, which covaried among the participants. The continuum is depicted in Figure 17.1.

←— Less   AUTONOMY   More —→

JOB VARIETY

JOB SATISFACTION

HHNs, PHN (new graduate), PHN (newcomer), PHN (old-timer), tribal nurse

HHN = Home health nurse; PHN = Public health nurse

Figure 17.1 A continuum of autonomy, job variety, and satisfaction.

HHNs

The three HHNs experienced the least autonomy, job variety, and job satisfaction because of constraints of home health regulations and concerns regarding insurance coverage and Medicare reimbursement. Homebound status regulations limited their flexibility in providing care. A vast amount of paperwork took time away from patient care and resulted in decreased job satisfaction. An example is depicted in the following HHN interview excerpt:

> Admissions were lengthy with paperwork taking two-and-one-half hours and now it takes 4 hours to do with the OASIS form. If you transfer a patient to the hospital there's more paperwork. If they go home you have to do the OASIS all over again even if you haven't had them off services for a week yet. There's another form to do when a patient gets discharged. There's just a lot of paperwork. And starting July 1, 1999 they passed a 15 minute increment billing deal, where now you have to track all the time in the home. You don't start counting until you've been in the home 8 minutes. If there's any interruption greater than 3 minutes, you're supposed to subtract time if they're in the bathroom or on the phone or whatever. It's an asinine regulation. I think all the staff feels bogged down with paperwork requirements.

PHNs

The PHN who was a new graduate thought she had a lot of autonomy but felt uncomfortable with the lack of set priorities in her job description. She mainly focused on school nursing, immunizations, and well-child clinic work. As time progressed, she stated she was becoming more comfortable in starting new programs in the community.

A second PHN was labeled a newcomer because she was new to her community and had only recently started her public health position. Previously, she worked for a home health agency in an adjacent county and felt comfortable in seeing clients in their homes as a PHN. She and her co-PHN were developing policies and procedures for their office and had the freedom to develop programs based on the needs of the community. As a newcomer to public health nursing she felt she was still growing in the role. She stated she was very pleased with the variety and flexibility of the job and her ability to do what is needed to promote positive health outcomes in her county.

The third PHN had worked for a long time in public health and lived most of her life in her community. She reported that a few years ago, county officials tried to combine the public health and home health nursing offices. Because she did not want to learn all of the home health regulations and paperwork guidelines, she restructured her position so that it would not be combined with home health. Her restructuring plan focused on meeting the public health needs of the community. She reported feeling highly satisfied in seeing the effect of her practice on all age levels in the community. However, because she lives a long distance from a major health center, she fills gaps and serves as a safety net, providing care to clients who otherwise would not qualify for home health or other programs.

Tribal Nurse

The widest variety in roles and tasks was seen with the tribal public health and home health nurse. She structured her job to best meet the needs of the tribe she serves. She performed classic public health activities as well as coordination of home health or hospice care for tribal members. Because of the isolation, poverty, lack of home phones, and lack of cell phone coverage on the reservation, she made decisions independently, often dealing with acutely ill patients in the home. She expressed great satisfaction with nursing; she thought using flexibility and ingenuity worked to improve the lives of clients.

DISCUSSION

The community-based nurses' descriptions reflected similarities and differences to Scharff's (1998) definition of rural nurse generalist. The nurses incorporated different roles and worked in different areas of nursing within the same work day, a key characteristic of the rural generalist reported in the literature (Bigbee, 1993; Weinert & Long, 1991).

In comparing the findings for the first ANA code *intersection,* both hospital and community-based nurses met, interfaced, and extended their practice into other professional areas of practice. However, differences existed in intersection between the two groups. Hospital-based nurses overlapped with pharmacy and medicine, particularly in emergency situations, whereas the community-based nurses' overlap occurred with mental health and social work. With regard to *dimension,* the rural hospital nurses performed roles, responsibilities, and skills specific for individual patients within the hospital setting. The community-based nurses were more likely to perform a variety of roles, responsibilities, and skills that focused on the needs of individuals and groups within the community. The *core* of nursing, dealing with human responses to health or illness, was the same for rural hospital and community-based nurses. The *boundary* (combination of intersection, dimension, and core) was similar for the rural hospital and community-based nurses in that both changed their boundaries in response to the variety of clinical or health care situations experienced. The differences between the two groups were the environments in which the boundaries were changed, the hospital or the community.

The findings of this study validated those from the single community-based nurse in Davis' (1991) study of rural nursing. Davis explored the rural nurses' domains of practice; the community nurse described a broader scope of practice within the community as compared with the practice of the rural hospital nurses in Davis' sample.

The continuum of autonomy, job variety, and job satisfaction was supported by the findings of a study of job satisfaction between PHNs and HHNs in a rural midwestern state (Juhl, Dunkin, Stratton, Getler, & Ludtke, 1993). The study findings demonstrated that PHNs were more satisfied than HHNs with their task requirements. The PHNs reported more diverse role expectations, and the HHNs indicated they had considerable more documentation of tasks for reimbursement purposes.

Rural community-based nurse novices need to attain a wide variety of knowledge, to learn what resources are available, and to learn how to access these resources. Personal traits, such as enjoying variety, may lead to experiencing more satisfaction as a rural community-based nurse. Flexibility is required when alternating between working with individuals and then with groups, particularly for PHNs.

Holistic nursing practice was exemplified in the study by the numerous insights related about their clients' environmental and social situations. The holistic view was fostered by the increased opportunities for social interaction with the client and their family and friends at their home and in the rural community. Often, these community-based nurses had taken care of the family or friends of the client and had a nearly complete picture of their health situation.

NURSING IMPLICATIONS

Based on the findings of this study, the ability to work as a generalist is required in the practice of the rural community-based nurses. More needs to be done to facilitate meeting the educational needs of rural community-based nurses. The importance of the work of rural community-based nurses should be recognized and efforts made at local, state, and national levels to improve their staffing conditions. The burden of the large amount of paperwork in home health nursing needs to be addressed. Nurses need to keep aware of changes occurring in the health care system and participate in designing policy and other changes that promote adequate care for clients in the rural setting in and out of the hospital.

Rural community health nurse novices need to develop a network of resources to assist them when starting their practice. Because a baccalaureate education is considered the entry level education for community nurses, associate degree prepared nurses would benefit from continuing their academic education; spending time as a student in a rural community-based setting with an experienced community-based nurse would be beneficial (Ide, 1992).

Limitations of this study were its small sample size and the possibility of regional bias. These findings cannot be generalized to other rural community-based nurses; however, the implications may be applicable if community nurses are employed in similar working circumstances in sparsely populated areas.

RECOMMENDATIONS

Replication of this study in other areas of Montana and similar sparsely populated areas is recommended. Replication is needed that compares larger samples of home health, public health, and tribal nurses. Further research is needed to verify or refute the concepts presented in the continuum of autonomy, job variety, and job satisfaction.

Further research needs to be done on the financial and regulatory constraints on the delivery of home health services in rural settings and how these affect job satisfaction of HHNs in other regions. Many home health agencies are closing in the region of Montana where this sample of nurses was employed largely because of changes in Medicare reimbursement occurring since 1997. The consequences of this decrease in services to clients and their community needs to be examined. The practice of PHNs filling the gap when home health offices close in these areas and other locations warrants further study.

REFERENCES

American Nurses Association (ANA). (1980). *Nursing: A social policy statement* (No. NP-63 20M 9/82R). Kansas City, MO: Author.

Bigbee, J. L. (1993). The uniqueness of rural nursing. *Nursing Clinics of North America, 28* (1), 131–144.

Center for Health Services and Policy Research. (1998). *Outcome and Assessment Information Set (OASIS)*. Denver: Author. Retrieved August 14, 2004, from http://www.hcfa.gov

Davis, D. J. (1991). *A study of rural nursing: Domains of practice-characteristics of excellence*. Unpublished master's thesis, University of Nevada, Reno.

Dunkin, J., Stratton, T., Movassaghi, H., & Kindig, D. (1994). Characteristics of metropolitan and non-metropolitan community health nurses. *Texas Journal of Rural Health, 7*, 18–27.

Ide, B. A. (1992). A process model of rural nursing practice. *Texas Journal of Rural Health, 9*, 18–27.

Juhl, N., Dunkin, J. W., Stratton, T., Getler, J., & Ludtke, R. (1993). Job satisfaction of rural public and home health nurses. *Public Health Nursing, 10*, 42–47.

Long, K. A., & Weinert, C. (1989). Rural nursing: Developing the theory base. *Scholarly Inquiry for Nursing Practice: An International Journal, 3*, 113–127.

Mayring, P. (2000, June). Qualitative content analysis. Forum: *Qualitative Social Research, 2*. Retrieved October 7, 2004, from http://www.qualitative-research.net/fqs-texte/2–00/200mayring-e.htm

Mish, F. C. (Ed.). (1989). *The New Merriam-Webster Dictionary*. Springfield, MA: Merriam-Webster.

Scharff, J. (1987). *The nature and scope of rural nursing: Distinctive characteristics*. Unpublished master's thesis, Montana State University, Bozeman.

Scharff, J. (1998). The distinctive nature and scope of rural nursing practice: Philosophical bases. In H. J. Lee (Ed.), *Conceptual basis for rural nursing* (pp. 19–38). New York: Springer.

Stratton, T. D., Dunkin, J. W., Juhl, N., & Geller, J. M. (1995). Retainment incentives in three rural practice settings: Variations in job satisfaction among staff registered nurses. *Applied Nursing Research, 8* (3), 73–80.

Troyer, L. E. (2000). *Rural generalist: Community-based nursing*. Unpublished master's thesis, Montana State University, Bozeman.

Weinert, C., & Long, K. A. (1991). The theory and research base for rural nursing practice. In A. Bushy (Ed.), *Rural nursing* (Vol. 1, pp. 21–38). Newbury Park, CA: Sage.

18 Men Working as Rural Nurses: Land of Opportunity

CHAD O'LYNN

A growing body of literature suggests that rural residency is associated with poorer health outcomes than urban residence (Center on an Aging Society, 2003; Goins & Mitchell, 1999; Kumar, Acanfora, Hennessy, & Kalache, 2001; National Institute of Nursing Research [NINR], 1995). The suggested reasons for this disparity generally relate to barriers of access to health services because of distance and lack of available providers in rural areas. One strategy to address the health disparities in rural settings is to recruit and to retain and then to support health care providers, including nurses. However, amidst the rural health literature, relatively little has been published describing the experiences of nurses who care for rural dwellers.

This gap in the literature is significant, in that recruitment and retention of nurses in rural practice is challenging and more difficult than in urban practice because of rural wages, paucity of jobs for spouses, and the negative perceptions of rural nursing (Bushy, 2002; Hopkins & Domrose, 2001; Long, 2000; Trossman, 2001; Vukic & Keddy, 2002). This challenge serves as an overlay for an already well-documented nationwide nursing shortage. To meet projected vacancies, the profession has begun to implement general recruitment strategies targeting groups such as ethnic minorities and men (Buerhaus, Staiger, & Auerbach, 2000; Gordon, 2002). Increasing the number of men in the nursing profession will assist in meeting the demands for future nurses and in improving the diversity of the nursing workforce (American Association of Colleges of Nursing [AACN], 1997, 2001; Anders, 1993; Davis & Bartfay, 2001; Sullivan, 2000; Villeneuve, 1994). However, virtually nothing is known about the experiences of men in rural nursing and the recruitment strategies that might be appropriate to attract men to practice in rural settings.

Because men only comprised 5.4% of the U.S. registered nurse (RN) workforce in 2000, one may assume that there is opportunity for increased recruitment (Spratley, Johnson, Sochalski, Fritz, & Spencer, 2001). However, there is some suspicion that men leave nursing shortly after entering the profession at higher rates than do women (Davis & Bartfay, 2001). The reason for this is unclear. O'Lynn (2004) noted that men in nursing felt that their basic nursing education program did not prepare them well for working primarily with women coworkers.

To recruit and retain men into rural nursing practice, a better understanding of rural nursing from the masculine perspective is needed. This understanding will assist in the development of gender-appropriate strategies to recruit men to critical shortage areas, as well as assist in the development of gender-appropriate supports to retain men in rural nursing. My purpose in this study was to examine the experiences and perspectives of men working as rural nurses. I asked two research questions: What are the experiences of men working as rural nurses? What would be appropriate strategies to recruit and retain men in rural nursing practice?

BACKGROUND AND SIGNIFIGANCE

Limitations of the Literature on Rural Male Nurses

Houde (2002) and Thompson (2002) report that invisibility of men occurs when researchers do not include men in study samples or when data generated from men are folded into the data generated by a majority of women. Most studies noted in this book do not include men. As such, the findings from these studies have questionable generalizability to men working or considering working in rural nursing. No study located for review described rural nursing practice from a male perspective. In the current study, I addressed this gap by providing an initial understanding of the experiences of men in rural nursing practice and how men may be recruited and retained to work in rural communities.

Significance

The implications of the invisibility of men in the nursing literature are profound. A review of literature by O'Lynn (2004) showed that men experience nursing education and nursing practice differently than women do. These differences stem from a variety of reasons, including historical discrimination of men in nursing, differing gender roles, and different approaches to caregiving. If men are to be recruited and retained in rural practice settings, strategies developed from the current understanding of rural nursing practice may not be gender appropriate.

METHODS

I used the hermeneutic phenomenology in the Heideggerian tradition for this study. According to Koch (1995) and Benner (1999), hermeneutic phenomenology assumes a constructivist reality, in which people encounter phenomena with uniquely individualized preunderstanding and historical knowledge that cannot be stripped away. Phenomena are experienced and understood in a highly contextualized and interpreted world. Consequently, reality is not absolute and cannot be reduced to essential truths, although individuals may have many similar experiences (Koch, 1995; Lincoln & Guba, 2000). From an epistemological perspective, hermeneutic phenomenology assumes that knowledge is cocreated among individuals. The researcher cannot be an objective observer, but rather serves as a vehicle through which understanding occurs from transactions with others and existing world contexts can only be corrected and modified (Benner). Hermeneutic phenomenology is a research approach appropriate for exploration of poorly understood phenomena and the meaning they hold for persons.

Procedure

I used open-ended interviews with six men working as RNs in frontier communities in Montana. Inclusion criteria for participation were (a) RN licensure in Montana, (b) employment in a frontier county and a community of less than 5,000 residents, and (c) the ability to speak English. I obtained informed consent from all participants. The Human Subjects Committee of Montana State University–Bozeman and the Institutional Review Board of Oregon Health & Science University approved this study. I completed the study as partial requirement for research practicum credit at Oregon Health & Science University.

I recruited a purposive sample of participants from a list of all RNs licensed in Montana supplied by the State Board of Nursing. This list provided only the names and residential addresses of the nurses. It provided no indication of the nurse's sex, ethnicity, or race. I examined the list for names of nurses believed to be male residing in frontier counties. If more than one nurse resided in a community, one name was highlighted for enrollment. The rationale for this procedure was to ensure maximum representation of rural communities in the sample. From the screening of the list, I identified 30 potential participants and sent letters in the spring of 2004 inviting them to participate. Seven letters were returned stamped "No longer at this address/No forwarding address." Of the 21 remaining potential participants, seven agreed to participate. However, one withdrew from the study prior to his interview.

The six men in the sample were Caucasian. The men's age ranged was 34–58 years (m = 40.7 years). Their years of experience as a nurse was less than 1 to 30 years (m = 11.4 years). All had some nursing experience in an urban setting at some point during their careers. The range of time spent working as rural nurses was less than 1 to 20 years (m = 7.7 years). Five worked in rural hospitals as staff nurses. The sixth worked as a nurse practitioner in a primary care clinic. Nursing was a second career for all of the participants.

The size range of communities in which the men worked was 940–2,874 residents (m = 1,668; U.S. Bureau of the Census, 2002). Two of the six communities were located on or near Indian reservations. The major economic activity of five of the communities was ranching and farming. One community relied on tourism, as it was located near a national park.

Two participants lived in the communities in which they worked. The other four participants commuted 340, 129, 53, and 35 miles one-way to the agencies where they worked. The participants working in hospitals not in their communities grouped their shifts, staying in town either at the hospital or in a motel and returning home during their off days. One participant had been doing this for 20 years.

The hospitals in which five participants worked were designated critical access hospitals (CAHs) with a range in beds of 4–15. All had long-term care facilities either attached to the hospital or located next door. None of the participants worked as staff nurses in these long-term care facilities at the time of the interviews. All hospitals were served by volunteer ambulance services. As such, local ambulance availability was not guaranteed on a 24-hour basis. Participants noted that it was not uncommon for patients to present to the emergency department (ED) who had transported themselves or were transported by family or friends or by the local sheriff. The nearest emergency services from these hospitals were located 23 to 65 miles away (m = 37 miles). However, the hospital located 23 miles from another emergency facility was accessible only by secondary roads, with a usual driving time of 45 minutes in the best of weather. All hospitals had access to helicopter transport to a regional medical center. Although some had improved heliport pads nearby, one helicopter service was seven miles away. However, if needed, there was a grassy area next to the hospital upon which a helicopter could land in good weather. For the helicopter to land safely, the participant needed to ensure that the area was clear of debris and turn on the outdoor lights if it was dark.

Data Collection and Data Analysis

I conducted interviews over the telephone at a time and date selected by the participants that lasted 45 to 100 minutes in length. Consistent with phenomenological methods, I used loosely structured interview questions, which allowed for free discussion of topics in which the participant or I deemed relevant. I asked some general (grand-tour) questions of all the participants to obtain information on rural nursing, gender, and recruitment. These questions included: (a) What is rural nursing? (b) What is your typical work day like? (c) What is it like being a man working in rural nursing? (d) Why do you work in a rural area? and (e) What would attract men to work as rural nurses?

I audio taped all interviews, and then transcribed them. I analyzed transcripts sequentially as each interview occurred. I read transcripts in total to gain a general perspective. I then analyzed each transcript section-by-section for codes. I used direct quotes when possible for codes to represent the participants' responses. I then organized codes into categories that represented emerging themes. I compared categories and themes from each transcript to each other to determine similarities and differences among the transcripts.

After I completed and analyzed interviews with four participants, I noted a redundancy in themes. However, the transcript of one participant, the nurse practitioner, included details of his duties and work day that were very different from the other transcripts. These differences were most likely reflective of the fundamental differences between the nurse practitioner and the staff nurse role. On the other hand, his discussion of other aspects of rural living and his rural clientele generated findings similar to the transcripts of the rural staff nurse participants. Because of this, I decided to include the transcript but did not pursue further exploration of the practice characteristics of rural advanced practice nurses.

After I conducted the first four interviews, I gave copies of the uncoded transcripts to two experienced rural nurse researchers and a graduate student who resided in a rural community. These peer auditors, working independently, examined these interviews for categories. They contrasted categories with the categories from the original data analysis. Although there were slight differences in the wording of the categories, the meaning of the categories were similar.

With redundancy in the transcripts and similarity in the categories derived from the peer auditors, I enrolled two additional rural hospital staff nurses and interviewed them to seek saturation of the themes. The findings were consistent with the previous findings and I did not conduct any more interviews.

RESULTS

Generally, the participants painted a very positive view of rural nursing and the rural environments in which they worked. For the men who were seasoned nurses, all were happy with rural nursing and had no plans for relocation. The men who were relatively new to rural nursing demonstrated a general excitement and enthusiasm with the characteristics and challenges of rural nursing practice. Although opportunities did not appear in the transcripts, it was an overarching theme. The term reflected the positive accounts provided by the participants and may reflect the desired perspective of a potential nurse recruiter looking to fill vacant nursing positions in rural communities. The specific themes of opportunities include (a) expanded practice, (b) autonomy, (c) meaningful relationships, (d) challenge, (e) rural rewards, and (f) recruitment.

Opportunity for Expanded Practice

All men described rural nursing as generalist practice that extended beyond the typical generalist practice employed by float or resource pool nurses in larger facilities. Typically, in larger hospitals, nurses who work on multiple units develop generalist skills for select patient populations. Rarely do nurses working in a larger hospital care for all the types of patients seen in that hospital. In rural nursing, the men stated that they take care of pediatrics to geriatrics, emergency care to long-term care, all within the same shift, every shift. The term *jack-of-all-trades* was used by several of the participants. One participant described his typical shift this way:

> Well, I guess a good example would be not too long ago, we had a serious motor vehicle accident involving a motorcyclist that we were stabilizing and trying to transport elsewhere. At the same time, we had a mom and a newborn baby . . . postpartum patient, and then with all that, we had an ambulance call with an 89-year old patient who had respiratory distress who died on us that night. . . . In the meantime, we had two or three patients down the hall, one was on a cardiac monitor, while another was just . . . I don't remember what the other one was, but you know, it's every night, you can see everything all in one night.

Four participants stated they were the only RN on duty, accompanied by a nurse's aide. As such, they completed all skilled procedures and care coordination for all of the patients present during their shifts.

In addition to the expanded patient population of the rural nurse, all participants described the expanded role of the rural nurse. The specific duties of each of the participants varied depending upon his workplace, but all discussed the completion of roles typically done by ancillary staff in larger hospitals. These roles included emergency department assistant, respiratory therapist, ward clerk, billing clerk, phlebotomist, electrocardiograph technician, security officer, central supply clerk, pharmacy technician, community educator, social worker, and ambulance personnel. The men noted that as the nurse on duty, they were the "only game in town." One participant described the time-consuming task of taking inventory of all medications and treatments provided to a patient during the previous 24-hour period for billing purposes. Another participant indicated that the RN also served as the hospital's security officer. Another participant provided the following description:

> Of course, in that facility, we do all the paperwork. We do the patient charts, we write out the lab slips. Sometimes if lab's not there, we go ahead and do the blood draw[.] . . . We basically do all the ward clerk duties. We do

all the transfer paperwork. We dispense medications from what we call the pharmacy. We don't have a pharmacy. . . . Well, actually, we have the hospital pharmacy, but we're it as far as dispensing and keeping track of what we have and what needs ordering and that kind of stuff. Of course, there's a lot of paperwork there involved in tracking, you know, what medication is going to what patient and that kind of thing. . . . We copy paperwork. We make sure we have insurance information. We do all the HIPPA privacy paperwork, you know, I mean we'll cook the meals if need be. We pretty much are there to do whatever needs doing.

The men discussed a blending of the roles noted earlier, but in particular, the blending of roles between medicine and nursing. This blending occurred most frequently in the ED and involved tasks such as initiating treatments and diagnostic work while waiting for the physician to arrive. However, all participants noted that they were practicing within their scope of practice as defined by the State of Montana.

Despite the seemingly overwhelming burden patient diversity and expanded roles might create, participants noted the benefits (and hence, opportunities) of these characteristics of rural nursing. One participant stated that working in a rural hospital was "less frustrating" than a larger hospital because he did not have to wait on other health care personnel to come and do their task for a patient before he could move forward with nursing care. "Instead," stated another participant, "you just do it yourself." Several participants described the expanded roles as a way to become more involved with their patients, and thus, become more knowledgeable about their individual care needs. They indicated that nurses might treat a patient in the ED, admit that patient to a hospital bed, take comprehensive and holistic care of that patient for several days, then work with that patient as they transition to a swing bed or are discharged to the community. The participants criticized the care received by patients in larger hospitals as being disjointed and poorly coordinated, because patients receive care by numerous providers and disciplines as they progress through a hospital stay. As such, the participants felt that the patients in rural hospitals receive more personalized care.

Opportunity for Autonomy

All participants described the increased level of autonomy enjoyed by rural nurses compared with their nonrural colleagues. Several of the men specifically used the term *autonomy*, whereas others used the terms *independence, having more leeway,* or *freer to make decisions.* One participant noted that rural nursing is a "self-driven practice." All described increased autonomy as a benefit of rural nursing practice.

Autonomy was categorized in two ways: (a) greater freedom to make decisions affecting patient care, and (b) greater freedom to use one's own work routines. The participants described using nursing judgment in revising an individual patient's plan of care more freely than they had experienced while working in larger hospitals. Several noted that rural nurses are able to request needed supplies, initiate protocols, or deliver necessary treatments that were once commonplace in nursing practice, but are now becoming increasingly dependent upon the decisions of other professionals (e.g., respiratory therapist required to initiate incentive spirometry). The greater autonomy described by the participants suggests greater integrity of the domains of collaborative and independent nursing practice, whereas the trend in larger hospitals may be increasing the domain of dependent nursing practice.

Some participants described the freedom to set one's own schedule and routines on any given shift as a positive experience. Because they usually worked with only one other individual, how and when specific tasks were to be accomplished during a shift was negotiated. The freedom to set work routines was not only desirable, but also necessary to provide the flexibility for unpredicted ED visits and patient admissions. On hospital units with more staff, an individual nurse has much less freedom for establishing routines, as these types of decisions will impact a larger group of workers and may conflict with preestablished unit routines and cultures. It is interesting that with a perceived increased level of autonomy, none of the participants noted autonomy-based conflicts with coworkers. Instead, the participants described how staff worked together better than in larger hospitals, hence, described relationships that are more meaningful with coworkers.

Opportunity for Meaningful Relationships

All participants described at length the improved ability to develop and maintain positive and meaningful relationships in rural practice settings with coworkers, clients, and the community. With coworkers, the men described the higher level of teamwork than they had experienced in urban settings. One participant noted,

> Basically, the biggest thing I found with rural nursing is the teamwork. When I worked in [urban setting] for so many doctors, you never really got to know any of them. I mean, there were some that were easier to work with than others, but you didn't get to know them very well. And in a rural community, your doctors and nurses really work together as a team. They have to because there are only so many of you.

This teamwork not only included nurses and physicians, but all health care workers. Several participants praised the nurse's aides with whom they worked. Because they were sometimes busy in the ED, participants relied upon their aides to "keep an eye on the other patients" for them. They noted the skill and dedication of their aides. The reliance upon and admiration for their aides led to a higher level of trust than they had experienced with the aides with whom they had worked in larger hospitals.

Because there were fewer employees and more frequent contact with other employees, participants stated that they really "got to know" the people with whom they worked. Teamwork was demonstrated by everyone "pitching in and helping out" and doing whatever it takes to "get the job done." As one participant explained,

> If we have something major going on, generally the ambulance crew is there to help. They can do CPR, help start IVs. Usually if it's something major, when the ambulance crew brings them in, they will stay and help.

All participants had access to an on-call nurse or nurse at the nursing home that they could call for assistance. Also, physicians and physician assistants were able to get to the hospital in a very short period of time when needed. This readiness to help each other was such that none of the participants felt isolated when working at the hospital.

Participants commented on how patient the staff and physicians were when asked questions and how willing they were to teach. This milieu facilitated teamwork and collaboration, maintained trust among the staff, created a climate of mutual respect, and enhanced camaraderie. Moreover, although two participants noted there were occasional conflicts ("everyone is human"), none reported troubled relationships with coworkers that eroded teamwork.

Another benefit of working in a rural practice is direct access to management. Small numbers of staff in the hospitals meant few, if any, layers of middle management that separated frontline workers from hospital administration. One participant sat on the hospital's foundation board;

he stated he was able to bring representation directly from the patient care staff to hospital decision makers. Such access can translate into beneficial power that directly affects the nurses' work environments.

All participants talked about meaningful relationships with their patients and with the communities in which they worked. Relationships with patients and communities have been described as inherently different from those in urban settings because of the lack of anonymity many rural health care providers experience (Lee, 1998). Lack of anonymity makes it difficult for rural health care providers to maintain professional role boundaries (Lee; Scharff, 1998). However, all participants in this study described familiarity with their patients as a benefit and improved their ability to provide quality care. One participant stated,

> Generally, patients coming in . . . if they recognize somebody, if they know somebody, then they are more confident. They feel more comfortable, you know, and more confident in the care. I don't know how many times that I've had people say that. They come into the ER or they're patients in the hospital and they go, "Oh, it's so nice to see someone I recognize." You know, but it's actually a real benefit for the patients.

Rural nurses "treat generations of families." For example, a woman may be admitted to the hospital. One month later, her son may come to the ED with an injury. Several months later, a grandmother is admitted, and so on. Because of the small population, each rural nurse can affect a relatively large percentage of the community, and, unlike urban settings where nurses may never see their patients again, in rural areas a nurse may encounter former patients several times a week at the store, a high school sporting event, and so forth. Participants did not seem burdened by off-duty contacts from the community.

Several participants remarked how supportive the community was of the hospital. Examples of the support included voluntarily raising taxes to support the local hospital, holding fundraisers to purchase an up-to-date ambulance, stopping by to visit patients and cheer them up, and volunteering a few hours to "do anything that we might need help getting done."

Opportunities for Challenge

All participants remarked that rural nursing was challenging. One stated, "The first eight months were tough. . . . REALLY tough." Most challenges stemmed from the realities of working with an expanded patient population and in an expanded practice role. In addition, the increased accountability required by working in multiple roles created additional challenges that the men felt were not as pronounced in nonrural practice settings. Such challenges require that rural nurses be flexible, have excellent triage and prioritization skills, and have broad-based nursing knowledge supplemented by emergency, critical care, and trauma certifications. Preparation for the unexpected was seen as crucial by the participants. One noted, "You don't see a lot of everything, but you see a little bit of everything a lot."

However, despite the challenges of rural nursing, all participants expressed a sense of pride in their accomplishments and their skills. One noted that when urban nurses come to a rural setting, they are amazed at the talent and versatility of rural nurses. Another who was new to nursing commented on how much better trained and skilled he was than his former classmates who were working in highly specialized urban practices. Another noted that because of his skill set and experience, he could go "just about anywhere" and be an asset to a potential employer.

Another challenge mentioned by the participants was maintaining confidentiality. As stated previously, some community members are actively involved in hospital activities. In addition, one participant commented that the stereotypes of small towns as "everyone knowing everyone's business" and "there are no secrets in a small town" are true. However, maintaining patient confidentiality was not particularly difficult, as long as nurses stayed vigilant. One participant stated, "You just know that you don't talk about certain things. If someone is persistent in finding out information, you just say 'I'm sorry, I can't share that information.'"

Opportunities for Rural Rewards

I asked each participant why he chose to work in a rural practice. Some commented on the ability to gain diverse nursing experiences, and two reported financial incentives. The nurse practitioner reported receiving a higher salary from the Public Health Service for working in an underserved rural area. The participant just out of nursing school discussed a federally funded loan repayment program available to him for agreeing to work in a critical (rural) shortage area. In addition, all commented on the beneficial aspects of a rural lifestyle. These aspects included picturesque surroundings, less stressful lifestyle, lower crime rate, and friendly people in the rural communities. However, most important were the close proximity to outdoor activities, such as hunting and fishing, and the family-friendly environments of the rural communities. One participant commented,

> Basically, the lifestyle in the small community is more conducive to family. Schools are closer. You have more involvement with the children in school. You can take the kids to the park, or they can go out on their own to the park and play. . . . So you don't have as much concern in a small town. The kids have much more freedom . . . a better way to grow up.

Gender and the Opportunities for Recruitment

Participants did not feel that nursing practice differed between male and female rural nurses. In addition, all felt well received and respected by their employers and their local communities. One participant said, "They told me they were excited to have a male nurse." Men provide physical strength and were able to provide balance to an all-female nursing staff. One participant felt he was able to confront belligerent males in the ED better than his female coworkers. He stated,

> I think that in the emergency room . . . sometimes just seeing a male quiets them down a little bit. They don't act quite as offensive. . . . [Although] some of the [female] nurses are pretty tough, some of them will get a little intimidated and walk out and ask me to take care of the patient or ask me to help settle them down.

Other participants stated that their experience with team sports provided a sound foundation for the teamwork necessary for effective rural practice.

All participants felt that rural nursing would be attractive for men. When I asked them about recruitment strategies, the participants stated that autonomy and diversity of experiences are particularly attractive for men. Two noted that, in their experience, men tend to like emergency and trauma nursing and believed that rural nursing would routinely provide these experiences. However, a number of participants pointed out that salaries are lower in rural areas than in urban areas and believed that rural hospitals need to be competitive with larger hospitals to attract men to rural practice.

DISCUSSIONS AND IMPLICATIONS

The findings from the current study support those of other studies describing rural nursing practice that primarily used the perspectives of female samples. In particular, the current study found similar descriptions of increased autonomy, collaboration, role expansion, patient diversity, challenges, and lack of anonymity as characteristics of rural nursing practice. Consistent with other studies, the men in this study also reported the need for flexibility, extensive generalist knowledge, emergency and trauma certifications, and a "can-do" attitude to be effective in rural nursing. Not found in the current study was the theme insider or outsider. Generally, the men were well received as they came to work in their rural communities.

The study provides new insight on the positive aspects of rural nursing practice (Hegney, McCarthey, Rogers-Clark, & Gorman, 2002; Rosenthal, 1996; Scharff, 1998). The men described potentially negative aspects of rural nursing, such as lack of anonymity and the diversity of patients, as benefits and attractions to rural nursing. The positive depiction of rural nursing provided by the men supports the term *opportunity* as a connecting theme. The participants in the current study took pride in their accomplishments at meeting the challenges of rural nursing and felt that their experiences in rural nursing made them better nurses overall.

In terms of recruitment, the findings are somewhat different from those noted by Australian researchers (Hegney et al., 2002). In both studies, factors that attracted and retained nurses to rural practice focused on the positive aspects of a rural lifestyle (Hegney et al. did not include outdoor recreation) and on positive relationships rural nurses have with coworkers and members of the community. However, the Australian study did not include the diversity of experiences offered in rural nursing—the increased autonomy available to rural nurses, the challenges of rural nursing practice, or the pride felt in meeting those challenges as attractions to rural nursing. Also, the Australian study identified the emotional and physical demands of rural nursing as key factors in causing nurses to leave rural nursing. The men in the current study did not mention emotional or physical demands as part of their practice. In fact, several indicated their physical strength was of benefit in the practice setting. The only negative aspect of rural nursing mentioned by the current study participants that might dissuade someone from rural nursing practice are the lower wages offered by most employers.

According to participants in the current study, nurse recruiters hoping to fill vacancies in rural settings by accessing the under-tapped male nurse labor pool should highlight the following in their marketing strategies: (a) increased autonomy; (b) increased opportunity for diverse patient experiences including emergency and trauma nursing; (c) more meaningful relationships with coworkers, patients, and the community; and (d) the outdoor recreation and family-friendly environments.

LIMITATIONS AND RECOMMENDATIONS FOR FURTHER RESEARCH

The sample size of the study was small. However, consistent with phenomenology, sample sizes are generally small, but data are rich from lengthy interviews (Creswell, 1998; Patton, 2002). Because I obtained saturation of the themes in the study, expanding the sample size may not have contributed additional themes. Consistent with qualitative studies, findings from this study cannot be generalized to rural nursing populations (Creswell; Patton). Yet, because the findings of this study are consistent with the findings of other qualitative studies of rural nursing practice, the findings may have high transferability to other nurses working in rural hospitals.

Another limitation is self-selection of the participants. It is possible that men working as rural nurses who had very different perspectives chose not to participate in the study. In addition, all of the participants are Caucasian. It is unclear how many male nurses of ethnic minority background are working in rural Montana communities because the State Board of Nursing did not provide this information with its list of RNs. However, there was some diversity within the sample in terms of years of nursing and rural nursing experience and of the types of communities in which they worked. Further research is needed to understand the experiences of men in other rural locations and practice settings, particularly in long-term care and in advanced practice, and men of other ethnic backgrounds.

CONCLUSION

My purpose in the current study was to examine the experiences and perspectives of men working as rural nurses. The findings indicate that men find rural nursing practice a very positive experience that can be described as a land of opportunities. These include the opportunities for expanded practice, autonomy, meaningful relationships, challenges, and rural rewards. Nurse recruiters trying to attract men to rural nursing should emphasize the positive aspects of rural nursing, the opportunities for outdoor recreation, and the family-friendly environments offered by rural communities.

ACKNOWLEDGMENTS

This research was funded by Montana State University–Bozeman College of Nursing Block Grant Program. The author acknowledges Helen J. Lee and Charlene A. Winters for their assistance with this study.

REFERENCES

American Association of Colleges of Nursing (AACN). (1997). *Diversity and equality of opportunity.* Retrieved March 12, 2002, from http://www.aacn.nche.edu/Publications/positions/diverse.htm

American Association of Colleges of Nursing (AACN). (2001, December Issue Bulletin). *Effective strategies for increasing diversity in nursing programs.* Washington, DC: American Association of Colleges of Nursing.

Anders, R. L. (1993). Targeting male students. *Nurse Educator, 18* (2), 4.

Benner, P. (1999). Quality of life: A phenomenological perspective on explanation, prediction, and understanding in nursing science. In E. C. Polifroni & M. Welch (Eds.), *Perspectives on philosophy of science in nursing: An historical and contemporary anthology* (pp. 303–314). Philadelphia: Lippincott.

Buerhaus, P. I., Staiger, D. O., & Auerbach, D. I. (2000). Implications of an aging registered nurse workforce. *JAMA, 283,* 2948–2954.

Bushy, A. (2002). International perspectives on rural nursing: Australia, Canada, USA. *Australian Journal of Rural Health, 10,* 104–111.

Center on an Aging Society. (2003, January). Data profile: Rural and urban health. *Challenges for the 21st century: Chronic and disabling conditions,* 1–6. Georgetown University: Institute for Health Care Research and Policy.

Creswell, J. (1998). *Qualitative inquiry and research design: Choosing among five traditions.* Thousand Oaks, CA: Sage.

Davis, M. T., & Bartfay, W. J. (2001). Men in nursing: An untapped resource. *Canadian Nurse, 97* (5), 14–18.

Goins, R. T., & Mitchell, J. (1999). Health-related quality of life: Does rurality matter? *Journal of Rural Health, 15,* 147–146.

Gordon, S. (2002). *A hemorrhage in the hospitals.* Retrieved June 4, 2002, from http://www.latimes.com/la-000038996jun03.story

Hegney, D., McCarthy, A., Rogers-Clark, C., & Gorman, D. (2002). Why nurses are attracted to rural and remote practice? *Australian Journal of Rural Health, 10,* 178–186.

Hopkins, M., & Domrose, C. (2001). *Remote control.* Retrieved January 11, 2004, from http://www.nurseweek.com/news/features/01–04/rural.asp

Houde, S. C. (2002). Methodological issues in male caregiver research: An integrative review of the literature. *Journal of Advanced Nursing, 40,* 626–640.

Koch, T. (1995). Interpretive approaches in nursing research: The influence of Husserl and Heidegger. *Journal of Advanced Nursing, 21,* 827–836.

Kumar, V., Acanfora, M., Hennessy, C. H., & Kalache, A. (2001). Health status of the rural elderly. *Journal of Rural Health, 17,* 328–331.

Lee, H. (1998). Lack of anonymity. In H.J. Lee (Ed.), *Conceptual basis for rural nursing* (pp. 76–88). New York: Springer.

Lincoln, Y. S., & Guba, E. (2000). Paradigmatic controversies, contradictions, and emerging confluences. In N. K. Denzin & Y. S. Lincoln (Eds.), *Handbook of qualitative research* (2nd ed., pp. 163–188). Thousand Oaks, CA: Sage.

Long, C. (2000, October 9). *Rural communities feel sting of nursing shortage.* Retrieved November 28, 2004, from http://community.bouldernews.com/news/statewest/091nurs.html

National Institute of Nursing Research. (1995). *Chapter 2: Rural America: Challenges and opportunities.* Retrieved April 9, 2003, from http://ninr.nih.gov/ninr/research/volq/chapter2.htm

O'Lynn, C. E. (2004). Gender-based barriers for male students in nursing education programs: Prevalence and perceived importance. *Journal of Nursing Education, 43,* 229–236.

Patton, M. Q. (2002). *Qualitative research & evaluation methods* (3rd ed.). Thousand Oaks, CA: Sage.

Rosenthal, K. (1996). *Rural nursing: An exploratory narrative description.* Unpublished Dissertation, University of Colorado, Denver.

Scharff, J. (1998). The distinctive nature and scope of rural nursing practice: Philosophical bases. In H. J. Lee (Ed.), *Conceptual basis for rural nursing* (pp. 19–38). New York: Springer.

Spratley, E., Johnson, A., Sochalski, J., Fritz, M., & Spencer, W. (2001). *The registered nurse population March 2000: Findings from the National Sample Survey of Registered Nurses.* Washington, DC: U.S. Department of Health and Human Services, Bureau of Health Professions, Division of Nursing.

Sullivan, E. J. (2000). Men in nursing: The importance of gender diversity. *Journal of Professional Nursing, 16,* 253–254.

Thompson, E. (2002). What's unique about men's caregiving? In B. J. Kramer & E. Thompson (Eds.), *Men as caregivers: Theory, research, and service implications* (pp. 20–50). New York: Springer.

Trossman, S. (2001, July/August). Rural nursing anyone? Recruiting nurses is always a challenge. *The American Nurse, 1,* 18–19.

U.S. Bureau of the Census. (2002). *U.S. summary: 2000* (Census profile No. C2K-PROF/00–US). Washington, DC: U.S. Department of Commerce.

Villeneuve, M. J. (1994). Recruiting and retaining men in nursing: A review of the literature. *Journal of Professional Nursing, 10,* 217–228.

Vukic, A., & Keddy, B. (2002). Northern nursing practice in a primary health care setting. *Journal of Advanced Nursing, 40,* 542–548.

19 Continuing Education and Rural Nurses

LORI HENDRICKX

The availability of continuing education (CE) is essential for maintaining skilled, competent nurses in the practice setting. Access to CE programming has been an issue for nurses practicing in rural and frontier areas, yet rural nurses have reported their desire and commitment to remain current through CE (Hendrickx, 1998). Rapidly changing technology, advances in health care, and the complexity of patients make it necessary for nurses in general to keep abreast of new information. In rural areas, complex situations may occur less frequently and nurses may often be working alone or with minimal support staff, making it even more imperative that these nurses remain current and have access to CE.

The rural health care environment provides nurses with an opportunity to practice as a generalist. Although the generalist role is ideal for those who appreciate a variety of experiences, some nurses are challenged by the concern that there is too much to know when caring for a diverse population of patients (Trossman, 2001). Bigbee (1993) identified a unique challenge of rural nursing as the multiple functions and generalist orientation. As a generalist, a rural nurse might practice in labor and delivery, medical, surgical, pediatric, or emergency departments, often within the same shift and with limited numbers of other nurses or support staff available. Limitations on nurses' time and the financial constraints facing rural hospitals have contributed to the increasing difficulty of maintaining proficiency for nurses in a generalist practice.

Providing high quality care in rural health care facilities is essential if rural facilities are to remain open. Moscovice and Stensland (2002) indicated that rural dwellers often perceived higher quality care existed in more metropolitan hospitals. Although this perception is often based on nonempirical evidence, patients may decide to bypass the local rural provider in favor of a larger facility. A key component in providing quality health care in the rural area is ensuring that rural nurses are up-to-date and have access to current knowledge through CE. The lack of CE opportunities or other barriers to obtaining CE have been identified as factors in nurses' decisions to work in nonrural areas (Hendrickx, 2001; Richards, 2008).

LITERATURE REVIEW

The nursing shortage has been well publicized; however, geographic areas experience the shortage in differing ways. Historically, rural areas felt the impact with larger numbers of shortage areas in the United States being in rural counties (Stratton, Dunkin, & Juhl, 1995). In a study examining nursing workforce issues in rural and urban settings, LaSala (2000) found that when major vacancies existed, they were greater in rural areas (19.2%) than urban areas (2.7%). Trossman (2001) stated that rural facilities face enormous challenges when trying to fill a registered nurse (RN) vacancy and that the nursing shortage is making recruitment of nurses to rural areas more difficult. Cramer, Nienaber, Helget and Agrawal (2006) found that RN shortages continue to be greatest in rural areas and that the shortage of rural nurses has been underestimated.

It is not uncommon to find that nurses residing in nonmetropolitan counties travel to metropolitan areas to work, further compounding the problem of recruiting nurses to rural areas. Even though salaries in both urban and rural areas have improved, rural administrators reported that urban areas continue to draw rural nurses by offering higher salaries (LaSala, 2000). Daniels, VanLeit, Skipper, Sanders, and Rhyne (2007) reported that supporting a family and income potential continue to be important considerations in recruitment and retention in rural areas. In addition to salary differences, other issues related to recruitment and retention of rural nurses have been identified. In studies describing nurse recruitment and retention concerns in rural areas, the lack of CE opportunities has often been identified as problematic related to the ability to recruit or retain nurses (Farmer & Richardson, 1997; Hendrickx, 1998, 2001).

For rural nurses, several deterrents to participation in CE have been identified. The most commonly identified factor has been distance to travel (Hedman & Lazure, 1990; Hegge, Powers, Hendrickx, & Vinson, 2002; Hendrickx, 1998, 2001; Richards, 2008). Hegge et al. (2002) reported that 39 participants in a study related to competence and CE indicated they traveled greater than 200 miles to obtain CE. In that same study, 75% of the participants had not attended a national conference in the past 2 years, 63% had not attended a regional conference, and 40% had not attended a local conference.

South Dakota is not a state that requires CE credits to renew nursing licensure. However, given the distribution of the respondents in a study across several specialty areas and among different areas within nursing, the need for continued exposure to current practice literature and education is important. In a study (Hendrickx, 2001) of barriers to CE experienced by rural nurses, I asked study participants to identify reasons they did not attend CE activities. Seventy percent ($n = 28$) responded that distance to travel was the major reason they had not attended more CE. Other reasons for not participating in CE were (a) cost, (b) difficulty getting time off from work, (c) topics not of interest, (d) not being able to be away from family, or (e) not knowing about possible CE activities being offered (Hendrickx). Several respondents also chose to add comments related to their CE activities. Comments often related to distance or cost. One respondent noted, "Many times I would have to travel 6–8 hours to receive 2–4 hours of CE. The cost of that is prohibitive, not to mention the time." Another respondent wrote,

> Usually they [CE] are too far away and if they're more than one day I need motel and food money since it takes another day to drive there and back. There aren't enough nurses at the hospital I work to cover me for that many extra days and I don't want to use my vacation days for that (Hendrickx, 2001).

In the same study, I reported that 12 (26.5%) respondents indicated they had not attended any CE activities during the previous year. Twelve (26.5%) had attended 1–5 hours of CE, 12 (26.5%) had attended 6–10 hours, 1 had attended 11–15 hours, and 11 (22.4%) had attended more than 15 hours. Nurses were also asked to indicate the distance they had traveled to attend CE. Only 5 (10.2%) nurses indicated they had been able to attend CE activities offered less than 50 miles from their homes. Six (12.2%) traveled 51–100 miles, 12 (24.5%) traveled 101–150 miles and 20 (41%) indicated they traveled greater than 150 miles to attend CE. In a replication of this work, Richards (2008) found that rural Montana nurses experienced similar barriers to obtaining CE. Richards reported distance, getting time off from work, and cost as the top three reasons for lack of participation in CE. Additionally, 78.3% of her respondents indicated they traveled greater than 50 miles to attend CE.

In addition to distance issues, nurses have identified the lack of financial resources to support CE attendance, limited transportation opportunities, weather, and inability to get time off from work as deterrents to obtaining CE (Hedman & Lazure, 1990; Hendrickx, 2001). The American Nurses Association (ANA) also has reported that reduced access to advanced education and CE was one of several challenges that face rural and frontier nurses (Weinert, Fuszard, Wasem, et al., 1996).

INCREASED OPPORTUNITIES THROUGH COMPUTER EDUCATION

The use of computers has been proposed as a solution to alleviate the barrier of distance related to CE (Hegge et al., 2002). Bushy (2002) indicated that a potential benefit of online courses is the reduction or elimination of commuting time. In addition, technological advances have been purported to be a possible solution to the isolation of rural nurses. Dunkin (2002) noted,

> With the advances in technology that have occurred in the last 10 years, isolation from other nurses is no longer a necessary part of rural nursing. While geography has not changed, there are many resources available to rural and remote nurses, primarily through the Internet. (p.1)

Although nurses have identified advantages, such as the convenience of taking courses from home and the increased variety of Internet topics, I reported that rural nurses use computers but not for CE (Hendrickx, 2001). In a study of 559 nurses, Hegge et al. (2002) reported that although 72.5% of respondents had computers at home and 76% of respondents had computers at work, only 100 of the nurses (17.9%) had used computers for CE. Reasons those nurses did not use computers for CE included (a) lack of knowledge about computer CE programs, (b) lack of access to a computer, (c) lack of Internet access, (d) lack of time, (e) discomfort using computers, (f) preference for books or other written material, or (e) that CE was not required (Hegge et al.).

I conducted a study (Hendrickx, 2003) examining the level of involvement and factors that influence professional development of rural nurses. I also asked these nurses ($n = 49$) whether or not they use a computer and if they had ever used a computer for CE. Eighty-six percent ($n = 42$) reported they had used a computer but only two of those had ever used a computer to obtain CE. One of those two reported she was in an online baccalaureate of science in a nursing completion program, so she was taking all her classes over the Internet.

More recently, Richards (2008) reported that computer use among rural nurses has increased from previous studies. In her study, 90.9% of respondents indicated they used computers and 51.8% had used computers to obtain CE.

Although the Internet has provided a new method for obtaining CE, there are other methods, such as interactive video conferencing, audio conferencing, Web-based seminars (Webinars) and the use of telemedicine networks that have been developed in rural areas. Telemedicine systems have been used in rural areas for some time to deliver health care services to rural dwellers. Telemedicine has been defined by the Institute of Medicine as "the use of electronic information and communications technologies to provide and support health care, when distance separates the participants" (Geyman, Norris, & Hart, 2001, p. 250).

Nurses in rural areas have used telemedicine systems to deliver CE to other nurses with distance barriers. The American Association of Critical Care Nurses (AACN) recently awarded the 2004 Outstanding Chapter Communication System Award to the Siouxland Chapter of AACN for its use of a telemedicine network to deliver their annual meetings and CE offerings to nurses across the state of South Dakota. In their exemplar submitted for the award, the Siouxland Chapter indicated that South Dakota is a state with only one AACN Chapter, located in the extreme southeast corner of the state and accessible to only a portion of the state's AACN members and critical care nurses. The Siouxland Chapter committed itself to reaching out to AACN members in South Dakota and critical care nurses without physical access to AACN through the use of the Avera McKennan TeleHealth Network. Chapter members established an interactive distance communication method using the TeleHealth network. Monthly meetings and CE then became available through the network to critical care nurses in several towns across South Dakota.

The Siouxland Chapter interactive system allows remote attendees to see and listen to meetings and contribute to discussions, while the local site attendees also see those at remote sites. Microphones stationed throughout the room allow attendees to talk to attendees at other sites and ask questions. All of the speaker's materials, such as slides or videos, are sent via the network to distant sites and available in real time. The Siouxland Chapter communication system has enabled several critical care colleagues to attend meetings and earn CE while in their own communities, reducing travel time and time away from work and families.

> The American Nurses Association envisions that telemedicine systems for nursing (termed *telenursing*) are especially relevant for nursing education through distance learning. For rural nurses, this technology has the potential for use "for formal coursework, continuing education, attendance at televised conferences, or participation in clinical teaching rounds." (ANA, 1997, p. 2)

The increase in distance delivery formats for education will be effective only if the education providers increase awareness and support for the use of distance education among rural nurses. Training programs will have to be developed for use in the professional educational setting as well as in CE that assist the learner with the technology.

ACADEMIC EDUCATION

Rural nurses have limited access to advanced academic programs. In rural areas, there tends to be a greater community college presence rather than university presence, making continuing academic education difficult for those nurses interested in completing a baccalaureate or graduate degree (Szigeti, 2000). The emergence of distance learning programs at universities has greatly expanded the availability of academic programming at the baccalaureate level and higher for rural nurses. Many nurses are demanding greater flexibility in educational programming, and for some rural nurses, a distance education program is the only type that allows nurses to complete or continue their education (McPeck, 2001). The most prevalent distance programs are the completion programs, which enable RNs with an associate degree or diploma in nursing to earn a bachelors or graduate degree in nursing.

A recent Internet search netted over 100 online graduate degree programs in nursing in the United States. This number will continue to increase as more colleges of nursing become aware of the advantages of distance learning for nurses. Szigeti (2000) reported that at a Doctoral Conference sponsored by the American Association of Colleges of Nursing, "Faculties in colleges of nursing are aware that it is difficult for many nurses to be on a university campus to earn a doctoral degree. They are developing doctoral programs for these potential students" (p. 2). As more online programs are developed, it is important that prospective students closely consider issues such as accreditation and available student resources (Stanton, 2007).

At South Dakota State University, since its inception in 2001, the Online Master's Degree Program has admitted the maximum number of students (15) and has had a waiting list each year. For Fall 2004, an additional section of students was added so that two groups of online students could be admitted, accommodating the increased number of applicants. Most applicants have been from South Dakota and neighboring states—Minnesota, Iowa, Nebraska, and Montana; however, the college also had applicants from North Carolina, Missouri, Michigan, Wisconsin, Texas, and overseas (S. Bunkers, personal communication, November 11, 2008).

For the RN wishing to obtain a baccalaureate degree (BSN), the online RN-to-BSN programs have increased the availability of this option. Programs that used traditional approaches to RN-to-BSN education have moved to online delivery with substantial increases in enrollments. The University of Kansas saw dropping enrollment in its traditional RN-to-BSN program. A change to an online program resulted in a 53% increase in enrollment (McPeck, 2001). Similarly, at South Dakota State University, enrollment numbers in the RN-to-BSN program were around 8–12 students prior to initiation of online course delivery. The change to online delivery has resulted in increased enrollment, and there are currently over 200 students taking either nursing courses or pre-nursing support courses. In 2004, 34 nursing students graduated from the RN-to-BSN program, and nearly twice that many graduated in 2008 (S. Rosen, personal communication, November 6, 2008).

Another area that has seen increased growth related to distance delivery of CE is RN and licensed practical nurse (LPN) refresher courses. These refresher courses have successfully facilitated the return of many retired and inactive nurses to the workforce (Blankenship, Winslow, & Smith, 2003). Rural nurses that are interested in reentering the nursing

Table 19.1

ENROLLMENT IN REFRESHER COURSE AT SOUTH DAKOTA STATE UNIVERSITY

YEAR	RN PROGRAM, *n*	LPN PROGRAM, *n*
2000	65	46
2001	61	53
2002[a]	117	71
2003	168	81
2004	135	91
2005	103	54
2006	94	53

[a]Online delivery began.

workforce and need a refresher course for licensing have also taken advantage of online programs. Since 2002, the RN and LPN refresher courses at South Dakota State University saw a substantial increase in enrollment with the development of online delivery. Enrollment numbers remain higher than enrollment prior to online delivery (see Table 19.1; M. Bohn, personal communication, November 20, 2008).

PROFESSIONAL NURSING ORGANIZATIONS

Numerous professional organizations have now added online CE content to their Web sites. For example, ANA and Sigma Theta Tau International offer online CE on a variety of topics for a minimal fee, while other organizations offer a number of free CE units as a membership benefit. Additionally, complete online educational programs have been made available for purchase, such as the Essentials of Critical Care Orientation (ECCO) program available through the AACN (2004). The ECCO program has been beneficial to rural hospitals that do not have the resources to support an education department. This online educational program is useful for hospitals who want to deliver a standardized orientation program to nurses, or when a hospital educator's time needs to be "freed up to focus on learning transference, supplemental information development, and learner's educational needs" (Berke & Wiseman, 2004, p. 80). Practicing nurses can then attend the orientation program on their own time or from home, balancing the didactic portion with the hands-on orientation in the practice setting.

The Rural Nurse Organization offers a variety of services for the professional development of nurses specifically interested in rural issues. Its Web site (www.rno.org) provides a newsletter, information about the organization, and access to the *Online Journal of Rural Nursing and Health Care.*

SUMMARY

Rural nurses are committed to maintaining quality care in their practice environments but often find that physical distance from programming and other barriers limit their ability to attend CE or academic programs. It is essential that rural health institutions, those responsible for the delivery of CE, and those in academia recognize and address the challenges that rural nurses face with regard to CE. With creative use of technology and commitment by all those involved, rural nurses need not be isolated from activities that will help them maintain current, competent practice.

REFERENCES

American Association of Critical Care Nurses (AACN). (2004). *Essentials of critical care orientation.* Retrieved June 9, 2004, from http://www.aacn.org
American Nurses Association (ANA). (1997). Telehealth: A tool for nursing practice. *Nursing Trends & Issues, 2* (4), 1–7.
Berke, W., & Wiseman, T. (2004). The e-learning answer. *Critical Care Nurse, 24*(2), 80–84.
Bigbee, J. (1993). The uniqueness of rural nursing. *Nursing Clinics of North America, 28* (1), 131–144.
Blankenship, J. S., Winslow, S. A, & Smith, A. U. (2003). Refresher course for inactive RNs facilitates workforce entry. *Journal for Nurses in Staff Development, 19,* 288–291.
Bushy, A. (2002). Cyber-learning: A primer to get you started. *Online Journal of Rural Nursing and Healthcare, 2* (2). Retrieved March 11, 2004, from http://www.rno.org
Cramer, M., Nienaber, J., Helget, P., & Agrawal, S. (2006). Comparative analysis of urban and rural nursing workforce shortages in Nebraska hospitals. *Policy, Politics, & Nursing Practice, 7* (4), 248–260.
Daniels, Z. M., VanLeit, B. J., Skipper, B. J., Sanders, M. L., & Rhyne, R. L. (2007). Factors in recruiting and retaining health professionals for rural practice. *Journal of Rural Health, 23* (1), 62–71.
Dunkin, J. (2002). Isolation: Real or perceived? *Online Journal of Rural Nursing and Healthcare, 2* (1). Retrieved March 11, 2004, from http://www.rno.org
Farmer, J., & Richardson, A. (1997). Information for trained nurses in remote areas: Do electronically networked resources provide an answer? *Health Library Review, 14* (2), 97–103.

Geyman, J. P., Norris, T. E., & Hart, L. G. (2001). *Textbook of rural medicine*. New York: McGraw-Hill.

Hedman, L., & Lazure, L. (1990). Extending continuing education to rural nurses. *Journal of Continuing Education in Nursing, 21*, 165–168.

Hegge, M., Powers, P., Hendrickx, L., & Vinson, J. (2002). Competence, continuing education, and computers. *Journal of Continuing Education in Nursing, 33*, 24–32.

Hendrickx, L. (1998). Attitudes of rural nurses toward computers: Implications for continuing education. *Dissertation Abstracts International, 59*(03A), 0690.

Hendrickx, L. (2001, March). *Continuing education needs and perceived barriers of South Dakota nurses in geographically isolated areas*. Paper presented at the Sigma Theta Tau Twelfth Annual Nursing Research Symposium, Brookings, SD.

Hendrickx, L. (2003, March). *Level of involvement and factors that influence professional development of rural nurses*. Paper presented at the Sigma Theta Tau Fourteenth Annual Nursing Research Conference, Brookings, SD.

LaSala, K. (2000). Nursing workforce issues in rural and urban setting: Looking at the difference in recruitment, retention, and distribution. *Online Journal of Rural Nursing and Healthcare, 1* (1). Retrieved March 11, 2004, from http://www.rno.org

McPeck, P. (2001, July 9). Education evolution: Nursing education models take a tech turn as students demand greater flexibility. *Nurseweek*. Retrieved June 1, 2004, from http://www.nurseweek.com/news/features/01–07/evolution.html

Moscovice, I., & Stensland, J. (2002). Rural hospitals: Trends, challenges, and a future research and policy analysis agenda. *Journal of Rural Health, 18* (Suppl.), 197–210.

Richards, C. (2008). *Learning needs and barriers to continuing education among rural Montana nurses*. Unpublished master's thesis, South Dakota State University.

Stanton, M. (2007). Online learning. *Online Journal of Rural Nursing and Health Care, 7* (2), 2. Retrieved December 15, 2008, from http://rno.org

Stratton, T., Dunkin, J., & Juhl, N. (1995). Redefining the nursing shortage: A rural perspective. *Nursing Outlook, 43*, 71–77.

Szigeti, E. (2000). Education at a distance. *Online Journal of Rural Nursing and Healthcare, 1*(3). Retrieved March 11, 2004, from http://www.rno.org

Trossman, S. (2001). Rural nursing anyone? Recruiting nurses is always a challenge. *The American Nurse, 33* (4), 1, 18–19.

Weinert, C., Fuszard, B., Wasem, C., Haldane, S., Yocum, D., & Schultz, C. (1996). *Rural/frontier nursing: The challenge to grow*. Washington, DC: American Nurses Association.

Rural Nurses' Attitudes and Beliefs Toward Evidence-Based Practice

20

BRENDA D. KOESSL, CHARLENE A. WINTERS, HELEN J. LEE, and LORI HENDRICKX

Evidence-based practice (EBP) is a hallmark of professional nursing practice and high quality patient care (Case, 2004). Melnyk, Fineout-Overholt, Feinstein, Sadler, and Green-Hernandez (2008) defined EBP as a "problem-solving approach to the delivery of care that incorporates the best evidence from well-designed studies in combination with a clinician's expertise and patient preferences and values" (p. 8). EBP is further characterized by the American Nurses Association (ANA, 2004) as practice that occurs within the context of available resources. Evidence-based nursing de-emphasizes ritual, isolated and unsystematic clinical experiences, ungrounded opinions, and tradition as a basis for practice. It stresses the use of research findings and other operational and evaluation data, the consensus of recognized experts, and affirmed experience to substantiate clinical practice (American Nurses Credentialing Center [ANCC], 2005). Most nursing leaders would agree that EBP should be usual and customary in their organizations (Munroe, Duffy, & Fisher, 2006). As a case in point, the Joint Commission (JC) requires the use of evidence in practice to ensure safe patient care (2008).

Nurses constitute the largest group of health care providers and their care directly influences patient outcomes (Aiken, Clarke, Cheung,

Sloane, & Silber, 2003). Numerous authors writing about EBP clearly support the premise that nurses need to be knowledgeable about how to access and use research (Funk, Champagne, Wiese, & Tornquist, 1991; Olade, 2004; Parsons, Merlin, Taylor, Wilkinson, & Hiller, 2003; Pravikoff, Tanner, & Pierce, 2005; Taylor, Wilkinson & Blue, 2001). However, a growing number of research studies (Estabrooks, Midodzi, Cummings, & Wallin, 2007; Funk et al., 1991; Hommelstad & Corne-lia, 2004; Olade, 2003; Taylor et al., 2001) have identified barriers that interfere with the ability of nurses to utilize evidence-based nursing in practice. Barriers include lack of (a) accessibility to research, (b) organizational and peer support for using research, (c) knowledge of research methods, (d) access to technology, and (e) time.

A small body of research literature has focused on nurses' attitudes and beliefs about research to explain nurses' use of evidence for practice (Olade, 2004; Melnyk, Fineout-Overholt, Feinstein, et al., 2004; Morrison, 1998; Smirnoff, Ramirez, Kooplimae, Gibney, & McEvoy, 2007). An attitude is a mental position with regard to fact or state (Merriam-Webster, 2007), while a belief can be considered a conviction held in the absence of evidence (Rawnsley, 2003). Rizzuto, Bostrom, Suter, and Chenitz (1994) reported that nurses with positive attitudes and beliefs toward EBP are more likely to utilize research and incorporate it into practice than nurses whose attitudes and beliefs toward EBP are negative.

Implementing EBP is especially important in rural and remote practice, to ensure the best outcomes for populations in areas with limited health care choices and resources (Taylor et al., 2001). However, limited literature exists regarding rural nurses' access and use of research in practice (Olade, 2004; Winters, Lee, Besel, et al., 2007). Professional isolation, limited access to colleagues with research backgrounds, and lack of administrative support for staff involvement in research affects rural nurses' use of research (Olade, 2003). Furthermore, limited budgets for continuing education (CE) and lack of medical libraries and technology resources place rural nurses at a disadvantage when it comes to an environment supportive of nurses' access and use of research (Olade). The further one ventures away from large urban medical centers, the less one hears about research utilization activities for EBP in nursing (Olade, 2004). Isolation from colleagues who are involved in research coupled with lack of research specific to rural nursing (Winters et al., 2007) are factors that could influence rural nurses' attitudes and beliefs about research.

PURPOSE OF THE STUDY

A gap exists between the time research findings are reported and the time they are incorporated into practice. If rural nurses are not familiar with research or how to access research, or do not value research, this gap may be exaggerated, putting patients at a disadvantage. If nursing is to be an evidence-based profession, improving the use of research findings in clinical practice must occur within urban and rural settings (Olade, 2004). The purpose of the study was to explore factors that influence rural nurses' attitudes and beliefs toward EBP. The research questions were:

1. What are rural nurses' attitudes and beliefs about research and evidence-based practice?
2. Do rural nurses find research easy to understand?
3. Do rural nurses believe the results of the research that they read?
4. Does number of years of experience as a nurse affect rural nurses' attitudes and beliefs about research?
5. Does level of education influence rural nurses' attitudes and beliefs toward research?
6. Does the size of facility that a rural nurse works in affect attitudes and beliefs toward research?
7. Does the role of a rural nurse within his or her facility affect attitudes and beliefs toward research?

THEORETICAL PERSPECTIVE

Rural nursing has been defined as the provision of health care by professional nurses to persons living in sparsely populated areas (Long & Weinert, 1989). Rural nursing is "a special variety of nursing in which the nurse must have a wide range of advanced knowledge and ability, in combination with commitment, to practice proficiently in multiple clinical areas simultaneously along the career trajectory" (Scharff, 1998, p. 37). Rural nursing theory (RNT), a descriptive middle range theory originally published by Long and Weinert was developed so that researchers would have a framework for describing, explaining, and predicting phenomena within the rural nursing culture (Lee & McDonagh, 2006).

The theory includes three statements regarding (a) a rural person's definition of health, (b) rural health seeking behaviors, and (c) the lack of anonymity and role diffusion experienced by rural health care providers. The third statement was specifically used to guide this study because it is the role diffusion coupled with the context in which rural nurses practice that makes use of evidence so critical to rural practice.

Role diffusion may also contribute to rural nurses' attitudes and beliefs toward EBP. Rural nurses function in many roles that may include pharmacist, dietician, respiratory therapist, and medical records clerk. Rural nurses often have to make do with what is available (Scharff, 1998), rely on information from colleagues to inform their practice (Ouzts, 2005; Winters et al., 2007), and may not be as easily influenced by what research or evidence supports or does not support. Exploring rural nurses' attitudes and beliefs about the use of evidence in their practice will provide insight into rural nursing and direction for nursing educators, managers, and health care administrators.

METHODOLOGY

This study was a secondary analysis of data collected to explore rural nurses' access and use of research (Luparell, Winters, Lee, O'Lynn, Shreffler-Grant, & Hendrickx, 2006a). A descriptive, cross-sectional survey design was used in the parent study to address the following research questions: To what extent are research findings available to rural nurses? What resources do rural nurses use to obtain research findings? To what extent do rural nurses find research relevant to their practice? How do rural nurses use research findings in their practice? What strategies would improve accessibility of research/information to rural nurses?

Data Collection

Participants were nurses practicing in rural settings in three northwestern states in the United States (U.S.) selected from mailing lists of all registered nurses (RNs) obtained from the Board of Nursing in each state. The lists were separated into rural and nonrural areas based on each nurse's county of residence using the Rural–Urban Commuting Codes developed by the Economic Research Service (ERS) of the United States Department of Agriculture (USDA, 2007). For purposes of the study, counties meeting the criteria for Codes 6–9 were considered rural. From the list of nurses residing in rural counties, 800 were selected at random; 300 names from each of two of the states and 200 names from the third. A cover letter describing the study and the questionnaire were mailed to each of the 800 nurses with a stamped return envelope. Nonresponders were mailed a reminder card three weeks after the initial mailing. There were 263 surveys returned, representing a 35.3% return rate. Overall response rates were similar for the three states. After the removal of respondents who declined to participate in the survey, provided incomplete zip code information, or lived in rural areas but commuted to urban facilities for work, 224 surveys were available for analysis.

Instrument

The questionnaire was a nine-page, 42-question survey adapted from surveys created by other researchers (Eastabrooks, 1996; Funk, Tornquist, & Champagne, 1995; McKenna, Ashton, & Keeney, 2004) and modified for an American sample based on a pilot study of 52 nurses conducted in one of the study states (Winters et al., 2006). The final survey contained questions to assess six areas of interest: (a) availability of resources, (b) sources of information, (c) access and use of the Internet, (d) use of research findings, (e) attitudes toward research-based practice, and (f) demographics. Some questions were structured to require a *yes* or *no* response, while answers to other questions were provided using a five-point Likert-type scale (strongly agree, agree, unsure, disagree, and strongly disagree). Respondents were also given the opportunity to provide comments contributing to qualitative data. Reliability of individual items ranged from a Chronbach's alpha of 0.643 to 0.863. In order to decrease any potential confusion, the study tool defined research utilization as the use of any kind of research finding, in any kind of way, in any aspect of work as a health care practitioner. Data for the study reported here included demographic information and responses to questions related to attitudes and beliefs (see Table 20.1).

Data Analysis

Data were displayed using the Statistical Package for Social Sciences (SPSS, version 16, Graduate Pack) and analyzed using descriptive statistics to determine item frequencies and measures of central tendency. Comparisons between naturally occurring groups were conducted to

Table 20.1

RESEARCH QUESTIONS AND RELATED QUESTIONNAIRE ITEMS

RESEARCH QUESTIONS	PARENT QUESTIONNAIRE ITEMS
1. Do rural nurses find research easy to understand?	Q22 a, b, & c. a. I feel confident in my ability to evaluate the quality of research papers. b. I find that research articles are not easily understood. c. I believe that I should take a course to help me understand research effectively.
2. Do rural nurses believe the results of the research that they read?	Q22 d & e. d. I believe the results of the research that I read. e. I would feel more confident if there was an individual experienced in research to supply me with relevant information.
3. Does number of years experience as a nurse affect rural nurses' attitudes and beliefs about research?	Q38. Total years of practice as a nurse? Q39. Total years of practice in a rural setting?
4. Does level of education influence rural nurses attitudes and beliefs toward research?	Q27. What is your basic nursing education? Q28. Year of graduation from basic nursing program? Q29. What is your highest educational achievement? Q30. Year of graduation from highest degree program?
5. Does the size of facility that a rural nurse works in affect attitudes and beliefs toward research?	Q35. What is your current, or most recent, practice setting? Q36. If applicable, number of beds in your facility?
6. Does the role of a rural nurse within their facility affect attitudes and beliefs toward research?	Q37. What is your primary position?

Source: Luparell et al. (2006b).

further explore the data. Tables and graphs were designed to visually aid in the interpretation of the survey results.

RESULTS

Sample

The majority of the 224 respondents were female (92.3%; n = 203), 41 to 60 years of age (62.7%; n = 136; m = 50.5), employed in health-care (94.1%; n = 207), and worked full-time (65.5%; n = 135). The most common place of employment was a hospital (46.4%; n = 84) and the most common position was that of a staff nurse (55.6%; n = 105). Most described their highest educational achievement as the bacca-laureate degree (48.2%; n = 105). Sample demographics are shown in Table 20.2.

Do Rural Nurses Find Research Easy to Understand?

In response to the question, "I feel confident in my ability to evalu-ate the quality of research papers," the sample was divided into two nearly equal groups. Forty-eight percent (48%) of the nurses (n = 108) agreed/strongly agreed with this statement. However, just slightly more (49.4%; n = 110) either disagreed or were unsure of their ability to evaluate quality.

To the question, "I find that research articles are not easily under-stood," the sample was similarly divided. Almost one-half (49.1%; n = 110) of the nurses agreed/strongly agreed with the statement, and nearly an equal number disagreed/strongly disagreed or were unsure (48.6%; (n = 109).

The participants were divided into three groups when it came to responding to the statement, "I believe that I should take a course to help me use research effectively." Just over one-third of the nurses agreed/strongly agreed with the statement, one-third disagreed/strongly disagreed, and 27.7% (n = 62) were unsure.

A majority of the nurses (63%; n = 114) indicated they would feel more confident if an individual experienced in research provided them with rel-evant practice information. Surprisingly, most of the nurses (58.0%; n = 130) were unsure if they "believed the results of the research that they read," and 12.9% (n = 29) reported they did not believe; only one-quarter (25.0%; n = 56) reported they believed the research they read.

Table 20.2

SAMPLE DEMOGRAPHICS

RESPONSE		NUMBER OF CASES	% OF TOTAL SAMPLE
Gender (*n* = 220)*	Female	203	92.3%
	Male	17	7.7%
Age (*n* = 217; *x* = 50.5 years)*	<30	17	7.8%
	31–40	43	19.8%
	41–50	71	32.7%
	51–60	65	30.0%
	>60	21	9.7%
Level of Highest Educational Preparation (*n* = 224)	Diploma	21	9.6%
	Associate Degree	66	30.3%
	Baccalaureate Degree	105	48.2%
	Master's Degree	26	11.9%
Employment Setting (*n* = 181)*	Hospital	84	46.4%
	Critical Access Hospital	33	18.2%
	Private Practice	4	2.2%
	Community/Public Health	20	11.0%
	Home Health	8	4.4%
	School of Nursing	2	1.1%
	Health Clinic	14	7.7%
	Nursing Home	16	8.8%
Primary Position (*n* = 189)*	Staff Nurse	105	55.6%
	Charge Nurse	34	18.0%
	Clinical Nurse Specialist	3	1.6%
	Nurse Practitioner	11	5.8%
	Nurse Midwife	3	1.6%
	Manager	23	12.2%
	Administration	5	2.6%
	Education	5	2.6%

**n does not equal 224 because some respondents did not answer this question.

Does Number of Years' Experience as a Nurse, Type of Role, or Size of Facility Affect Rural Nurses' Attitudes and Beliefs About Research?

To assess the influence of years of experience, type of role, and size of facility on rural nurses' overall attitudes toward research, it was necessary to generate composite scores for nurses' attitudes and then divide the scores into quartiles. The following labels were applied to the quartiles: (a) worst attitudes for scores in the first quartile, (b) below average attitudes for scores in the second quartile, (c) above average attitudes for scores in the third quartile, and (d) best attitudes for scores in the fourth quartile. The new composite attitude score was then analyzed using the independent variables of total years of practice as a nurse, total years of practice in a *rural setting*, type of role, and size of facility.

Years of Experience

The largest portion of nurses with 1 to 5 years of experience (50%; n = 6) and 5 to 10 years of experience (35.5%; n = 11) were in the "above average" attitude group, while the largest portion of nurses with 10 to 20 years of experience (35.1%; n = 27) and more than 20 years of experience 29.1%; n = 30) were in the "best" attitude group (see Table 20.3). It is interesting to note that the second largest segment of nurses with greater than 20 years of experience (28.2%; n = 29) were in the "worst" attitude group. Similar results were obtained when reviewing the data for

Table 20.3

TENURE COHORTS						
ATTITUDE	MISSING (*n* = 1)	1 TO 5 YEARS (*n* = 12)	5 TO 10 YEARS (*n* = 31)	10 TO 20 YEARS (*n* = 77)	MORE THAN 20 YEARS (*n* = 103)	TOTAL (*n* = 224)
Worst	100.0%	0.0%	22.6%	19.5%	28.2%	23.2%
Below Average	0.0%	25.0%	22.6%	23.4%	23.3%	23.2%
Above Average	0.0%	50.0%	35.5%	22.1%	19.4%	24.1%
Best	0.0%	25.0%	19.4%	35.1%	29.1%	29.5%
Total	100.0%	100.0%	100.0%	100.0%	100.0%	100.0%

ATTITUDES AND ROLE

Table 20.4

	STAFF NURSE (n = 105)	CHARGE NURSE (n = 34)	CLINICAL NURSE SPECIALIST (n = 3)	NURSE PRACTITIONER (n = 11)	NURSE MIDWIFE (n = 3)	MANAGER/ SUPERVISOR (n = 23)	ADMINISTRATOR/ EXECUTIVE (n = 5)	EDUCATOR/ INSTRUCTOR (n = 5)	TOTAL (n = 189)
Worst	22%	38%	0%	18%	0%	22%	20%	0%	23%
Below Average	17%	32%	67%	18%	0%	22%	20%	40%	22%
Above Average	29%	15%	0%	9%	100%	22%	20%	60%	25%
Best	32%	15%	33%	55%	0%	35%	40%	0%	30%
Total	100%	100%	100%	100%	100%	100%	100%	100%	100%

years of experience as a nurse in a *rural setting* with one exception. Rural nurses with greater than 20 years of experience were equally divided between the "worst attitude" and the "best attitude" groups (28.2%, 29.1%, respectively; *n* = 18 in each group).

Role

When assessing the influence of *role* on rural nurses' overall attitudes toward research (see Table 20.4), the largest percent of nurses in the "best" attitude group were nurse practitioners (55.0%; *n* = 6), while the greatest number in this group were staff nurses (32.0%; *n* = 23). Of the nurses falling into the "worst" attitude group, the largest percent were hospital charge nurses (38.0%; *n* = 13). The greatest number in this group were staff nurses (22.0%; *n* = 23).

Practice Setting

Similarly, the largest percent of nurses whose primary *practice setting* was public/community health fell into the "best" attitude group (50%; *n* = 10) and the greatest number worked in hospitals (36.9%; *n* = 31). Interestingly, the largest segment of nurses in the "worst" attitude group were also hospital based (27.4%; *n* = 23). The majority of nurses practicing in Critical Access Hospitals (CAH) fell into the "below average" attitude group.

Does Level of Education Influence Rural Attitudes and Beliefs Toward Research?

In order to assess the influence of level of education on rural nurses' overall attitudes toward research, the previously described composite attitude scores were cross-tabulated with the level of education variable (see Table 20.5). The largest portion of nurses with a diploma were in the "below average" attitude group (33.3%; *n* = 7). Nurses with an associate's degree were evenly divided between the "worst" attitude group and the "best" attitude group (30.3%; *n* = 20 in each group). The largest portion of nurses with a baccalaureate degree were in the "below average" attitude group (29.5%; *n* = 31), and the largest segment of nurses with a master's degree were in the "best" attitude group (38.5%; n=10).

Table 20.5

ATTITUDES AND EDUCATION

ATTITUDES	DIPLOMA ($n = 21$)	ASSOCIATE DEGREE ($n = 66$)	BACCALAUREATE DEGREE ($n = 105$)	MASTER'S DEGREE ($n = 26$)	TOTAL ($n = 218$)*
Worst	19.0%	30.3%	19.0%	15.4%	22.0%
Below Average	33.3%	12.1%	29.5%	19.2%	23.4%
Above Average	19.0%	27.3%	23.8%	26.9%	24.8%
Best	28.6%	30.3%	27.6%	38.5%	29.8%
Total	100.0%	100.0%	100.0%	100.0%	100.0%

*n does not equal 224 because some respondents did not answer this question.

DISCUSSION

Nearly one-half of the respondents agreed with the statement "I feel confident in my ability to evaluate the quality of research papers"; yet almost one-half reported that ". . . research articles are not easily understood." Of equal concern was the finding that nearly 71% of the participants either disbelieved or were unsure if they believed research findings. This doubt in the veracity of research findings may relate to the clarity and writing level of the research reports. It may also indicate a lack of research related to rural patients or rural nursing practice (Olade, 2004) making interpretation and application of findings difficult. If research articles are not written clearly, written above a staff nurse's level of understanding, or on unfamiliar topics, rural nurses may find the research difficult to evaluate and therefore question their ability to believe the findings. Information literacy is the ability to (a) decide that information is needed about a subject, (b) access credible and understandable information about the subject, and (c) use the information to effectively solve a problem or make a decision (Tanner, Pierce, & Pravikoff, 2004). The lack of access to credible and understandable information is an important barrier to research utilization (Tanner et al.). It is also apparent from the available literature that nurses who believe EBP can and will enhance their practice are more likely to utilize research and incorporate it into practice than nurses whose attitudes and beliefs toward EBP are negative (Rizzuto et al., 1994). Encouraging researchers and publishers to provide research reports that are easily interpreted and available in widely circulated practice-oriented journals may aid rural nurses' access and understanding of reports.

Positive attitudes toward research have been found to directly relate to educational levels and participation in research (Smirnoff et al., 2007). A logical implication is to design baccalaureate level research courses that focus on skills needed to access, read, interpret, and evaluate research, and include the opportunity to participate in research. However, in this study, there were nearly equal numbers of nurses who believed as disbelieved that a course could help them use research effectively. This finding may be explained by the fact that more than one-half (60.1%) of participants had at least a baccalaureate degree. Baccalaureate prepared nurses were likely to have at least one course in research included in their curriculum. The baccalaureate prepared nurses who believed a course would be useful may value CE more than the associate degree or diploma prepared nurses (Goode, Pinkerton, McCausland, et al., 2001). The baccalaureate prepared nurses who answered that they were unsure about taking a research course to help them use research effectively may have answered that way because their education was long enough ago that research was not included in their curriculum; the research course(s) taken was not adequate in helping them understand research effectively; or they believed the course(s) was sufficient and questioned the need for further instruction. Additional research is needed to explore the relationship between completion of a research course, course design, and nurses' ability to use research findings effectively.

Most respondents indicated that they would like a research-experienced person to provide them with information. One hundred fourteen (114) respondents (51%) agreed with this statement and 27 (12%) strongly agreed. Olade (2003) reported that only 20% of the nurses she surveyed considered themselves adequate in regard to research, and several investigators (Kosteniuk, D'Arcy, Stewart, & Smith, 2006; Olade; Pravikoff et al., 2005; Winters et al., 2007) reported that respondents identified nursing colleagues as the information source most used even though professional isolation and distance can affect rural nurses' access to research knowledgeable colleagues.

Connecting rural nurses with knowledgeable research experts could be accomplished using the Internet; however, nurses who practice in rural settings are more likely to have inequitable access to information technology than their urban counterparts (Bushy, 2002; Winters et al., 2007). Rural nurses have indicated that their computer and Internet availability is limited because of computer location, lack of overall general computer knowledge (Winters et al.), and limited time to search for information (Olade, 2003; Winters et al.). Lack of time may also result from the variety of roles fulfilled by rural nurses during a typical work shift.

Isolation and distance are barriers that are a constant factor in rural nursing (Long & Weinert, 1989) and asking a coworker for his or her opinion on how to perform a task may be the most efficient way to complete the task. Role modeling the use of evidence by nursing leaders has been shown to influence rural nurses' use of research (Winters et al., 2007). Hospital administrators and nursing leaders in rural and remote facilities must become proactive in encouraging the use of evidence, perhaps through practice policies and procedures, affiliation with larger institutions or universities, and assignment of research mentors or collaborators, and by making access to evidence readily available to nursing staff through professional journal subscriptions, journal clubs, and accessible technology resources.

Nurses with differing levels of experience and education were included in the study reported here. In assessing attitudes and beliefs about research based on years of *rural nursing* experience, the nurses with the "worst" attitudes in this group were the nurses with more than 20 years of experience. The "worst" attitude finding may have resulted from research not being a part of their nursing curricula or the culture of rural nursing. It may also reflect lack of research applicable to rural nursing, the nurses' difficulty understanding research reports, and their preference for receiving information from peers rather than reading the literature. The "best" attitudes were found in the nurses with 1 to 5 years of experience, which may reflect their exposure to research content in their nursing programs.

When measuring attitudes and beliefs, those nurses with diploma, associate, and baccalaureate degrees were found to have similar attitudes (the "worst") and nurses who were master's prepared had the "best" attitudes. This may be due to the fact that most diploma and associate degree programs have little or no research education included in their curriculum, and, although baccalaureate level programs do require at least one research course, it may not be enough for a nurse to develop an appreciation of the importance of research or the skills required to understand and incorporate research into practice. Further study is needed to understand the relationship between years of experience and attitudes toward research.

The results of this study suggest that nurses working in the direct patient care roles, such as staff nurse or charge nurse, had the "worst" attitudes about research, and those nurses whose roles were more autonomous, such as that of nurse practitioner, public health nurse, manager/ supervisor, or executive, had the "best" attitudes. Perhaps nurses working in these latter roles have more access to technology, professional journals, and more time to utilize such resources. Providing access to research and a culture of expectation that practice is based on evidence is needed in order to move from a practice based on tradition to one based on evolving facts. More research is needed to explore nursing role and attributes such as autonomy and control as they relate to attitudes and beliefs about research.

Study Limitations

The statistics used for this study were descriptive. The sample size used for this secondary data analysis and the cohorts based on education, practice location, and years of experience are small, perhaps limited by the use of one reminder to complete the survey. Therefore, caution is required when drawing conclusions or generalizing the findings to all rural nurses. Because this was a secondary data analysis, no further information was obtained from participants and there was no control over the sample or how the original data were collected. More information could be gleaned from studying additional groups and cohorts. The nurses included in this study were persons living in the western United States, with the preponderance residing in Montana. This geographical location could have influenced the results because of differing socioeconomic issues, cultural differences, and varying distances to larger cities.

CONCULSIONS

The results of this study support the findings from others (Bushy, 2002; Kosteniuk et al., 2006; Olade, 2003) who reported that access to technology, education, and role are factors that affect rural nurses' attitudes and beliefs toward EBP. Further research is needed to explore the role that baccalaureate education plays in determining rural nurses' attitudes and beliefs toward EBP, specifically the type and number of research courses needed in a nursing curriculum in order for a nurse to be able to properly assess and critique research information. The results also suggest that although the nurses felt confident in their ability to evaluate the quality of research papers, they did not find research articles easy to understand and were unsure if they believed the results of the research that they read. Based on these findings, it is important for nursing educators teaching in universities and CE courses alike to include more education with respect to how to assess data for credibility and how to interpret research information.

Findings from this study support the need for research that examines the length of rural and nonrural experiences, and nursing position (i.e., staff nurse and charge nurse) on attitudes toward EBP. Findings from such studies will improve our understanding of rural nursing practice.

Furthermore, the results of this study support the relationship between master's education and attitudes and beliefs about EBP. These findings are in line with recommendations from the JC (Elements of Performance NR.2.10. B) for CAHs and other hospitals that educational factors be considered when appointing the nurse executive. If required of facilities, the element (EPs 2–6), "Whether the prospective nurse executive possesses the knowledge and skills associated with a master's degree in nursing or a related field or another appropriate postgraduate degree, or has a written plan to obtain these qualifications" (Joint Commission, 2006) may significantly impact rural nurses' attitudes and beliefs about research and increase the amount of practice that is evidence-based.

Nurses working in environments with a more positive culture, strong leadership, and lower rates of patient and staff adverse events report significantly more research utilization than nurses working in less positive environments (Estabrooks, Midodzi, Cummings, & Wallin, 2007). Given that nurses constitute the largest group of health care providers and their care influences patient outcomes (Aiken et al., 2003), the pressure on the nursing profession to strengthen the importance of EBP for all RNs is crucial.

REFERENCES

Aiken, L. H., Clarke, S. P., Cheung, R. B., Sloane, D. M., & Silber, J. H. (2003). Education Levels of Hospital Nurses and Surgical Patient Mortality. *The Journal of the American Medical Association, 290* (12), 1617–1623.

American Nurses Association (ANA). (2004) *Scope and Standards for Nurse Administrators* (2nd ed.). Washington, DC: nursesbooks.org

American Nurses Credentialing Center (ANCC). (2005). *Magnet Recognition Program for Recognizing Excellence in Nursing Services: Application Manual.* Washington, DC: Author.

Bushy, A. (2002). International perspectives on rural nursing: Australia, Canada, U.S.A. *Australian Journal of Rural Health, 10,* 104–111.

Case, B. (2004, April 1). Evidence-based practice: The future of nursing. *rn.com.* Retrieved September 2, 2007, from http://www.rn.com

Estabrooks, C. A. (1996). *Research utilization in nursing: Factors influencing the utilization and non-utilization of research by nurses.* Edmonton: University of Alberta.

Estabrooks, C. A., Midodzi, W. K., Cummings, G. G., & Wallin, L. (2007). Predicting research use in nursing organizations: A multilevel analysis. *Nursing Research, 56* (4, Suppl. 1), S7.

Funk, S. G., Champagne, M. T., Wiese, R. A., & Tornquist, E. M. (1991). Barriers to using research findings in practice: The clinician's perspective. *Applied Nursing Research, 4* (2), 90–95.

Funk, S. G., Tornquist, E. M., & Champagne, M. T. (1995). Research utilization: Reconnecting research and practice. *AACN Clinical Issues, 6,* 105–109.

Goode, C. J., Pinkerton, S., McCausland, M. P., Southard, P., Graham, R., & Krsek, C. (2001). Documenting chief nursing officers' preference for BSN-prepared nurses. *Journal of Nursing Administration, 31* (2), 55–59.

Hommelstad, J., & Cornelia, R. (2004). Norwegian nurses' perceived barriers and facilitators to research use. *AORN Journal, 79* (3), 621–634.

Joint Commission (JC). (2006, November). *Joint Commission Perspectives, 26* (11), 10–11.

Joint Commission (JC). (2008). *Accreditation Programs: Hospital National Patient Safety Goals.* Retrieved March 1, 2009, from http://www.jointcommission.org/PatientSafety/NationalPatientSafetyGoals/09_hap_npsgs.htm

Kosteniuk, J. G., D'Arcy, C., Stewart, N., & Smith, B. (2006). Central and peripheral information source use among rural and remote registered nurses. *Journal of Advanced Nursing, 55* (1), 100–113.

Lee, H. J., & McDonagh, M. K. (2006). Examining the rural nursing theory base. In *Rural nursing concepts, theory, and practice* (2nd ed., pp. 17–26). New York: Springer.

Long, K.A., & Weinert, C. (1989). Rural nursing: Developing the theory base. *Scholarly Inquiry for Nursing Practice: An International Journal 3,* 113–127. New York: Springer.

Luparell, S., Winters, C., Lee, H., O'Lynn, C., Shreffler-Grant, J., & Hendrickx, L. (2006a). *Rural nurses' access to and use of research in practice.* Unpublished raw data.

Luparell, S., Winters, C., Lee, H., O'Lynn, C., Shreffler-Grant, J., & Hendrickx, L. (2006b). *Rural nurses' access to and use of research in practice* (pp. 1–9) [Questionnaire].

McKenna, H., Ashton, S., & Keeney, S. (2004). Barriers to evidence-based practice in nursing and healthcare. *Journal of Advanced Nursing, 45* (2), 178–189.

Melnyk, B. M., Fineout-Overholt, E., Feinstein, N. F., Li, H., Small, L., Wilcox, L., et al. (2004). Nurses' perceived knowledge, beliefs, skills, and needs in regarding evidence-based practice: Implications for accelerating the paradigm shifts. *Worldviews on Evidence-Based Nursing, 1* (3), 185–193.

Melnyk, B. M., Fineout-Overholt, E., Feinstein, N. F., Sadler, L. S., Green-Hernandez, C. (2008). Nurse practitioner educators' perceived knowledge, beliefs, and teaching strategies regarding evidence-based practice: Implications for accelerating the integration of evidence-based practice into graduate programs. *Journal of Professional Nursing, 1,* 7–13.

Merriam-Webster. (2007). *Merriam-Webster Medical Dictionary.* New York: Merriam-Webster.

Morrison, E. (1998). Erroneous beliefs about research held by staff nurses. *Journal of Continuing Education in Nursing, 29* (5), 196–203. Abstract retrieved July 29, 2007, from http://eric.ed.gov/ERICWebPortal/cU.S.tom/portlets/recordDetails/detailmini. jsp?_nfpb=true

Munroe, D., Duffy, P., & Fisher, C. (2006). Fostering evidence-based practice in a rural community hospital. *Journal of Nursing Administration, 36* (11), 510–512.

Olade, R. A. (2003). Attitudes and factors affecting research utilization. *Nursing Forum, 38* (4), 6–15.

Olade, R. A. (2004). Evidence-based practice and research utilization activities among rural nurses. *Clinical Scholarship, 36* (3), 220–225.

Ouzts, K. (2005). Evidence-based practice and information literacy skills in rural nurses [Abstract]. *Communicating Nursing Research, 38* (13), 287.

Parsons, J. E., Merlin, T. L., Taylor, J. E., Wilkinson, D., & Hiller, J. E. (2003). Evidence-based practice in rural and remote clinical practice: Where is the evidence? *Australian Journal of Rural Health, 11* (5), 242–248.

Pravikoff, D. S., Tanner, A. B., & Pierce, S. T. (2005). Readiness of U.S. nurses for evidence-based practice. *American Journal of Nursing, 105* (9), 40–51.

Rawnsley, M. M. (2003). Dimensions of scholarship and the advancement of nursing science: Articulating a vision. *Nursing Science Quarterly, 16* (1), 6–15.

Rizzuto, C., Bostrom, J., Suter, W. N., & Chenitz, W. C. (1994). Predictors of nurses' involvement in research activities. *Western Journal of Nursing Research, 16* (2), 193–204.

Scharff, J. E. (1998). The distinctive nature and scope of rural nursing practice: Philosophical bases. In H.J. Lee (Ed.), *Conceptual Basis for Rural Nursing* (pp. 19–38). New York: Springer.

Smirnoff, M., Ramirez, M., Kooplimae, L., Gibney, M., & McEvoy, M. (2007). Nurses' attitudes toward nursing research at a metropolitan medical center. *Applied Nursing Research, 20* (1), 24–31.

Tanner, A., Pierce, S., & Pravikoff, D. (2004). Readiness for evidence-based practice: Information literacy needs of nurses in the United States. *MEDINFO 2004, 936*–940. Retrieved August 24, 2008, from http://www.cmbi.bjmu.edu.cn/news/report/2004/medinfo2004/pdffiles/papers/4770Tanner.pdf

Taylor, J., Wilkinson, D., & Blue, I. (2001). Towards evidence-based general practice in rural and remote Australia: An overview of key issues and a model for practice. *Rural and Remote Health, 1* (106). Retrieved October 21, 2007, from http://rrh.deakin.edu.au

United States Department of Agriculture (USDA) Economic Research Service. (2007). *Measuring rurality: Rural urban continuum codes.* Retrieved September 3, 2007, from http://www.ers.usda.gov/Briefing/Rurality/RuralUrbCon/

Winters, C. A., Lee, H. J., Besel, J., Strand, A., Echeverri, R., Jorgensen, K. P., et al. (2007). Access to and use of research by rural nurses. *Rural and Remote Health 7,* 758. Retrieved August 24, 2008 from, http://www.rrh.org.au

Winters, C. A., Lee, H. J., O'Lynn, C., Schreffler-Grant, M. J., Edge, D., McDonagh, M., et al. (2006). [Health research: Accessible, applicable and useable for rural & remote health practitioners.] Unpublished raw data.

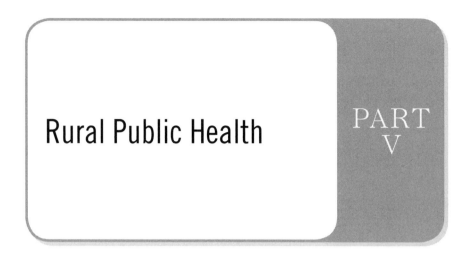

Rural Public Health

PART
V

Public Health Emergency Preparedness in Rural or Frontier Areas

21

SANDRA W. KUNTZ, JANE SMILIE, and
MELANIE REYNOLDS

Preparedness for public health emergencies, including intentional, technological, or natural disasters has become a continuing national initiative in small and large communities across the United States following the September 11, 2001, terrorist attacks. Although one of the six goals of public health includes "response to disasters and assistance to communities in recovery" (Public Health Functions Steering Committee, 1994, p. 1), most local public health agencies prior to the World Trade Center attack and subsequent anthrax events had few resources and limited specific directives for addressing the disaster objective (Department of Justice [DOJ], 2000; Henderson, 1998; Wetter, Daniell, & Treser, 2001). Early efforts to bolster the sagging public health infrastructure included reprioritizing the critical need for "response" and "assistance" and adding "preparedness" of the public health system and workforce to increase response capacities during significant events (Gebbie, 2002; Koplan, 2001).

Congressional funding and focused local and national efforts have resulted in gradual but significant public health infrastructure improvements since the 2001 incidents. However, despite the positive changes, the American Public Health Association (2002) noted the following unmet service needs in some communities: "[C]oordination at a regional (and local) level is still lacking . . . preparation in rural areas falls behind the level of preparedness in major metropolitan areas" (p. 3). To learn more about local preparedness capacities, the Centers for Disease Control and Prevention (CDC) funded states to conduct an assessment of local public health agencies (counties and tribes) to determine the current preparedness status and needs. The central aim of this chapter is to examine the qualitative description of challenges and benefits encountered by local public health agencies in Montana when they partner for preparedness with local emergency planning committees (LEPCs) and tribal emergency response commissions (TERCs). There is general agreement that a coordinated response is required in order to address natural events such as pandemic influenza or a hurricane; technological disasters such as a plane crash or mining accident; or, an intentional biological, radiological, or chemical event.

BACKGROUND AND SIGNIFICANCE

In 1986, Congress passed the Emergency Planning and Community Right to Know Act, also known as the Superfund Amendments and Reauthorization Act (SARA). The intent of this law was in part to develop community-based local emergency planning committees to protect the public's health and safety and the environment from chemical hazards (U.S. Code, 1986). Fifteen years after the SARA legislation, Lindell and Perry (2001) questioned the status of implementation of SARA at the local level including the required LEPC. Landesman and Leonard (1993) found that when an LEPC existed in a community, hospitals and public health agencies were often not included or had simply failed to become active in LEPC meetings and activities.

Public health emergency preparedness requires an all-hazard approach and a wide-range of sustainable public health workforce skills and competencies. Officials of the CDC's 2002 Public Health Practice Program Office stated that "establishing relationships among public health system partners is likely the most critical aspect of emergency (preparedness) and response" (p. 1). Evidence of dynamic, transforming, and often synergistic outcomes related to intersectoral partnerships and complex community problems (substance abuse, teen pregnancy, violence) is documented by researchers (Florin, Mitchell, Stevenson, & Klein, 2000; Lasker, Weiss, & Miller, 2001; Mattessich, Murray-Close, & Monsey, 2001; Polivka, Dresbach, Heimlich, & Elliott, 2001). For the Community Tracking Study, McHugh, Staiti, and Felland (2004) collected data through telephone and in person semistructured interviews from 12 metropolitan statistical areas. Results show that readiness was related to (a) previous experience with public health emergencies, (b) adequate funding, (c) successful collaboration, and (d) strong leadership. These themes could help guide policy and funding decisions as federal and state agencies search for the most efficient and effective preparedness tools and methods.

No study to date has described the qualitative aspects of the rural preparedness experience. The categorical differences between frontier spaces and urban places create a great divide in capacity to mobilize, educate, and sustain the workforce. In some rural areas, a volunteer workforce partners for emergency preparedness and other public health concerns (Reynolds & Leahy, 2002). Cowie, Elder, and Leibowitz (2000) made the following observations regarding local emergency response capacity: "Frontier facts are simple. There are probably no or few paid responders, outdated or nonexistent equipment, no tax base, no time to train, and possibly no active local emergency planning committee (LEPC) as required by law" (p. 6).

In Montana, 45 of 56 (80%) counties are classified as *frontier* with a population density of 6 or fewer people per square mile, and 10 of 56 (18%) counties are categorized as *rural* with more than 6 but fewer than 50 people per square mile. Yellowstone County is the only urban county with 51.9 people per square mile. Just three counties include metropolitan areas with at least one city with 50,000 or more inhabitants; these cities are Billings, Missoula, and Great Falls (Montana County Profiles, 2004). The public health workforce consists of a variety of professionals employed by counties and tribes including nurses (47%), sanitarians (32%), health educators (16%), and registered dieticians (5%) (Montana County Profiles, 2004). In large and small counties, nurses serve in a range of roles from health officer to public health caseworker. In some frontier counties, the nurse is the only part-time or full-time public health employee.

According to the Montana Department of Public Health and Human Services (MDPHHS) (2003) statewide capacity assessment report, 26% of respondent counties reported they had been a member of a LEPC for less than 6 months; 19% had been members for under one year; and 10% were not currently members but were considering joining a committee. Most of the "new member" respondents were from the smallest frontier counties with total populations under 10,000. Most of the respondents who had been members of a LEPC for over 1 year were from large counties with populations over 20,000. With over half of Montana's counties in the early stages of partnering for preparedness, exploring public health perception regarding the collaborative experience is timely and could inform future development and sustainability efforts. Therefore, the question for this study was: How does the rural Montana public health workforce perceive the challenges and benefits of partnering for preparedness?

METHOD

The 2002 Montana Public Health Emergency Preparedness and Response Capacity Assessment (PHEPRCA) conducted by the MDPHHS (2002) provided the data for this study. Lead local public health agency officials, their designee, or a selected team of individuals with expertise from inside and outside the agency completed the assessment. The paper and pencil, 61–page survey came with a projected time commitment of approximately 24 hours. The University of Montana Technical Assistance Center provided help, answered questions, and supplied local technical assistance to counties and tribes across the state throughout the assessment time period. An initial training session was held to explain the purpose, process, and expectations of the PHEPRCA to local officials. At the end of the day-long session, the survey was distributed with full instructions, technical assistance contact information, and a 12–week time period for submitting the completed survey for contract reimbursement. The overall PHEPRCA response rate was 84% with 50 of the 56 counties (89%) and three of seven tribes (43%) participating in the capacity assessment.

The extensive PHEPRCA data set provided opportunity for four types of analyses. First, data were entered into SPSS version 11.5 for Windows, and analyzed by the University of Washington, Northwest Center for Public Health Practice generating descriptive counts, frequencies, and means. These results were reported in regional and statewide summaries. In addition, each local agency received an individual jurisdiction report. Second, the data were analyzed by Smilie (2003) and Kuntz (2004) to investigate preparedness levels and establish a matrix for scoring preparedness. Third, Kuntz investigated the relationship between preparedness and collaboration. The fourth study and the focus of this chapter emerged from two qualitative PHEPRCA questions. The two open-ended questions included in the survey helped to identify key components of the preparedness experience in rural and frontier areas. The first qualitative question asked, "What is the greatest challenge your agency has experienced in joining or leading a LEPC?" The second question queried, "What is the greatest benefit your agency has experienced in joining or leading a LEPC?"

Data Analysis

We used textual discourse analysis (Denzin & Lincoln, 1998) to identify "themes, issues and recurring motifs" (p. 43). Data from the two questions were entered into a Microsoft Access database. In the first analysis phase, we identified primary themes. In the second phase, we sorted themes based on county population data. For this study, we stratified counties by population number rather than population density (see Table 21.1). This designation allowed for greater stratification of the frontier counties. The three population categories included 33 small frontier counties (population < 10,000), 8 medium frontier counties (population between 10,000 and 20,000), and 9 rural counties (population > 20,000). We incorporated reservation data into the county counts to avoid the possibility of identifying specific Native American groups. All seven Indian Nations have population numbers of fewer than 10,000 people so we counted them with the small frontier groups for this research.

Table 21.1

RESPONDENT CHARACTERISTICS: POPULATION DENSITY, AGENCY STAFFING

CHARACTERISTIC	ALL JURISDICTIONS REPORTING ($n = 50$)	SMALL FRONTIER ($n = 33$)	MEDIUM FRONTIER ($n = 8$)	RURAL ($n = 9$)
Population (M)	16,358	4,663	12,840	66,746
Agency Staff FTE				
Range	0–90.0	0–13.2	0–10.0	6.0–90.0
M	8.8	2.7	4.4	38.8
SD	18.32	2.81	3.01	31.95

Note: Small frontier = < 10,000 in jurisdiction; medium frontier = 10,000–20,000; rural = > 20,000; FTE = full-time equivalent. From MDPHHS (2003).

FINDINGS

Two primary themes emerged from the thematic analysis. Respondent answers to both open-ended questions could be categorized as either agency-based or partnership-based perceptions related to both challenges and benefits. Agency-based perceptions referenced internal organizational issues. Partnership-based perceptions alluded to the external collaborative formed with other agencies to address preparedness issues. Four themes in each category of "challenges" emerged. Table 21.2 shows the challenges cited by all respondents according to the themed responses made by small frontier (< 10,000), medium frontier (10,000–20,000) and rural (> 20,000) local public health agencies. Table 21.3 identifies the primary themes related to benefits of partnering for preparedness and differentiates the themed responses made by small frontier (< 10,000), medium frontier (10,000–20,000), and rural (> 20,000) local public health agencies. Because frontier agencies (both small and medium) outnumber rural agencies by 4:1 and respondent agencies listed different numbers of challenges and benefits, our intent of Tables 21.2 and 21.3 focuses on acknowledging differences rather than serving as a comparison between jurisdiction types.

Table 21.2

PREPAREDNESS CHALLENGE RESPONSES OF ALL AGENCIES STRATIFIED BY LOCAL PUBLIC HEALTH AGENCY

	JURISDICTION SIZE		
TYPE OF CHALLENGE	SF	MF	R
Agency-Based			
Time Constraints (*n* = 11)	7	2	2
Human Resources (*n* = 11)	8	3	—
Generating Interest or Overcoming Apathy (*n* = 8)	6	—	2
Fiscal Resources (*n* = 11)	10	1	—
Partnership-Based			
Organizational Coordination (*n* = 19)	9	5	5
Communication (*n* = 4)	2	1	1
Turf (*n* = 5)	1	3	1
Roles and Inclusion (*n* = 8)	8	—	—

Note: SF = small, frontier < 10,000 population in jurisdiction (*n* = 30); MF = medium, frontier 10,000–20,000 population in jurisdiction (*n* = 7); R = rural > 20,000 population in jurisdiction (*n* = 9).

Table 21.3

PREPAREDNESS BENEFIT RESPONSES OF ALL AGENCIES STRATIFIED BY
LOCAL PUBLIC HEALTH JURISDICTION SIZE

	JURISDICTION SIZE		
TYPE OF BENEFIT	SF	MF	R
Agency-Based			
Networking (*n* = 18)	11	3	4
Recognition or Respect (*n* = 15)	10	4	1
Increased Disaster Awareness (*n* = 8)	7	1	—
Partnership-Based			
Effort Synergy (*n* = 14)	6	35	—
Resource Sharing (*n* = 12)	9	1	2
Education/Training (*n* = 9)	7	2	—

Note: SF = small, frontier < 10,000 population in jurisdiction (*n* = 30); MF = medium, frontier
10,000–20,000 population in jurisdiction (*n* = 7); R = Rural > 20,000 population in jurisdiction (*n* = 9).

Perceptions Related to Challenges

Coordinating efforts among partners, time constraints, and the need
for fiscal and human resources represented the most commonly cited
challenges to partnering for preparedness in Montana (see Table
21.2). With so many pressing public health issues, generating interest,
overcoming apathy, and establishing a sense of commitment aimed
toward preparedness efforts confronts local agencies. Turf, role, and
inclusion surfaced as issues with comments indicating some public
health representatives search for purpose and identity in previously
organized groups. Some comments related to frontier agency status
included few employees covering numerous mandates with limited
funding. Respondents from frontier counties most often mentioned
agency-based challenges, whereas participants from larger rural counties with normally more fiscal and human resources named partnership-based issues as the primary point of concern. The following
comments are representative of the challenges related to partnering
for preparedness:

> [It is difficult to] maintain momentum between perceived threats. (Rural)
> Our agency has a kind of "New Kid on the Block" feeling but the LEPC
> [the local emergency planning committee] seems willing to accept public
> health. (Small, Frontier)

Difficult communication between public health and the DES [department of emergency services] coordinator. (Rural)

The RN in the Health Department works part time. All emergency group members work full time and volunteer countless hours as EMTs, firemen, etc. There isn't much time for more group meetings. (Small, Frontier)

Our involvement is in the early stages—everything is challenging. (Small, Frontier)

We have been attending these meetings for ten years. We feel like a part of their meetings. No challenges at the moment. (Rural)

Educating the group about the role public health plays in emergency preparedness is a big challenge. (Small, Frontier)

Public health has not been recognized as a "player" and I've had difficulty determining my role in the group [i.e., what I can offer]. I have progressed but I still need role/responsibility clarification. (Small, Frontier)

LEPC seems to be a back-burner item in our county. Public health has been sharing bioterrorism information but no LEPC meetings have been held despite requests by this agency for the same. (Small, Frontier)

The same people are involved in many organizations and everyone is involved in too many things to attend. Also, it is challenging to avoid stepping on someone else's toes. (Small, Frontier)

Perceptions Related to Benefits

The most prevalent theme from the benefits question was the perception that synergy was possible through joining forces to develop preparedness plans—opposed to going it alone (see Table 21.3). Several agency respondents mentioned that preparedness partnering seemed to strengthen cooperation and coordination among agencies on other community issues. Although garnering respect for public health contributions was noted as a challenge, the act of participating in partnership activities helped raise recognition of and respect for public health contributions so was listed as a benefit by some agencies. Another important acknowledged benefit is the advantage gained when public health personnel train alongside emergency response personnel and other providers.

Sample comments representative of the benefits question posed to local agency personnel include the following:

Networking with other agencies strengthens each participating agency in preparedness as well as other community projects. (Medium, Frontier)

Becoming a partner and networking; experiencing some nontraditional partnering. (Small, Frontier)

Legitimacy as a player in the emergency response field—also access to individuals for follow-up. (Medium, Frontier)

Introduction to all agencies and person's responsible for agencies; knowing resources available from each agency. (Small, Frontier)

Brainstorming with others and having a local group resource base to work with coalition building. (Small, Frontier)

Getting to know key contacts in case of an emergency; fostering better communication between LEPC and public health; sharing resources and information; learning from drills and follow-up critiques. (Small, Frontier)

Our ability to respond seamlessly and well to the community's public health needs in an emergency on all levels [county, tribal, state, and federal]. (Rural)

System for gaining access to resources from other agencies. (Rural)

DISCUSSIONS AND RECOMMENDATIONS

Data collected through the open-ended questions on the Montana PHEPRCA provide beginning insight into key challenges and benefits associated with public health agency partnering for preparedness. Gray (1989) characterized collaboration as "a process through which parties who see different aspects of a problem can constructively explore their differences and search for solutions that go beyond their own limited vision of what is possible" (p. 5). Although collaboration is a complex process, survey participants acknowledged the possible synergistic effects of interagency collaboration. Networking opportunities improved public health disaster response infrastructure and contributed to other community-based projects. Although not specifically mentioned, joint training and educational opportunities help professionals develop a common language and an appreciation for the skills, knowledge, contributions, and points of view of others (Butler, Cohen, Friedman, Scripp, & Watz, 2002).

We captured several differences between frontier and rural counties in this investigation. First, the test faced by frontier counties to meet a wide range of service area needs, including the complexities of preparedness, may help explain statements regarding the burden disaster preparedness puts on limited fiscal and human resources. This reality might support sharing resources in a regional approach to preparedness planning and response while maintaining and preserving local identity and unique needs. Secondly, larger rural jurisdictions are more likely to be an established partner in a LEPC. Partnering is a dynamic and transforming process but requires time, skill, commitment, and interest. As more local public health agencies become active contributors in a LEPC, the potential synergistic effects could raise awareness and help identify ways of extending the public health effort toward disaster and other critical issues. Finally, additional qualitative research focusing on public health professionals and their partnership experiences in rural and frontier communities is needed to learn more about successful efforts to strengthen response to disasters and public health essential service number 4, "mobilize community partnerships to identify and solve health problems" (Public Health Functions Steering Committee, 1994, p. 1).

REFERENCES

American Public Health Association. (2002). *One year after the terrorist attacks: Is public health prepared? A report card from the American Public Health Association.* Retrieved October 19, 2002, from http://www.apha.org/united

Butler, J., Cohen, M., Friedman, C., Scripp, R., & Watz, C. (2002). Collaboration between public health and law enforcement: New paradigms and partnerships for bioterrorism planning and response. *Emerging Infectious Disease, 8* (10). Retrieved December 2002 from http://www.cdc.gov/neidod/EID/ Vol8no10/02–0400.htm

Centers for Disease Control and Prevention (CDC). (2002). *Local public health preparedness and response capacity inventory: A voluntary rapid self-assessment* (Local Version 1.1). Retrieved December 2002 from http://www.phppo.cdc.gov/od/ inventory/

Cowie, F., Elder, M., & Leibowitz, R. (2000). *Realistic approaches to rural and frontier hazardous materials risk management.* Retrieved June 28, 2002, from http://www.state.mt.us/dma/des/Library/Frontier_HazMat.pdf

Denzin, N., & Lincoln, Y. (1998). *Collecting and interpreting qualitative materials.* Thousand Oaks, CA: Sage.

Department of Justice (DOJ). (2000). *Public health performance assessment: Emergency preparedness.* Retrieved September 5, 2000, from http://www.phppo.cdc.gov/Home-landsec6rants/Images/Do.15_41May4.pdf

Drexler, M. (2002). *Secret agents: The menace of emerging infections.* Washington, DC: Joseph Henry.

Florin, P., Mitchell, R., Stevenson, J., & Klein, I. (2000). Predicting intermediate outcomes for prevention coalitions: A developmental perspective. *Evaluation and Program Planning, 23,* 341–346.

Gebbie, K. (2002, November 12). *Bioterrorism and emergency readiness: Competencies for all public health workers* (Preview Version II). New York: Columbia University School of Nursing.

Gray, B. (1989). *Collaborating: Finding common ground for multiparty problems.* San Francisco: Jossey-Bass.

Henderson, D. (1998). Bioterrorism as a public health threat. *Emerging Infectious Disease, 4* (3), 1–6. Retrieved November 20, 2001, from http:www.cdc.gov/ncidod/eid/vol4no31/hendrsn.htm

Koplan, J. (2001, November). *Building infrastructure to protect the public's health.* Paper presented at the National Public Health Training Network [Satellite Downlink from Atlanta, GA].

Kuntz, S. (2004). Association between collaboration and bioterrorism preparedness in Montana: A local rural public health agency perspective. (Publication #: 3126263). Retrieved May 27, 2004, from http://www.hsls.pitt.edu/guides/histmed/researchresources/dissertations/dissertations.html?topic_id = 12&mmth = 2004/12

Landesman, L., & Leonard, R. (1993). SARA three years later. *Prehospital Disaster Medicine, 8* (1), 39–44.

Lasker, R., Weiss, E., & Miller, R. (2001). Partnership synergy: A practical framework for studying and strengthening the collaborative advantage. *The Milbank Quarterly, 79* (2), 179–205.

Lindell, M., & Perry, R. (2001). Community innovation in hazardous materials management: Progress in implementing SARA Title III in the United States. *Journal of Hazardous Materials, 88,* 169–194.

Mattessich, P., Murray-Close, M., & Monsey, B. (2001). *Collaboration: What makes it work* (2nd ed.). St. Paul, MN: Amherst H. Wilder Foundation.

McHugh, M., Staiti, A., & Felland, L. (2004). How prepared are Americans for public health emergencies: Twelve communities weigh in. *Health Affairs, 23,* 201–209.

Montana County Profiles. (2004). Retrieved January 15, 2005, from http://www.dphhs.state.mt.us/hpsd/pubheal/healplan/profiles/

Montana Department of Public Health and Human Services (MDPHHS). (2002). Montana's public health preparedness and response to bioterrorism and other public health threats and emergencies. Cooperative Agreement with the Centers for Disease Control and Prevention (U90/CCU816832–03–1).

Montana Department of Public Health and Human Services (MDPHHS). (2003). *An assessment of Montana's capacity to respond to a public health emergency: Statewide report.* Seattle: University of Washington, Northwest Center for Public Health Practice.

Polivka, B., Dresbach, S., Heimlich, J., & Elliott, M. (2001). Interagency relationships among rural early intervention collaboratives. *Public Health Nursing, 18,* 340–349.

Public Health Functions Steering Committee. (1994). *Public health in America.* Retrieved October 2001 from http://www.health.gov/phfunctions/public.htm

Reynolds, M., & Leahy, E. (2002). Developing a public health training institute through public health improvement efforts: Montana's story. *Journal of Public Health Management Practice, 8* (1), 83–91.

Smilie, J. (2003, May 2). *Using your preparedness capacity assessment results to conduct a gap analysis.* Paper presented at MDPHHS Public Health Emergency Preparedness and Response Program, Helena, MT.

U.S. Code. 1986. Title 42, Chapter 116. *Emergency planning and community right-to-know.* Retrieved June 28, 2002, from http://www4.law.cornell.edu/uscode/42/ch116.html

Weiss, E., Miller, R., & Lasker, R. (2001). *Findings from the national study of partnership functioning: Report to the partnerships that participated.* New York: Center for the Advancement of Collaborative Strategies in Health.

Wetter, D., Daniell, W., & Treser, C. (2001). Hospital preparedness for victims of chemical or biological terrorism. *American Journal of Public Health, 91,* 710–716.

22

Environmental Risk Reduction for Rural Children

WADE G. HILL and PATRICIA BUTTERFIELD

Rural living is often portrayed as inherently healthy and wholesome, with children enjoying the benefits of fresh air and clean water. The idealized view of rural life is perpetuated by what some have referred to as the "agrarian myth," in which youngsters thrive on living away from the artificiality and materialism of cities (Kelsey, 1994). However, the realities of rural living and their requisite patterns of environmental exposure are complex, dynamic, and multidimensional. Exposure risks to children vary by place, time, and age. The risks also vary by parents' occupations, seasonal changes, and jurisdictional policies addressing the use and disposal of local toxicants. Each of these factors, plus many more, creates a complicated web of exposures that influence current and future risks of disease. Exposure patterns in children are so multifaceted that it is not unusual to see very different measures of exposure among three or four children living under the same roof. Such are the challenges in understanding environmental health risks to children living in rural communities.

However, the challenges inherent in assessing complex exposures in children are, in many ways, dwarfed by the ability of the current health care system to document patterns of exposure in groups at risk. Neither exposures to biologic and chemical agents nor their potential health consequences (e.g., asthma, neurodegenerative diseases) are recorded systematically in medical databases. Health professionals have a superficial understanding of only the most prevalent exposures (e.g., lead) and are typically at a loss to answer clients' questions about other common exposure risks (e.g., pesticides, solvents, metals).

For more than 200 years, rural areas have been considered the "dumping ground" of a production-based economy. Items (e.g., nuclear waste, antiquated military supplies) and activities (e.g., mining, smelting) considered dangerous, distasteful, or requiring large plots of land have been preferentially located in remote parts of the country. Contaminants from such historic activities have left a legacy of risks for local residents. Because the contamination is not routinely discovered until decades later, the culpable group can no longer be located and the community must rely on federal resources for cleanup and remediation resources. Typically, rural municipalities lack both the financial, technical, and scientific expertise (e.g., laboratories, behavioral researchers) to understand local exposures and their commensurate health risks. Small county and regional health departments, which have been understaffed and over-mandated since September 11, 2001, often field questions about environmental risks in their area, but lack the time and money to fully pursue investigative efforts. Rural families who live in unincorporated areas may live adjacent to agricultural (e.g., combined animal feeding operations) and industrial facilities, but may be unaware of risks associated with such facilities.

Development

Despite risk patterns that may pose a threat to young children, contaminant patterns in rural communities are understudied and rural citizens are often underrepresented in environmental health research (Malcoe, Lynch, Keger, & Skaggs, 2002). Research in rural communities has focused almost exclusively on the sequelae from a specific agent (e.g., mercury, arsenic) or contaminant site (e.g., Environmental Protection Agency [EPA] Superfund site). Such research has provided an important foundation about the health consequences of living adjacent to a mine, railroad yard, or waste disposal site. However, examining environmental health risks from a single agent perspective provides a myopic view of risks to a family or community, rather than providing families with answers about their overall health risks and what they can do to minimize such risks.

Requirements of rural nursing practice necessarily follow trends in the health status of populations, demographic changes, and the dynamic nature of the determinants of health, illness, and safety. From a population view, perhaps no segment of our society requires more attention in promoting health than young children. It is known that the most rapid mental growth occurs during early childhood and that the early years are critical in the development of intelligence, personality, and social behavior (Bellamy, 2002). Equally important is an understanding that children are particularly susceptible to environmental exposures, as the exploratory behaviors of childhood are the principle ways that children learn (Moya, Bearer, & Etzel, 2004).

Rural nurses have a unique opportunity to identify and intervene in cases where environmental exposures to children exist. Despite commonly held notions that rural environments offer isolation from environmental contaminants, many rural areas offer the most potent environmental exposures in the United States. For example, the state of Montana currently has 11 sites of industrial contamination listed on the National Priority List (Superfund), and ranks among the top 20% of states in land releases of toxic contaminants (Scorecard.org, 2004). Although rural childhood environmental exposures may result from effluents of extractive industries or other industrial sites, many chronic environmental exposures occur within the home where caregivers and nurses have significant capacity for intervention. By employing common sense low-cost behaviors, caregivers of young children can prevent environmental exposures that may manifest in negative health outcomes.

ENVIRONMENTAL RISK REDUCTION THROUGH NURSING INTERVENTION AND EDUCATION

The Environmental Risk Reduction through Nursing Intervention and Education (ERRNIE) study is a 5-year project designed primarily to (a) determine the prevalence of multiple environmental exposures among rural children, and (b) deliver and evaluate environmental risk reduction education to rural households by public health nurses through a randomized controlled trial. Because nurses generally feel unprepared to manage environmental health issues (Van Dongen, 2002), the ERRNIE project will also evaluate the capacity and needs of public health nurses to integrate environmental health into their practice. The ERRNIE project capitalizes on the existing public health infrastructure that currently accesses at-risk populations through programs such as Women, Infants, and Children (WIC), immunization clinics, and the Head Start program, among others. Childhood exposures of interest in the ERRNIE study are those that occur in or around homes and include environmental tobacco smoke (ETS), radon, carbon monoxide (CO), lead, and impurities in well water. In the discussion that follows, we focus on the first objective of the ERRNIE study to determine the prevalence of multiple environmental exposures among rural children.

The conceptual basis for the ERRNIE project is the World Health Organizations Multiple Exposures Multiple Effects (MEME) model first described in the report, "Making a Difference: Indicators to Improve Children's Environmental Health" (Briggs, 2003). This model suggests that neither exposures nor health indicators can be interpreted in simple direct relationships and that health outcomes should be viewed in terms of actions and contexts as well as exposures. The MEME model proposes that the exposure and health outcome dichotomy exists within contextual conditions (e.g., social, economic, and demographic conditions) that may influence the nature of the relationship. This idea agrees with the assumption of the ERRNIE project that rural environments offer unique risk factors for environmental exposures, such as lack of municipal water, sewage treatment, and housing regulations. The MEME model also portrays the home environment as the most proximal location for employing preventive actions to limit exposures associated with health outcomes (see Figure 22.1).

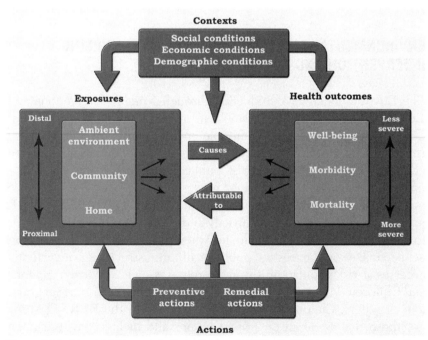

Figure 22.1. The MEME model. From Briggs (2003), © World Health Organization. Reprinted with permission.

METHODS

Design

Because Phase I of the ERRNIE project attempts to understand the prevalence of multiple environmental contaminants among rural children, the project staff used a cross-sectional correlational design. Project staff recruited eligible households through the local public health agency in Gallatin County, Montana. To be eligible for the study, each household had to be located in Gallatin County, be receiving public health services, have at least one child under six years of age, use a private or community well as the primary source of drinking water, and read or speak English fluently. Following referral from the local public health agency, ERRNIE project staff contacted each household to establish a date for home visitation and to establish a primary household respondent. Staff mailed questionnaires to each household prior to the home visit eliciting data on demographics, household characteristics, risk reduction behaviors, occupational risks, environmental exposure risk perceptions, and children's developmental and health histories. During the home visit ERRNIE staff collected consents and questionnaires from the household respondent and performed the necessary tests on five potential exposures of interest: (a) CO, (b) lead, (c) ETS, (d) well water contaminants, and (e) household radon.

Home and Biomarker Testing

Staff tested CO with a portable CO monitor (Series 450, Dwyer Instruments, Michigan City, IN) following an established protocol that included an assessment of primary and secondary gas heat sources, gas water heaters, gas range tops and ovens, and gas dryers. They tested individual appliances followed by a total system induction in which they turned on all gas appliances and tested each appliance. The staff established action level for CO exposures at 9 ppm and referred values at or above this level to the local health department and the client's health care provider. Additionally, staff advised clients not to use the appliance until it had been retested by the local fire department or energy provider (testing is free) and provided health education concerning the cause and health effects of CO exposure.

The project staff also tested each child in the household for exposure to lead and ETS. They accomplished lead testing by using blood lead collection filter paper (Tamarack Medical Lab, Centennial, CO) and a single finger-stick for each child. Action levels for lead exposure were set conservatively at 5 (μ)g/dL; staff retested all values at or above this level for confirmation and trend analysis and referred them to the local public health department and clients' health care providers for follow-up. They also collected urine samples (2–3 ml) from household children to assess ETS exposure through cotinine assay (Mayo Medical Laboratories, Rochester, MN). There was no established action level for ETS exposure, but staff provided education regarding health effects of passive smoke exposure for all positive findings.

Lastly, staff assessed possible contaminants from well water and household radon. They collected water samples from each household for a complete well screen (Montana Department of Public Health, Environmental Laboratory) including the assessment of bacteria, nitrates, metals (e.g., lead, arsenic), anions (e.g., sulfate, fluoride), petroleum, and pesticides or herbicides. Because of the complexity of water chemistry and the number of possible contaminants evaluated, a water quality expert evaluated each case independently and performed appropriate follow-up testing and referral for abnormal findings. Staff left a short-term charcoal radon test (DRHOMEAIR, Alpha Energy Laboratories, Carrollton, TX) with each household after reviewing the instructions for performing the test with the primary household respondent. Staff provided any household with a radon level exceeding 4 pCi/L (EPA established action level) a long-term radon test as well as referral back to the health department and their usual medical provider for follow-up.

FINDINGS

Sample Description

Thirty-one rural households were referred from the local health department in Gallatin County, Montana, and consented to participate in the ERRNIE project. Each household had an average of 2 adults (range 1–5) and 2 children (range 1–5) and the primary household respondents were female (100%), aged 21–40 (94%), and Caucasian (97%). Consistent with a population receiving public health services, 58% of the sample either had no source of health insurance or were receiving Medicaid and generally had total household incomes of less than $35,000 (68%).

Children's Exposures

Our findings indicate that rural children in Gallatin County experience preventable environmental exposures within the home and that some experience multiple exposures. Table 22.1 shows the number of households that had exposures exceeding action levels for ETS, radon, CO, lead, and impurities in well water.

About 13% ($n = 4$) of the households and 7% ($n = 4$) of the children in this sample had identifiable exposures to ETS. Urinary cotinine values among these 4 children ranged from 18 to 41 (μ)g/dL indicating that the children were moderately to heavily exposed to ETS (Pirkle, Flegal, Bernert, et al., 1996). In total, we found 10 households containing 18 children to have radon levels above the EPA action level of 4 pCi/L. Radon levels within the homes ranged from 4.10 to 24.10 with an average of 10.0 pCi/L (SD = 5.85). We found CO levels exceeding 9 ppm in a single house with a single child where a stovetop burner emitted 14 ppm CO with a spot-check.

We found blood lead levels exceeding 5 (μ)g/dL among 7 children (12.1 % of sample) in 6 households and ranged from 5.0 to 7.5 (μ)g/dL with an average of 5.9 (μ)g/dL. We identified well water quality issues as follows: 9 households with total coliform bacteria counts exceeding quality standards, 2 households that had chemical contamination,

Table 22.1

CHILDREN'S ENVIRONMENTAL EXPOSURES
($n = 31$ HOUSEHOLDS, 58 CHILDREN)

TYPE OF ENVIRONMENTAL EXPOSURE	HOUSEHOLDS n	%	CHILDREN n	%
Tobacco smoke[a]	4	12.9	4	6.9
Radon[b]	10	32.3	10	31.0
Carbon monoxide[c]	1	3.2	1	1.7
Lead[d]	6	19.4	7	12.1
Impure well water[e]	12	38.7	21	36.2
Multiple	8	25.8	16	27.5

[a]ETS exposure defined as any cotinine value above 5 ng/ml.
[b]Radon exposure defined by levels ≥ 4pCi/L.
[c]CO exposure defined by ≥ 9 ppm on any appliance.
[d]Lead exposure defined by ≥ 5 (μ)g/dL.
[e]Impure well water exposure was expert defined as any contaminant that may pose health risk.

and 1 household that had naturally occurring fluoride levels exceeding safe levels. In total, almost 39% of the households in this sample experienced some water quality issue that had the potential to affect health.

We found multiple household exposures among 16 children (27.5%) residing in 8 households (25.8%). Combinations of exposures that occurred most frequently included having radon and water quality problems (3 households), lead exposure and water quality problems (2 households), and ETS exposure and water quality problems (2 households). We found a single household containing 3 children to have 3 exposures, including lead, ETS, and water quality problems.

DISCUSSION

Data from Phase I of the ERRNIE project support the need for environmental risk reduction interventions among rural populations receiving public health services. These data indicate that many rural children likely experience potent exposures to environmental agents known to have health consequences. Although each exposure carries unique risk of health consequences, exposures that occur in or around the home may be prevented with simple low-cost solutions.

Behaviors aimed at reducing environmental health risks for children focusing in or around the home have been organized into five main categories: (a) environmental modification; (b) caretaker vigilance; (c) food; (d) home and personal hygiene; and (e) behavioral modification (Schneider & Freeman, 2000). Many of the behaviors within these categories require little to no resources and have the potential to yield significant benefits in risk reduction from exposure to environmental contaminants. Environmental modification includes actions, such as placing doormats at home entry areas to collect potential contaminants, designating places isolated from living areas where dirty clothes and shoes are stored, and keeping household chemicals out of reach of children. Caretaker vigilance requires adults who are responsible for children to consider issues such as the hygiene and food preparation practices of day care services and not allowing anyone to smoke in the presence of their children. Food, home, and personal hygiene simply direct adults to wash foods well, maintain safe food cooking and storage practices, and teaching children the importance of hand washing. Lastly, important aspects of behavioral modification with respect to children's environmental health include enforcing the use of utensils for eating and running tap water for a period of time before drinking.

ETS

Childhood exposures to ETS are known to cause health effects, such as middle ear disease, asthma, bronchitis, pneumonia, and impaired pulmonary function (DiFranza, Aligne, & Weitzman, 2004). Four children in four separate households within Phase 1 of this study were shown to have appreciable and significant exposures to ETS. National averages of serum cotinine for a nonsmoking population aged 3–11 years range from 0.109 to 3.37 ng/ml (National Center for Environmental Health, 2003). When adjusting for the differences between urinary and serum concentrations of cotinine (i.e., urinary levels are about 6 times greater; Benowitz, 1999), cotinine values for the children in this study ranged from 3.0 to 6.8 ng/ml placing these children in the top 10% of nonsmokers in the United States for this age group.

Household Radon

Significant radon exposure occurred in about a third of the sample for both households and children. Although acute effects of radon exposure in children are unlikely, regulatory agencies such as the EPA and International Agency for Research on Cancer have consistently classified radon as carcinogenic to humans (Frumkin & Samet, 2001). The average radon level within our sample was 10.0 pCi/L (SD = 5.85), which translates to a lifetime lung cancer risk of 56 out of 1,000 persons compared with 23 out of 10,000 persons with consistent lifetime exposures to radon at 0.4 pCi/l (U.S. EPA, 2003).

CO Poisoning

Effects of CO poisoning are well-known and include fatigue, headaches, dizziness, impaired vision and coordination, confusion, and possibly death. The U.S. National Ambient Air Quality Standards for indoor air limits CO concentrations to 9 ppm over an 8-hour period (U.S. EPA, 2004), although cumulative measurements over extended periods of time are difficult and costly. Because of this, measurement of CO for this study represents an effort to screen for possible malfunctioning appliances and the potential for harmful levels of CO to be present within the home. Despite finding only a single household with relatively low concentrations of CO (14 ppm) from a single appliance, possible acute health effects from exposure to CO warrant continued attention.

Lead Poisoning

Pediatric lead poisoning has remained a priority environmental health issue since the use of lead-based paints and lead additives to gasoline have brought exposures within close reach of children. Among adults, health effects from lead exposure, such as neurobehavioral abnormalities, tend to be reversible (Baker, White, Pothier, et al., 1985); however the more centralized nervous system effects occurring in children are not (Needleman, Schell, Bellinger, Leviton, & Allred, 1990). Although a 1991 CDC statement on childhood lead poisoning suggests 10 (μ)g/dL as a screening action guideline, a threshold value below which lead has no apparent adverse developmental effect has not been established (Bellinger, 2004). In fact, some evidence indicates that children with blood lead levels lower than 10 (μ)g/dL experience sustained effects of lower intelligence (IQ), academic achievement, and cognitive function (Bellinger, Stiles, & Needleman, 1992; Lanphear, Dietrich, Auinger, & Cox, 2000). Blood lead concentrations of 7 children (12.1%) in 6 households (19.4%) ranged from 5.0 to 7.5 (μ)g/dL and indicate that children in this sample were at risk for developmental effects from lead exposure.

Well Water Impurities

Impurities in well water can take many forms, each imparting a particular set of health risks. Because of the complexity of well water chemistry, a water quality expert evaluated analysis results from each water sample in this study to determine if health risks were present. Findings indicate that most (75%) well water contamination in this sample occurred as a result of total coliform counts exceeding safety standards. Total coliform is generally thought to be a nonspecific indicator of fecal contamination and may indicate the presence of more pathogenic bacteria, such as Escherichia coli, which is associated with acute gastrointestinal illness (Strauss, King, Ley, & Hoey, 2001). Other contamination findings include two households with chemical contamination thought to be related to solvents leaching from plumbing and one household with naturally occurring fluoride levels exceeding safe standards.

Solutions

Simple low to no-cost solutions exist for each of the five potential exposures of interest in the ERRNIE project. ETS can be easily avoided by designating a place outside of the home to smoke, not smoking in automobiles although children are not present, and ventilating the home well. Although full abatement for homes with high radon levels is costly, caretakers can locate sleeping areas for children on upper levels within the home and maximize ventilation. All homes with gas appliances should have CO detectors, which are fairly inexpensive (i.e., $20–$30), and malfunctioning appliances should be repaired or replaced. Exposures to lead can be limited or avoided by cleaning floors and walls to minimize dust, using doormats and areas of the home separate from living areas for soiled shoes and clothing, hand washing, and being aware of occupational risk factors where adults may carry lead into the home from work environments. Well water should be tested annually for contaminants, and testing is often subsidized by local health authorities. A number of solutions exist for unsafe well water depending on the type of contaminant involved. Bacterial contamination can usually be addressed cheaply by following a cleaning procedure using a diluted bleach solution within the well, and more complex problems can be addressed by various water cleaning and filtration systems of varying costs. The least costly solution may be to use a municipal source of water for drinking and cooking until more permanent solutions can be found.

CONCLUSIONS AND IMPLICATIONS FOR RURAL NURSING

Although many environmental health problems are necessarily addressed on a population level through policy and regulation, changes toward health protections can be slow and may often be at odds with other forces in the social milieu, such as economics. Although policy may be ideal for broad-based reform to prevent childhood exposures to environmental contaminants, nurses working at the household level have a significant capacity to assist families in understanding and identifying health risks and risk-avoidance strategies.

Families and communities often look to nurses for guidance on health risks, especially those associated with hazards at home or work (National Environmental Education and Training Foundation, 2002). Rural areas provide a context for increased risk of environmental exposures for children that may have both acute and long-term health consequences. Lack of resources, regulatory fragmentation, and the inadequacy of data and data systems contribute to this context (Center for Rural Health Practice, 2004), and rural nurses should become increasingly aware of how they can improve the environmental health of their communities.

ACKNOWLEDGMENT

This research was financially supported by NIH Grant No. 1 P20 RR17670-01, CEHS Faculty.

REFERENCES

Baker, E. L., White, R. F., Pothier, L. J., Berkey, C. S., Dinse, G. E., Travers, P. H., Harley, J. P., & Feldman, R. G. (1985). Occupational lead neurotoxicity: Improvement in behavioural effects after reduction of exposure. *British Journal of Industrial Medicine, 42* (8), 507–516.

Bellamy, C. (2002). Child health. In R. Detels, J. McEwen, R. Beaglehole, & H. Tanaka (Eds.), *Oxford textbook of public health* (4th ed., pp. 1603–1622). Oxford: Oxford University Press.

Bellinger, D. C. (2004). Lead. *Pediatrics* (Vol. 113, pp. 1016–1022). Washington, DC: American Academy of Pediatrics.

Bellinger, D. C., Stiles, K. M., & Needleman, H. L. (1992). Low-level lead exposure, intelligence and academic achievement: A long-term follow-up study. *Pediatrics, 90,* 855–861.

Benowitz, N. L. (1999). Biomarkers of ETS exposure. *Environmental Health Perspectives, 107,* Suppl. 2, 349–355.

Briggs, D. (2003). *Indicators to improve children's environmental health.* Geneva, Switzerland: World Health Organization.

Center for Rural Health Practice. (2004). *Bridging the health divide: The rural public health research agenda.* Pittsburgh, PA: University of Pittsburgh.

DiFranza, J. R., Aligne, C. A., & Weitzman, M. (2004). Prenatal and postnatal environmental tobacco smoke exposure and children's health. *Pediatrics* (Vol. 113, pp. 1007–1015). Washington, DC: American Academy of Pediatrics.

Frumkin, H., & Samet, J. M. (2001). Radon. *A Cancer Journal for Clinicians, 51* (6), 337–344, quiz 345–348.

Kelsey, T. W. (1994). The agrarian myth and policy responses to farm safety. *American Journal of Public Health, 84,* 1171–1177.

Lanphear, B. P., Dietrich, K., Auinger, P., & Cox, C. (2000). Cognitive deficits associated with blood lead concentrations < 10 microg/dL in US children and adolescents. *Public Health Reports, 115,* 521–529.

Malcoe, L. H., Lynch, R. A., Keger, M. C., & Skaggs, V. J. (2002). Lead sources, behaviors, and socioeconomic factors in relation to blood lead of Native American and White children: A community-based assessment of a former mining area. *Environmental Health Perspectives, 110* (Suppl. 2), 221–231.

Moya, J., Bearer, C. F., & Etzel, R. A. (2004). Children's behavior and physiology and how it affects exposure to environmental contaminants. *Pediatrics* (Vol. 113, pp. 996–1006). Washington, DC: American Academy of Pediatrics.

National Center for Environmental Health. (2003). *Second National Report on Human Exposure to environmental chemicals.* Retrieved July 28, 2004, from http://www.cdc.gov/exposurereport/2nd/pdf/secondner.pdf

National Environmental Education and Training Foundation. (2002). Nurses and environmental health: Success through action. In *Agency for toxic substances and disease registry* (Ed.), Washington, DC: Author.

Needleman, H. L., Schell, A., Bellinger, D., Leviton, A., & Allred, E. N. (1990). The long-term effects of exposure to low doses of lead in childhood. An 11–year follow-up report. *New England Journal of Medicine, 322,* 83–88.

Pirkle, J. L., Flegal, K. M., Bernert, J. T., Brody, D. J., Etzel, R. A., & Maurer, K. R. (1996). Exposure of the US population to ETS: The Third National Health and Nutrition Examination Survey, 1988 to 1991. *Journal of the American Medical Association, 275,* 1233–1240.

Schneider, D., & Freeman, N. (2000). *Children's environmental health: Reducing risk in a dangerous world.* Washington, DC: American Public Health Association.

Scorecard.org. (2004). *Land contamination report: Montana.* Retrieved July 26, 2004, from http://www.scorecard.org/env-releases/land/state.tcl?fips_state_code = 30#ej

Strauss, B., King, W., Ley, A., & Hoey, J. R. (2001). A prospective study of rural drinking water quality and acute gastrointestinal illness. *BMC Public Health, 1* (1), 8.

U.S. Environmental Protection Agency (EPA). (2003). *EPA assessment of risks from radon in homes.* Retrieved July 28, 2004, from http://www.epa.gov/radiation/docs/assessment/radon_in_homes.pdf

U.S. Environmental Protection Agency (EPA). (2004). *Sources of indoor air pollution—carbon monoxide (CO).* Retrieved July 28, 2004, from http://www.epa.gov/iaq/co.html

Van Dongen, C. J. (2002). Environmental health and nursing practice: A survey of registered nurses. *Applied Nursing Research, 15* (2), 67–73.

23

The Culture of Rural Communities: An Examination of Rural Nursing Concepts at the Community Level

NANCY FINDHOLT

In the late 1970s, faculty members and graduate students at Montana State University–Bozeman College of Nursing initiated a 6-year ethnographic study to explore the health beliefs and practices of rural Montana residents (Long & Weinert, 1989; Weinert & Long, 1987). Several of the concepts that emerged from this research were later validated by a quantitative survey and became the foundation for a theory of rural nursing. These concepts included work beliefs and health beliefs, isolation and distance, self-reliance, lack of anonymity, outsider or insider, and old-timer or newcomer. My purpose in this chapter is to describe how these concepts were manifested over two decades later and at the community level in three rural communities in Oregon.

The findings that I present here represent a portion of the results I obtained from a study (Findholt, 2004) examining the influence of rurality on community participation in a community health development initiative. Although many researchers have sought to identify the factors that influence community participation, most previous studies have focused on the characteristics of people who participate and those who do not, the reasons people choose to participate, or the characteristics of organizations that facilitate or hinder participation (Wandersman & Florin, 2000). Very few investigators have explored how community characteristics affect participation, yet these characteristics may have a significant effect on the forms or levels of participation that are possible, as well as on the outcomes of participation that can be achieved. This study of rural community participation was guided by a conceptual framework that posited that the ability of a rural community to participate in health development is both facilitated and hindered by factors in the culture, physical setting, and social structure of the community. Among the cultural factors included in the conceptual framework were three that were derived from the Montana State University–Bozeman research. These were (a) the priority given to health, (b) perceived efficacy of collective action, and (c) insider or outsider differentiation.

Priority Given to Health

Priority given to health was defined as the priority assigned to health programs as compared to economic programs at the community level. It corresponded to the concept of "work beliefs and health beliefs." The Montana State University–Bozeman study found that rural residents assessed their health needs in relation to work roles and work activities (Weinert & Long, 1987). Being productive in their role was of primary importance to these individuals, and health problems were often ignored unless they interfered with the ability to work. On the basis of these findings, I proposed in the current study that rural communities would place a higher value on economic development than on health development.

Perceived Efficacy of Collective Action

Perceived efficacy of collective action referred to the belief of community members in their ability to work together to solve problems. This cultural variable corresponded to the concept of "self-reliance." The Montana State University–Bozeman findings revealed that rural people were self-reliant in coping with personal and family health problems and preferred self-care, or care provided by family and friends, over professional care (Weinert & Long, 1987). Thus, in the current study I proposed that rural residents, as a whole, would have confidence in their collective ability to solve problems, including problems related to health.

Insider or Outsider Differentiation

Finally, insider or outsider differentiation was a phrase chosen to refer to the degree to which community members, as a group, accepted and trusted individuals based upon their tenure in the community. It was derived from the concepts of "insider or outsider" and "old-timer or newcomer." The ethnographic data collected in Montana suggested that rural people organized their social environment around these concepts and determined who to accept and who to trust based upon variables such as length of residence, family history, and type of occupation (Weinert & Long, 1987). Therefore, I anticipated that in a rural community a health development leader who was well-known to residents and perceived as an insider would be more likely accepted than a leader who was viewed as an outsider.

I did not include the concepts of "isolation and distance" and "lack of anonymity" in the conceptual framework for this study and, therefore, they were not among the cultural factors that I intentionally explored. However, as described in this chapter, some of the qualitative findings did provide insight into the presence of these characteristics in the rural communities.

METHODS

This research employed a multiple-case study design featuring three communities that were engaged in the Community Health Improvement Partnership, a health development initiative offered by the Office of Rural Health (ORH) (2003) in Oregon. Besides being selected for their involvement in the health development effort, the communities chosen as cases were required to meet specific criteria for rurality that were established using the Rural-Urban Commuting Area (RUCA) scale. The RUCA scale classifies census tracts based upon size and daily commuting patterns (Rural Health Research Center, 2002). Communities participating in this study were required to have a main town of no more than 9,999 people, no primary or secondary commuting flow greater than 5% to an urban area, and no secondary flow greater than 30% to a large town. I used these criteria to restrict the sample to communities with small populations that were unlikely to be influenced by urban culture. I labeled the three communities chosen for the sample as Communities A, B, and C.

I collected data reported in this chapter through key informant interviews and focus groups with community members. The key informants were health professionals or members of local health boards. The focus group participants included school administrators, small business owners, retirees, employees of social service organizations, and others from the non health sectors of the community. All of the respondents were participants in the health development planning team. I conducted 21 key informant interviews and six focus groups.

I designed the interview questions to solicit the respondents' perceptions of their community and of community members' views, rather than their personal opinions. To assess the priority given to health, I asked the respondents how their community ranked health in comparison with other concerns, such as the economy, environment, or infrastructure. I assessed perceived efficacy of collective action by asking the respondents whether most residents believed that by working together they could bring about general improvements in the community, and whether residents believed they had the collective ability to improve the community's health. I assessed insider or outsider differentiation by asking whether the leader of the health development initiative was perceived by residents as an insider and whether this perception had an effect on their acceptance of the leader.

I used semistructured interviews to facilitate comparability of the data across communities; however, I also encouraged the respondents to describe other community characteristics they believed had influenced participation in the health development initiative. It was through these opportunities that the comments concerning isolation and lack of anonymity emerged.

Data analysis occurred concurrently with data collection and consisted of three interwoven processes described by Miles and Huberman (1994). These were data reduction, data display, and conclusion drawing and verification. Data reduction involved simplifying and abstracting the raw data through a process of writing summaries, coding, and writing memos. Data display occurred as I compressed the data and organized it into matrices. I developed within-case displays first and later "stacked" these to create cross-case displays. I accomplished conclusion drawing and verification by making contrasts and comparisons across different communities and different data sources, looking for evidence of patterns and examining exceptions to patterns, following up on surprises, and looking for negative evidence.

DESCRIPTION OF THE COMMUNITIES

The communities that participated in this study were not towns, but were regions with boundaries that corresponded to the service area of the local hospital. The service area boundaries were delineated by the Office of Rural Health (2003) when the communities were chosen to participate in the health development initiative. Table 23.1 shows demographics of Communities A, B, and C.

Community A was, in many respects, the neediest and most rural of the three communities. It was a sparsely populated and isolated coastal region, 72 miles by winding roads from the county seat, with the oldest and poorest residents, and an economy that was floundering. The traditional industries of forestry and fishing had declined significantly in recent years, forcing many families to leave the area. An effort was being made to attract tourists and to recruit new businesses, but at the time of this study, the economy remained depressed.

Community B encompassed a large portion of a county located in the ranch and farm lands of eastern Oregon. Of the three communities included in the study, Community B was the farthest from a metropolitan area of 50,000 or more residents. However, its main town was over

Table 23.1

SELECTED DEMOGRAPHIC CHARACTERISTICS OF STUDY COMMUNITIES AS COMPARED WITH OREGON

COMMUNITY CHARACTERISTIC	COMMUNITY A	COMMUNITY B	COMMUNITY C	OREGON
Size	7,641 residents w/1 main town, population 4,230	14,266 residents w/1 main town population 9,840	44,479 residents w/2 main towns, populations 9,532 & 5,903	N/A
Median age	47.3	45	44	40
White	91.7%	94.3%	90.6%	82.7%
Below poverty	15.8%	14.4%	13.9%	11.6%
Population age 25+ without high school diploma	19.6%	20.0%	15.1%	14.9%

Note: From ORH (2003) and Portland State University (PSU), Population Research Center (2002).

twice as large as Community A's and a major interstate highway traversed the community. Besides agriculture, which was a large component of the economy, many people were employed in human services (health care, education, and social services) or in wood products manufacturing, an industry that had been developed to replace the loss of jobs in forestry. Demographic statistics for this region revealed a community that was older and poorer than the state as a whole, yet was younger and less poor than Community A.

Community C was the largest, least rural, and least needy of the study communities. This community was an entire county located on the coast in western Oregon. There were two main towns in the county, both of which were less than 60 miles from a major metropolitan corridor. The region was popular as a weekend and vacation retreat and as a retirement destination, and had an economy based on tourism. Residents described the community as having two populations: (a) the retirees, who were generally well educated and financially comfortable, and (b) the people who struggled to make ends meet by working in the tourist industry. Both groups were quite transient; the community had few long-term residents. Overall, the population was poorer, older, and less educated than the state as a whole, but was closer to the state demographic averages than either Communities A or B.

RESULTS

Priority Given to Health

The case study data revealed that the priority given to health matters, in comparison with the economy, was relatively high in these communities. Although some of the respondents believed that economic development or issues, such as infrastructure improvement and education, were more important to their community than health development, approximately half of the people from each study site said that health was one of their community's top concerns.

One reason that was cited for the high priority given to health was the change in the communities' demographics. Respondents explained that as the percentage of residents who were poor or old had increased, there had been a corresponding increase in the need for health care services, which in turn had placed a burden on the community, resulting in greater attention being given to health issues. In Communities A and C, the influx of retirees was also cited as a reason for the high priority given to health. It was noted that the retirees expected adequate health care services. Furthermore, respondents in all of the study sites observed that health had become a higher priority in their communities as local leaders learned that to recruit business and to attract newcomers, they needed to have a strong health care system.

Perceived Efficacy of Collective Action

The degree to which residents had confidence in their collective ability to improve the community varied across the study sites. Most of the respondents in Community A reported that residents believed that by working together they could achieve positive change. Similarly, in Community B it was noted that some, and possibly most, of the residents had confidence in collective action. However, in Community C over half of the people I interviewed stated that a large segment of the population was pessimistic or negative about community efforts.

In contrast to the varying degrees of confidence concerning general community improvement, the findings show that residents in all of the communities were quite skeptical about their ability to resolve community health problems. A primary reason given for the skepticism was that the complexity and magnitude of the rural health care crisis made the problems seem overwhelming. However, lack of experience in making health improvements and the failure of other social programs were also cited as factors that contributed to residents' skepticism.

Insider or Outsider Differentiation

In Communities A and C two people were identified as being the leader of the health development initiative. One of these was viewed as a community insider and the other as an outsider. In Community B only one person was identified as the leader. She was well-known among members of the agricultural sector, but was unknown to other residents.

Whether leaders were perceived as an insider or an outsider appeared to have little effect on how they were accepted by residents in any of the study sites. Although a few respondents said that familiarity was essential in establishing credibility and trust, most thought that the leader's skills and personality were more important. It is interesting that one theme that emerged across the communities was that having a leader who was unknown was beneficial to the health development effort in that it allowed the process to be perceived as unbiased and impartial. Respondents explained that in a small community where residents know the leaders' opinions on issues, they are apt to assume that planning projects led by a known leader will be slanted in favor of that leader's agenda.

Although the concepts of insider versus outsider and old-timer versus newcomer had little relevance in terms of the communities' acceptance of the health development leader, these concepts did emerge as factors that defined, and in some cases divided, the residents in two of the study sites. In Communities A and B individuals who had resided in these communities for as long as 24 years were described by themselves or by others as newcomers, a finding which suggests that they were not fully integrated into the community. In addition, many of the respondents in Community A reported that tension existed among the newcomers who were interested in changing the community, and the old-timers who wanted things to remain the same. On the other hand, in Community C several respondents commented that the concepts of old-timer and newcomer had little meaning because there were so many newcomers. As one person stated, "We're so used to different people. . . . It's not something that divides the community at all."

Lack of Anonymity

Lack of anonymity was mentioned only in Community A. Respondents there noted that one of the challenges of serving on a health planning team in a small community was that team members knew each other well and interacted often, thus they were reluctant to be confrontational or to express opinions that conflicted with others in the group. This had the effect of reducing openness during discussions. One person observed, "That's the thing that I think is the hardest part about this process in a small community, is the inability to . . . be frank about things."

Isolation and Distance

The comments concerning isolation and distance emerged during discussions of collective efficacy. Because of the distances that separated the study communities from larger communities, respondents perceived that they were isolated. For example, one individual from Community A observed that the next largest community was 70 miles away and "may as well be on the moon."

Some of the respondents believed that their community's isolation was a positive factor in that residents realized they needed to work together to solve problems. As one person explained, "We're just not sitting there, looking for someone else to solve the problems because, you know, we're out here in all this ground and there ain't no cavalry. There's no cavalry. We've just got to figure out what to do." However, it was also noted that isolation and distance contributed to a sense of collective depression, a sense of skepticism about whether positive change was possible, and a feeling of being disenfranchised. Furthermore, isolation made it difficult for rural communities to solve problems because their access to resources was very limited.

DISCUSSION

The discovery that health development was a rather high priority in these communities was unexpected in light of the earlier findings from Montana. One explanation for the inconsistency between this study's findings and those reported by Montana State University researchers might be that many of the Montana subjects were people who were still working, whereas the participants in the current study were from aging communities with many residents who were no longer working. Just as it is logical to assume that an individual's interest in health would increase with age, so too might a community's interest in health increase as its population ages. It is important to note, however, that one of the reasons cited for the high priority given to health in the Oregon communities was that health services were necessary for economic development. This perspective of health as a means to an economic end was very similar to the Montana observations.

The high level of skepticism among residents concerning their collective ability to resolve community health problems was also unexpected given that Weinert and Long (1987) had found that rural people had confidence in their ability to manage personal and family health problems. It is possible that Oregon residents had less confidence in their ability to address health concerns than Montana residents. However, it is also likely that solving community health problems was perceived by rural people as different, and perhaps more complex, than solving problems pertaining to their own health or the health of family members.

Another finding that was unanticipated was that the communities' acceptance of the health development leader was not, for the most part, influenced by residents' perceptions of the leader as an insider or an outsider. I had assumed that if the concepts of insider and outsider divided the community, which was clearly the case in Community A, then insider status would be a critical element in assuring that the leader was accepted. However, the respondents' comments suggested that in a small community where people know the local leaders and are aware of their opinions, familiarity might actually hinder residents' acceptance of the leader. This finding relates to lack of anonymity, which is discussed next.

The case study data pertaining to lack of anonymity were consistent with those obtained by Weinert and Long (1987). The comments made by respondents in Community A concerning the difficulties of serving on a planning team with people they knew well were very similar to remarks made by rural nurses who were part of the Montana sample. These nurses had reported that because their patients were often also their neighbors, friends, or family members, it was difficult for them to separate their professional and personal roles (Long & Weinert, 1989).

The findings pertaining to the residents' perception of their isolation were inconsistent with Weinert and Long's (1987) results. Although the Oregon respondents described their communities as isolated, Montana residents who lived outside of town and traveled more than 50 miles to receive routine health care did not view themselves as isolated (Long & Weinert, 1989).

In summary, only one of the concepts that were identified in the early Montana research was evident in the community level data collected in Oregon. This concept was lack of anonymity, a characteristic pertaining more to the small size of a community than to rurality per se.

CONCLUSION

These findings, drawn from a study of rural community participation in a health development initiative, provide insight into the culture of rural communities and serve to extend rural nursing theory by revealing how the concepts identified in the initial theory work were manifested at the community level in Oregon. The many inconsistencies between this study's findings and those of the early Montana research may be due to several factors, but one likely cause is that the culture of rural communities has changed in the 30-plus years since the initial data were collected. Given the loss of jobs in traditional rural industries, advances in telecommunications and transportation, relocation of retirees to rural areas, and other major social changes that have impacted rural communities, it follows that rural culture has been altered. The results of this study have relevance to all nurses who have an interest in improving rural health, and especially to those who practice in a rural setting. The health of rural Americans is closely linked to factors in the culture, economy, demography, and geography of rural places (Ricketts, 1999). Thus, to successfully impact the health of rural people, nurses need to have an understanding of rural communities. Furthermore, for nurses interested in community-based practice in a rural setting, it is important to understand community-level perspectives of health as well as community-level influences on health decision making.

The findings from this study were limited by several factors, including the small size and limited diversity of the sample, the potential for bias in the use of health development committee members as representatives of their community, and the lack of an urban comparison group. Further research is needed to explore whether the characteristics identified in this research are unique to rural communities, and to confirm their applicability in other rural settings.

REFERENCES

Findholt, N. E. (2004). *The influence of rurality on community participation in a community health development initiative.* Unpublished doctoral dissertation, Oregon Health and Science University, Portland.

Long, K. A., & Weinert, C. (1989). Rural nursing: Developing the theory base. *Scholarly Inquiry for Nursing Practice, 3* (2), 113–127.

Miles, M. B., & Huberman, A. M. (1994). *Qualitative data analysis* (2nd ed.). Thousand Oaks, CA: Sage.

Office of Rural Health (ORH). (2003). *Demographic, socioeconomic, and health status report.* Portland: Oregon Health and Science University.

Portland State University (PSU), Population Research Center. (2002). *Oregon population report.* Retrieved February 19, 2003, from http://www.upa.pdx.edu/CPRC/

Ricketts, T. C. (1999). Introduction. In T. C. Ricketts, III (Ed.), *Rural health in the United States* (pp. 1–6). New York: Oxford University Press.

Rural Health Research Center. (2002). *Rural–urban commuting area codes (RUCAs).* Retrieved February 3, 2003, from http://www.fammed.washington.edu/wwamirhrc/rucas/rucas.html

Wandersman, A., & Florin, P. (2000). Citizen participation and community organizations. In J. Rappaport & E. Seidman (Eds.), *Handbook of community psychology* (pp. 247–272). New York: Kluwer Academic/Plenum.

Weinert, C., & Long, K. A. (1987). Understanding the health care needs of rural families. *Family Relations, 36,* 450–455.

24

Community Resiliency and Rural Nursing: Canadian and Australian Perspectives

JUDITH C. KULIG, DESLEY HEGNEY, and DANA S. EDGE

"Resiliency is [a] community that's willing to pick up an issue, work with it, and decide what they want to do about it . . . without blowing the place apart."
—Community Resident

In the last several years, considerable discussion about the applicability of resiliency to understand and augment community functioning has occurred. Community resiliency is a process that describes change, provides an opportunity to focus on strengths, and offers opportunities for residents to be involved. Agencies, such as the Red Cross, have found that through the development of social capital and cross sectoral coalitions in communities that have experienced disasters, resiliency is enhanced (J. Walter, 2005). Within this chapter, examples of Canadian and Australian led research on community resiliency in Canada, Australia, and the United States illustrate how rural communities have dealt with adversity. The rural communities in the Canadian-led research discussed here were all under 10,000 in population size, which matches the rural and small town definition commonly used to describe communities of that size outside the commuting zones of large urban centers (du Plessis, Beshiri, Bollman, & Clemenson, 2001). Communities serve to satisfy their members' needs (MacMillan & Chavis, 1986) and are places where interactions and social relationships are tantamount (Bellah, Madsen, Sullivan, Swidler, & Tipton, 1996; Hawe, 1994). The community-based

385

research exemplars suggest how rural registered nurses (RNs) can enhance community resiliency, and ultimately improve the health status of rural residents and the sustainability of rural communities.

BACKGROUND TO RESILIENCY RESEARCH

Historically, resilience has been studied among individuals, particularly young children, who were living in challenging circumstances. Numerous scholars have used "resilience" to describe a trait held by individuals as a result of dealing with adversity. However, since the 1990s, resiliency has also been used to describe the "process" communities undergo when dealing with adversity. This process also refers to the ability of a community to strengthen and change despite the adversity encountered (Brown & Kulig, 1996/1997; Kulig, 1999, 2000; Kulig & Hanson, 1996). Various factors are important within the community resiliency process, including community infrastructure, such as health and social service departments and social capital, represented by neighborhood networks and associations (Breton, 2001). Events such as public fairs and festivals add to a sense of self, place, and community while also enhancing viability and vitality that contribute to the resiliency of communities (Porter, 2000).

There is no definitive answer about the relationship between individual and community resiliency. Although we speculate that "you can't have one without the other," it remains unclear if there are a certain number of resilient individuals required to ensure that community resiliency occurs or that there is a specific type of relationship between individual and community resiliency. Additional research is needed among a variety of rural communities in order to further our understanding of this and other issues related to community resiliency.

OVERVIEW OF RESEARCH STUDIES
ON COMMUNITY RESILIENCY

A series of studies on community resiliency based in Canadian, U.S., and Australian rural communities have been conducted in order to understand the concept. This brief overview provides highlights from the qualitative and focus group interviews conducted within the case studies. Interviews and analyses occurred simultaneously, with interviews continuing until data saturation occurred in each investigation. Trustworthiness was

Table 24.1

SUMMARY OF RESILIENCY STUDIES IN CANADIAN, U.S., AND AUSTRALIAN COMMUNITIES

COMMUNITY STUDIED	YEAR	# QUALITATIVE INTERVIEWS $n =$	# FOCUS GROUP INTERVIEW PARTICIPANTS $n =$
Crowsnest Pass, AB, Canada	1995	40	74
Southeastern Kentucky, USA	1997	23	
Crowsnest Pass, AB, Canada	1998	22	
Hinton, AB, Canada	2003	25	
Riverside Meadows, AB, Canada	2003	27	
Hardisty, AB, Canada	2003	30	
Crowsnest Pass, AB, Canada	2006–2007	30	
Barriere, BC, Canada	2007–2008	30	
La Ronge, SK, Canada	2007–2008	27	
Stanthorpe, Australia	2007–2008	11 (phase 1) 74 (phase 2)	20
TOTAL		339	94
		GRAND TOTAL	*$n = 433$*

established through member checking, independent audit of themes, and presentation of preliminary findings to residents (Creswell, 2007; Streubert, Speziale, & Carpenter, 2007). Principles of community development guided the conduct of the studies with community consultation prior to study commencement, establishment of community advisory teams, employment and training of local research assistants, and dissemination of findings back to community members (Labonte, 1993). Table 24.1 provides a visual presentation of the specific studies and their accompanying sample sizes.

Canadian and U.S. Exemplars

The initial studies on community resiliency (Brown & Kulig, 1996/1997; Kulig, 1999) were conducted in an amalgamated community, the Crowsnest Pass, in southern Alberta, Canada, with an approximate population of 6,000 (Statistics Canada, 2006). Before 1979, the amalgamated community had been a series of former coal-mining towns, hamlets, and improvement districts. In total, three studies that focused on resiliency have been conducted in this community.

The "Pass," which it is often referred to, has experienced a number of challenging events: (a) the Frank Slide, a well-known mountain slide that partially buried one of the hamlets in 1903, killing over 75 people; (b) the worst mine disaster in Canadian history, which led to the death of 189 miners and left 400 children fatherless in 1914; (c) community strife related to the coal industry, including strikes and lockouts; and (d) the resultant economic decline from the loss of underground coal mining in the late 1970s. Natural disasters continue to be common with severe windstorms leading to extensive damage to homes and businesses. Two recent natural disasters include the Lost Creek Fire in 2003 and the ice storm in 2005 that left numerous residents without power for up to 5 days.

The first study in the Pass dealt with the general history of the area and the participants' perspectives about how the aforementioned historical events shaped their community and contributed to its resiliency (Brown & Kulig, 1996/1997; Kulig & Hanson, 1996). The second study focused on the attempts to create a community health center and how this process actually damaged the community's resiliency (Kulig & Waldner, 1999). The third study addressed the community's response to the Lost Creek Fire, the worst wildfire experienced by the community which led to evacuations and the loss of 21,000 hectares (51,800 acres) of land (Kulig, Reimer, Townshend, Edge, Neves-Graca, Lightfoot, et al., 2007). In each study, regardless of the issue being addressed by the community, the individuals were interviewed about their perspectives regarding the functioning of the Pass, how the community faced the many challenges it had encountered, and their understanding of community resiliency.

Between the first and second investigations in the Pass, the first author conducted an interrelated study examining how community-based workers enhanced community resiliency in southeastern Kentucky in the United States (Kulig, 1999, 2000). The setting was chosen for study because of the similarities to the Pass, including a coal mining history with strikes and community unrest. The area in Kentucky was rural in nature with the towns having a few hundred to a few thousand residents in each. The findings from the studies conducted in the Pass and in Kentucky led to the beginnings of a community resiliency model in 1995, which has since been revised, and will be described in a subsequent section. Building upon the emerging community resiliency model, a pilot study explored whether community resiliency could be linked to health status in several resource-reliant central Alberta communities. Agricultural-based rural communities have experienced a number of economic and social challenges, including a decline in the number of family farms (Bollman & Rothwell, 2002) with a simultaneous increase in intensive livestock operations (ILOs) (Cole, Todd, & Wing, 2000; Wing & Wolf, 2000). Community tensions arise when plans are proposed to locate ILOs into farming communities. Conflicts can result as rural residents typically value family farm ownership over corporate owners, and rural beliefs of mutual respect and reciprocal exchange may not be respected (Schiffman, Miller, Suggs, & Graham, 1995; Thu et al., 1997). Similarly, natural resource communities, such as mining towns, experience competing interests of generating economic opportunities for residents and minimizing mining extraction environmental concerns.

Two rural communities in central Alberta were chosen for the pilot study. The agricultural-based community of Hardisty and surrounding communities successfully prevented the establishment of an ILO in their community. The second rural community was the mining community of Hinton, which dealt with a coal mining closure (Kulig, Edge, & Joyce, 2008a, 2008b). The urban neighborhood of Riverside Meadows was also included. This community was originally a French Canadian village, and at the time of the study was dealing with identity issues. These three communities were chosen because of the challenges that they were addressing.

Finally, the most recent and current studies on community resiliency focus on the relationship between the phenomenon and disasters (Kulig et al., 2007). Given the increased number of disasters worldwide and the impact of wildfire on residents in rural communities (Public Safety & Emergency Preparedness Canada, 2005), the current ongoing study is examining two communities that experienced wildfires which led to evacuations and property losses (Kulig et al.).

The communities Barriere (British Columbia, population 2,500) and La Ronge (Saskatchewan, population 5,700) are rural and remote communities, respectively (Statistics Canada, 2006). Both study sites are isolated from larger cities, with Barriere economically struggling while La Ronge has experienced a shortage of skilled workers for their currently booming mining industry. Both communities include aboriginal residents who participate in all sectors of community life. The fire in Barriere burned 26,420 hectares (65,257 acres), led to the evacuation of the entire community, and destroyed over 80 homes and businesses. In La Ronge, the fire burned over 8 kilometers, a partial evacuation of the community occurred, and 8 homes were destroyed. In each community, the wildfire disaster was seen as a potential stimulus for the community's resiliency.

Australian Case Studies

Between 2005 and 2007, a study was undertaken in the Australian town of Stanthorpe. The aim of the study was to work collaboratively with members of this rural community to develop, implement, and evaluate a model that enhances resilience in rural people and communities. Stanthorpe is located in southeast Queensland, and at the time of the study the town and its satellite communities had an area of 2,699 square kilometers and a population of 10,124 (Australian Bureau of Statistics, 2007). The main industries included fruit and vegetable production, wineries, and tourism. At the time of the study the area was experiencing a protracted drought, and in the previous 2 years it had also experienced "black" frosts, hail storms, and bushfires. The area was rated as highly disadvantaged on the National Index of Social and Economic Disadvantage (Australian Bureau of Statistics, 2006) with almost 60% of the population in the lowest 20th percentile.

The study was carried out in three phases. Phase 1 of the study involved face-to-face interviews with 11 people identified as being resilient. It was designed to explore key informants' conceptions of resilience, both as an individual and as a community characteristic (Hegney, Buikstra, Baker, et al., 2007). Phase 2 used a modified convergent interviewing technique (Dick, 1990) to interview six groups (service providers, those with special needs, youth, farmers, the commercial sector, and those "resilient" individuals identified from phase 1 of the study). A total of 74 people participated in the face-to-face interviews. Following data analysis of phase 1 and 2 data, resilient concepts were identified. These concepts were then evaluated using a modified photovoice exercise and a focus group of community members. The final product was 11 concepts that were seen to be linked to individual, group, or community resilience: (1) social networks and support; (2) positive outlook; (3) learning; (4) early experience; (5) environment and lifestyle; (6) infrastructure and support services; (7) sense of purpose; (8) diverse and innovative economy; (9) embracing differences; (10) beliefs; and (11) leadership. One of the products of the study was the development of a "toolkit," which explained each of the 11 concepts and gave examples of how the concept could be assessed and programs introduced to enhance the concept.

DEVELOPING THEORY ABOUT COMMUNITY RESILIENCY

The initial study that focused on community resiliency in the Pass led to the development of a model that illustrated that when specific variables combined and interacted, resiliency was the result (see Figure 24.1) (Kulig, 2000). These variables, which emphasize social interactions and relationships, include (a) the ability to cope with divisions, (b) leadership, (c) community togetherness, and (d) networks. In this version of the model, resiliency is seen as constantly fluctuating, depending upon the situation that was being addressed. However, it was also crucial that community cohesiveness be present, otherwise resiliency would not occur.

The subsequent study, conducted in Kentucky (Kulig, 1998) and supported by the second study in the Pass (Kulig, 1999), led to the revision of the original model (see Figure 24.2). The findings from these studies also confirmed that resiliency is a process that is influenced by variables such as the presence of community leadership, proactive members, and the ability to use a community problem-solving process. These variables contributed to the development of community cohesiveness, an important precursor to community resiliency. Community resiliency therefore implies three processes: (1) the community experiencing interactions as a collective unit, including "getting along" and "a sense of belonging"; (2) the development of a "sense of community," demonstrated by a shared

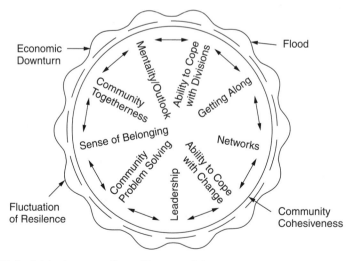

Figure 24.1. Original community resiliency model.

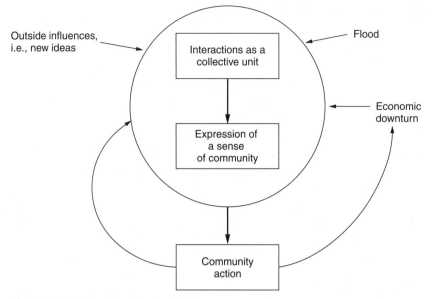

Figure 24.2. Revised resiliency model.

mentality and outlook and community togetherness; and (3) community action, shown by the coping with divisions, dealing with change in a positive way, the accompaniment of visionary leadership, and the surfacing of community problem solving. In order for community resiliency to develop, these internal processes are required, as well as the consideration and incorporation of new ideas from the outside.

Varying levels of resiliency were displayed by communities in the previous studies. For community-based workers, the findings suggest that there are different times when they can intervene to potentially enhance a community's resiliency. Being proactive was found to be very important to resiliency, as proactiveness signals a community's flexibility and openness to change and to new ideas. Finally, a sense of hope and community pride was noted as tantamount for resiliency to occur.

The central Alberta pilot study focused on the relationships between health status and community resiliency, not only with interviews, but also the examination of health databases (Kulig, Edge, & Joyce, 2008a). Residents in the urban neighborhood scored lowest on sense of belonging on the household survey compared to their rural counterparts in Hardisty and Hinton. This finding, along with the interview data, raised questions about the degree of resiliency present in the neighborhood, as a sense of community is associated with community resiliency. In addition, this neighborhood had higher proportions of self-reported physician-diagnosed depression and a corresponding increase in health care utilization for mental diseases. These results represent the first time that quantitative evidence has linked health status and community resiliency. Consequently, the community resiliency model was again revised (see Figure 24.3). In the latest revision, sense of belonging and community pride are results of a sense of community rather than the other way around.

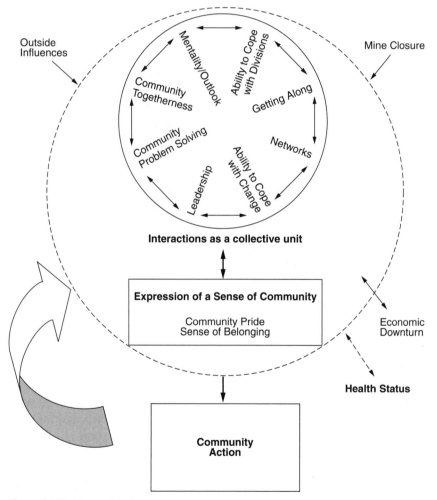

Figure 24.3. Updated resiliency model.

The characteristics of and barriers to community resiliency were further clarified in the central Alberta pilot study (Kulig et al., 2007). Community resiliency includes the following five characteristics: (1) positive infrastructure, such as a diverse economy and gathering places; (2) intact social infrastructure (i.e., residents honoring history); (3) constructive people characteristics exemplified by core leadership and people participating; (4) problem-solving processes that are transparent and collective in nature; and (5) helpful conceptual characteristics, such as being proactive, community pride, and "stick-to-itiveness." Barriers to resiliency consist of: (a) challenging events, such as the community dealing with a series of successive adverse events or dealing with a natural disaster; (b) negative infrastructure characteristics, for example an economic downturn or poor access to services; (c) harmful social infrastructure, such as a high crime rate and a lack of community spirit; (d) limited people infrastructure, including a lack of knowledge and education, a lack of participation, and a lack of leadership; (e) compromised conceptual infrastructure, for instance a failure to be proactive; and (f) attitudinal characteristics like complacency, rigidity, and individualism.

The most recent study conducted in the Pass focused on the impact of the Lost Creek Fire on community resiliency (Kulig et al., 2007) but did not lead to any additional changes in the model. With a focus on perceptions of risk, vulnerability, and community resiliency in a disaster, findings from the Lost Creek Fire investigation imply that vulnerability, at the individual and community level, tests resiliency and affects the community response to adversity. The challenge will be to examine the association between perceived vulnerability and community resiliency.

The ongoing study in Barriere and La Ronge has confirmed the importance of resiliency in explaining how these communities have dealt with the wildfires. The data analysis is still ongoing and thus no further changes to the model are available at this time.

In summary, community resiliency is a theoretical model that describes processes that rural communities undergo when dealing with adversity. It requires, at a minimum, informal leadership, community togetherness, and a positive proactive community outlook. Resiliency naturally fluctuates but can be positively influenced by residents and community-based workers. Given the threats to rural sustainability, it is vitally important to consider how rural RNs can assist in this process to positively influence the health of rural residents.

ROLE OF RURAL REGISTERED NURSES IN ENHANCING COMMUNITY RESILIENCY

Rural RNs assume a generalist role in their practice with rural communities (Kulig, MacLeod, Stewart, & Pitblado, 2008). By using the community resiliency model, rural nurses can collectively attend to the overall needs of the community while also supporting the health of rural residents. In practical terms, this is achieved by focusing on the model's separate components (see Figure 24.3).

Interactions as a Collective Unit

It is very clear that the threats to rural sustainability focus on the loss of infrastructure and the subsequent losses of opportunities for interactions and networking. This first aspect of the community resiliency model can be considered a "building phase" that requires the work of many to be successful.

Rural RNs assist in this process of strengthening infrastructure by enhancing networks that foster feelings of "getting along," and a sense of belonging through their professional roles and as community residents. At multiple levels of interchanges (C. Walter, 2005), rural nurses use a holistic approach that fosters interactions and exchanges between all community members regardless of gender, age, economic, religious, or ethnic backgrounds. In short, rural nursing requires working across sectors, with a variety of people. Rural nurses are typically very good at being "inclusive." Nurses in rural settings care for their neighbors, friends, and family members as their personal and professional roles are inseparable. Their worldview extends beyond the walls of the health care facilities or institutions where they practice and acknowledges the social and political dynamics of their community. All of this means that rural nurses can assist in enhancing community members' sense of belonging and networking. Using a holistic approach that incorporates community input and involvement, rural nurses can plan programs, activities, or initiatives that naturally result in increased community resiliency.

The negative effect of threats to rural sustainability can be mediated via rural nurses by working with community members to identify individual and community assets. This is the first step in addressing community need while also providing opportunities for engagement at the individual resident level. Working from a whole-community approach to health promotion, nurses can assist in creating partnerships and in fostering community champions. These actions can lead to an overall increase in a community's capacity. However, none of these steps will be effective unless the community is willing to be involved. Community involvement is not "expected" and requires time, trust, and mutual regard between rural RNs, rural residents, and other stakeholders within the community. Without community buy-in, planned initiatives will stall or fail.

Developing a Sense of Community

Frequently, rural nurses are at the front lines making decisions that influence the community in its entirety. Opportunities for visionary ideas and the action toward those goals require that nurses work with community residents. This activity alone is a positive step in the development of community togetherness and cohesion. Positive community spirit and hopefulness can be encouraged within the community in other ways. If the community has had success in developing interactions as a collective unit, then their sense of community will begin to expand. It can be further fostered by implementing activities that will augment community pride. For example, even a simple activity such as naming a "yard of the month" during summer when gardens are at their height can increase pride in one's physical community. This example demonstrates the importance of the link between community resiliency and a community's overall health.

Community Action

Being proactive is key to community resiliency. Given their professional presence in a rural community, nurses, along with others, can advocate for changes in public policy (Kulig, Nahachewsky, Thomlinson, MacLeod, & Curran, 2004). Local knowledge and skill in policy development among the nursing collective can be used to support rural residents in efforts to affect change. As interpreters of health information for the public, rural nurses have a responsibility to provide accurate information about local health issues. For example, rural RNs can help decipher information about potential environmental threats from ILOs on rural residents' health, or use their connections to bring experts to the community to share their knowledge on specific topics. Community processes can be employed to ensure that community residents' opinions are heard and are used in determining which specific actions need to be taken. One example is a community profile process that includes local individuals and community members at large being involved in the planning and generation of solutions for identified issues (University of New Hampshire, no date).

RECOMMENDATIONS FOR NURSING EDUCATION

In the past two decades, the relationship between social determinants of health and the well-being of communities has received renewed interest and exploration (Kawachi & Berkman, 2003). In undergraduate nursing programs, the examination of societal forces that influence health have typically been discussed in community health nursing courses (Vollman, Anderson, & McFarlane, 2008). Relatively new models, such as the Population Health Promotion Model, provide visual representations of the interconnections between the social determinants of health, the various populations to serve (e.g. individual, family, community, society), and components of the Ottawa charter (Hamilton & Bhatti, 1996). In particular the five components of the Ottawa charter—(1) strengthen community action, (2) build public health policy, (3) create supportive environments, (4) develop personal skills, and (5) reorient health services—should lead to enhanced community resiliency if enacted. The different components of the resiliency model allow for connections with the Population Health Promotion Model and provide further rationale for the link between community resiliency and health status. Educators can use the revised model of community resiliency as a starting point for student discussion about the underlying reasons why rural communities and urban neighborhoods may vary in how they deal with adversity.

RECOMMENDATIONS FOR FUTURE RESEARCH

Several recommendations for future research in community resiliency arise in this discussion. Suggestions include (a) focusing on communities that have dealt with different kinds of natural disasters (i.e., floods, hurricanes, tornadoes) in order to provide comparative data; (b) conducting mixed method studies to identify the components of resiliency; (c) establishing international studies to allow for further examination and comparison of the concept; (d) performing a systematic review to compare resiliency, empowerment, and social capital; and, (e) carrying out a meta-synthesis of community resiliency studies.

CONCLUSION

Community resiliency is the ability for communities to "bounce back" and deal with adverse situations that they face. When communities demonstrate resiliency they also display adaptability and the capacity to move forward. Communities with resiliency also reveal that they can maintain themselves as a strong, functioning, collective unit. Given that rural sustainability is a growing concern, resiliency gives hope to rural communities that are struggling. It also demonstrates an important role that rural RNs play in enhancing resiliency, and thereby potentially improving the health of all rural residents.

REFERENCES

Australian Bureau of Statistics. (2006). *Socio-economic index for areas*. Canberra: Commonwealth of Australia.

Australian Bureau of Statistics. (2007). *Australian Bureau of Statistics 2006 Census*. Canberra: Commonwealth of Australia.

Bellah, R., Madsen, R., Sullivan, W., Swidler, A., & Tipton, S. (1996). *Habits of the heart: Individualism and commitment in American life*. Los Angeles: University of California Press.

Bollman, R. D., & Rothwell, N. (2002). *Key features of Canadian agriculture. Presentation to the Workshop of "Structural Change in the Agribusiness Sector" organized by the Cooperative Program in Agricultural Marketing and Business*. Edmonton: University of Alberta.

Breton, M. (2001). Neighborhood resiliency. *Journal of Community Practice, 9* (1), 21–36.

Brown, D., & Kulig, J. (1996/1997). The concept of resiliency: Theoretical lessons from community research. *Health & Canadian Society, 4* (1), 29–50.

Cole, D., Todd, L., & Wing, S. (2000). Concentrated swine feeding operations and public health: A review of occupational and community health effects. *Environmental Health Perspectives, 108* (8), 685–699.

Creswell, J. W. (2007). *Qualitative inquiry & research design: Choosing among five approaches* (2nd ed.). Thousand Oaks, CA: Sage.

Dick, B. (1990). *Convergent interviewing*. Brisbane: Interchange.

du Plessis, V., Beshiri, R., Bollman, R., Clemenson, H. (2001). Definitions of rural. *Rural AND Small Town Analysis Bulletin, 3* (3), Catalogue #21 006 XIE. Ottawa: Statistics Canada.

Hamilton, N., & Bhatti, T. (1996). *Population health promotion: An integrated model of population health and health promotion*. Ottawa, ON: Health Promotion Development Division, Health Canada.

Hawe, P. (1994). Capturing the meaning of "community" in community intervention evaluation. *Health Promotion International, 9* (3), 199–210.

Hegney, D., Buikstra, E., Baker, P., Rogers-Clark, C., Pearce, S., Ross, H., et al. (2007). Individual resilience in rural people, a Queensland study, Australia. *Rural and Remote Health, 7,* 620 [online].

Kawachi, I., & Berkman, L. F. (Eds.). (2003). *Neighbourhoods and health*. Oxford: Oxford University Press.

Kulig, J. (1998). The enhancement of community resiliency by community-based workers in Central Appalachia. Lethbridge, AB: University of Lethbridge, Regional Centre for Health Promotion and Community Studies.

Kulig, J. (1999). Sensing collectivity and building skills: Rural communities and community resiliency. In W. Ramp, J. Kulig, I. Townshend, & V. McGowan (Eds.), *Health in rural settings: Contexts for action* (pp. 223–244). Lethbridge, AB: University of Lethbridge.

Kulig, J. (2000). Community resiliency: The potential for community health nursing theory development. *Public Health Nursing, 17* (5), 374–385.

Kulig, J., Edge, D., & Joyce, B. (2008a). Community resiliency as a measure of collective health status: Perspectives from rural communities. *Canadian Journal of Nursing Research. 40* (4), 92–110.

Kulig, J., Edge, D., & Joyce, B. (2008b). Understanding community resiliency in rural communities through multimethod research. *Journal of Rural and Community Development, 3* (3) [online].

Kulig, J., & Hanson, L. (1996). *Discussion and expansion of the concept of resiliency: Summary of a think tank*. University of Lethbridge: Final Report.

Kulig, J., MacLeod, M., Stewart, N., & Pitblado, R. (2008). Clients in rural areas. In L. Stamler & L. Yui (Eds.), *Community health nursing: A Canadian perspective* (2nd ed., pp. 301–310). Toronto, ON: Pearson.

Kulig, J., Nahachewsky, D., Thomlinson, E., MacLeod, M., & Curran, F. (2004). Maximizing the involvement of rural nurses in policy, *The Canadian Journal of Nursing Leadership, 17* (1), 88–96.

Kulig, J., Reimer, W., Townshend, I., Edge, D., & Lightfoot, N. (2007). *Resiliency in rural settlements that have experienced wildfires: Implications for disaster management and mitigation*. [Ongoing study]. Funder: SSHRC.

Kulig, J., Reimer, W., Townshend, I., Edge, D., Neves-Graca, K., Lightfoot, N., et al. (2007). *Understanding resiliency and risk: A final report of the Lost Creek Fire pilot study*. Lethbridge, AB: University of Lethbridge.

Kulig, J., & Waldner, M. (1999). Lessons in community development: Attempting to create a community wellness centre. *Journal of Community Development Society, 30* (1), 29–47.

Labonte, R. (1993). Community-based, community development programming. In *Health promotion and empowerment: Practice frameworks* (pp. 32–34). Toronto, ON: Centre for Health Promotion and ParticipACTION.

MacMillan, D. W., & Chavis, D. M. (1986). Sense of community: A definition and theory. *Journal of Community Psychology,* 14, 6–23.

Porter, M. K. (2000). Integrating resilient young into strong communities through festivals, fairs, and feasts. In S. Danish & T. Gullota (Eds.), *Developing competent youth and strong communities through after-school programming*. In: Child Welfare League of America.

Public Safety and Emergency Preparedness Canada. Fact sheets: National disaster mitigation strategy (NDMS). (2005). Retrieved June 21, 2005, from http://www.ocipep.gc.ca/info_pro/fact_sheets/general/P_NDMS_e.asp

Schiffman, S. S., Miller, E. A. S., Suggs, M. S., & Graham, B. G. (1995). The effects of environmental odours emanating from commercial swine operations on the mood of nearby residents. *Brain Research Bulletin, 37* (4), 369–375.

Statistics Canada. (2006). *Community profiles*. Retrieved March 3, 2009, from www. statcan.gc.ca

Streubert Speziale, H. J., & Carpenter, D. R. (2007). *Qualitative research in nursing: Advancing the humanistic imperative* (4th ed.). Philadelphia: Lippincott Williams & Wilkins.

Thu, K., Donham, K., Ziegenhorn, R., Reynolds, S., Thorne, P. S., Subramanian, P., et al. (1997). A control study of the physical and mental health of residents living near a large-scale swine operation. *Journal of Agricultural Safety and Health, 3* (1), 13–26.

University of New Hampshire Cooperative Extension. (no date). *Community profiles*. Retrieved August 15, 1999 from http://extension.unh.edu/CommDev/CommProf.htm

Vollman, A. R., Anderson, E. T., & McFarlane, J. (2008). *Canadian community as partner: Theory & multidisciplinary practice* (2nd ed.). Philadelphia: Lippincott Williams & Wilkins.

Walter, C. (2005). Community building practice: A conceptual framework. In M. Minkler (Ed.), *Community building and community organizing for health* (2nd ed., pp. 66–81). New Brunswick, NJ: Rutgers University Press.

Walter, J. (2005). *World disasters report 2004: Focus on community resilience*. Geneva: International Federation of Red Cross and Red Cross Societies.

Wing, S., & Wolf, S. (2000). Intensive livestock operation, health and quality of life among eastern North Carolina residents. *Environmental Health Perspectives, 108* (3), 233–238.

The Influence of the Rural Environment on Children's Physical Activity and Eating Behaviors

NANCY E. FINDHOLT, LINDA JEROFKE, YVONNE MICHAEL, and VICTORIA W. BROGOITTI

Since the 1980s, the prevalence of childhood obesity has tripled, making this one of the nation's most serious public health threats (Ogden, Carrol, Curtin, et al., 2006). Rural populations appear to be especially vulnerable to obesity. Several studies have identified higher rates of obesity among rural children and adolescents than among their urban or suburban counterparts (Joens-Matre, Welk, Calabro, et al., 2008; Lewis, Meyer, Lehman, et al., 2006; Lutfiyya, Lipsky, Wisdom-Behounek, & Inpanbutr-Martinkus, 2007).

Why obesity prevalence is higher among rural youth is not completely clear at this time, but some evidence suggests that the rural environment presents challenges to obtaining physical activity and healthy foods. One recent study found that a dispersed residential layout, lack of an attractive town center, threats to personal safety (e.g., fear of drug dealers or child molesters), and lack of accessible open spaces were barriers to physical activity for children in some rural communities (Yousefian, Ziller, Swartz, & Hartley, 2008). A second study found that rural schools and schools with many low-income students were less likely than urban or wealthier schools to have policies that promoted physical activity and healthful nutrition—a characteristic which could impede the establishment of healthy behaviors among students in these schools (Nanney, Bohner, & Friedrichs, 2008). Also, research involving adults has shed light on factors within the rural environment that may be hindrances

401

to physical activity and healthy eating habits among children. Previous studies have found that rural adults perceived fewer places available to them for exercise than urban or suburban adults (Parks, Housemann, & Brownson, 2003; Wilcox, Castro, King, Housemann, & Brownson, 2000). Also, rural adult women were more likely than urban women to report street-related hazards, such as absence of sidewalks and unattended dogs, as impediments to walking (Wilcox et al.). Furthermore, Liese, Weis, Pluto, Smith, & Lawson (2007) identified many barriers to obtaining healthful and inexpensive foods in rural areas, including a preponderance of convenience stores as compared to large grocery stores.

Identifying the factors within rural schools and communities that affect children's physical activity and eating patterns is imperative for the development of interventions that are likely to be effective in preventing obesity among rural children. In this chapter, we present the findings of a study that explored the perceptions of rural children concerning environmental influences on their physical activity and food choices.

METHODS

This research was an exploratory study using qualitative methods. Data were collected through focus groups with rural children. The study setting was Union County, Oregon, a sparsely populated agricultural region in the northeast part of the state with a predominately Caucasian population (94.3%). The sample was drawn from fifth-grade classes in four (out of eight total) public elementary schools in Union County. These schools were selected because they represented the variability in size and socioeconomic status that existed among schools in the county. Total school enrollment ranged from 102 to 467, and the percentage of students eligible for free or reduced-price lunches ranged from 39% to 77%. Two of the schools were located in Union County's largest community (population 12,540) and two were located in communities of 1,670 and 490 residents, respectively.

Two focus groups, segregated by gender, were conducted in each of the four schools. Of the 41 children who participated, 22 were girls and 93% were Caucasian. Discussion topics included (a) the adequacy of physical activity resources in the school and community; (b) the ease or difficulty of being active during and outside of school; (c) satisfaction with school meals and the mealtime experience; (d) access to and utilization of convenience markets and fast food outlets; and (e) adult influences on children's physical activity and food choices. Each focus group lasted approximately one hour and was audio taped and transcribed verbatim. The transcripts were analyzed using a modified version of focused coding and grounded theory methods (Miles & Huberman, 1994; Strauss & Corbin, 1990). Study procedures were approved by the Institutional Review Boards at Oregon Health & Science University and Eastern Oregon University.

RESULTS

The data analysis revealed several barriers to physical activity and healthy food choices within the rural schools and communities. However, factors that promoted healthy behaviors were identified as well. The following represents the major themes and insights gained from the focus groups.

Barriers to Physical Activity

Unsafe streets emerged as a major hindrance to walking or bicycling to school or for pleasure. Several students commented on the lack of bike lanes and expressed concern about bicycling on the streets. Others reported that the speed of traffic kept them from using the streets. For example, one student said, "[My street] is really dangerous because cars go really fast. But our neighbors have a big driveway, so I just go up and down that." Long distances between home and school and adverse weather conditions were also cited as impediments to walking or bicycling to school.

Inadequate facilities for exercise and play were identified as a barrier to physical activity within the schools. Problems included insufficient gym space (i.e., too many classes sharing a gym and/or gyms that also served as the school cafeteria); limited playground equipment; and a shortage of balls and jump ropes. Similarly, inadequate facilities and equipment were an impediment to physical activity outside of school, especially in the smallest community. Students in this town said that there was just one small park with almost no playground equipment. Students living in Union County's largest community were generally satisfied with the city parks, although some said that there should be more resources, such as ice skating rinks and skateboard facilities.

Several students expressed concern about the quality and quantity of physical education (PE). Approximately half indicated that they received PE only twice per week, and some noted that PE classes were not vigorous. One girl stated, "I think that [PE] is . . . too easy. We don't get a whole lot of exercise because . . . people just sit around and stuff." Furthermore, many students reported that denial of recess was commonly used as a disciplinary measure: "Sometimes, if you get in trouble or you don't bring your homework back, you don't get to go to recess. . . . Or, if you go to the bathroom during class." ["Then you don't get to go to recess?"] "Yeah, because you are wasting your class time."

Factors that Supported Physical Activity

The availability of non curricular sports programs emerged as a facilitator of physical activity outside of school. A variety of team sports were offered to children of both genders and participation in sports appeared to be common, particularly among boys. The male students told us that they and their peers were involved in many sports. One said that he participated in at least five sports per year, and another stated, "I get about two hours of activity every day almost. I'm in wrestling and other things." The female students mentioned participating in sports less often than did the male students, which may indicate that fewer girls participated.

Union County's natural environment (e.g., the mountains, forests, and open spaces) was also commonly cited as a factor that supported physical activity. One student explained, "I believe the environment we live in around here . . . you know, we have great ski mountains and camping areas. Since we live in an area like [this], it makes it easier to get to a place where you can get good exercise but still have fun with it." Many students reported activities such as hiking, hunting, skiing, playing in creeks, and climbing trees. The community's sociocultural norms also appeared to support outdoor activity, as evidenced by this quote: "There are many ranchers here and people that go hunting, and being outdoors is really important to this community."

Adults were generally perceived as a good influence in regard to physical activity. Several students reported that their teachers and other adults were active (e.g., walked, bicycled, or skied), and that many coached or attended children's sports events. Others said that their parents and teachers urged them to play outdoors, participate in sports, or both, and that teachers played with them during recess and physical education. A few students, however, did not believe that physical activity was important to adults in their community, and noted that many adults were overweight and sedentary.

Barriers to Healthy Food Choices

Poor quality school meals, specifically the entrées, emerged as a primary impediment to a healthy diet. Students reported that most of the entrées were prepackaged rather than homemade, and that the food tasted "artificial" and was salty and greasy. This comment was typical: "[S]ometimes [the school food] is really gross. They say it is healthy, but some chicken . . . you can open it and you can see all the grease. . . ." It was also noted that fast-food choices were served frequently. One student said, "Sometimes they have pizza and then that week they make just stuff out of pizza, like pizza sticks and then maybe pizza again. . . . Sometimes they have breakfast pizza that is basically leftover pizza that they put meat on it with eggs."

Limited cafeteria space and an unpleasant cafeteria environment were also reported as hindrances to healthy eating. Many students said that lunchtime was rushed because a large number of classes had to be accommodated in a small cafeteria. Others said that cooks or other school personnel often scolded them for talking during lunch or for not finishing their meal, and that the cafeteria was very noisy. Students further noted that teachers often did not model healthy eating habits. One said, "[T]hey are always putting . . . brownies and cookies in the teachers' lounge." Others observed that teachers "drink soda right at their desk" even though students were not permitted to have soda.

The presence of convenience stores near many elementary schools emerged as a barrier to healthy food choices outside of school. The students reported that they and their peers frequently purchased snacks from these stores. Common snack items included energy drinks, pop, beef jerky, cheese sticks, candy, chips, and deep-fried deli foods.

Factors that Supported Healthy Food Choices

Gardening appeared to be a social norm that promoted healthy diets. Many students said that their families had gardens, fruit trees, or both, and most said that they commonly ate fresh fruits and vegetables when these were in season. For example, when asked how often he ate fresh fruit, one student said, "Every time I can get to the tree. I like going down to my tree and getting a plum off of it." However, it appeared that most family gardens were small and that preserving produce was an uncommon practice.

Hunting also emerged as a community norm that may support healthful eating, and fishing was common as well. Many students reported eating game regularly, and some stated that all of their meat was obtained through hunting or fishing.

Despite the comments about teachers drinking soda and eating sweets, most of the students said that nutrition was important to adults in their school. Several noted that teachers and food service personnel encouraged them to select fruits and vegetables from the salad bar, and that the teachers often ate salads themselves. Some also observed that the school staff had removed the soda machine and had stopped giving out candy in the classroom. Others said that their teachers had invited nutritionists to speak in their classes.

Finally, it was reported that salad bars were available in the school cafeterias. However, the type and quality of the foods offered appeared to be variable. Some students said that their school's salad bar included a variety of fresh fruits and vegetables, such as broccoli, carrots, beets, cauliflower, apples, and oranges. Others, however, observed that foods such as Jell-O and desserts were available. In addition, several students said that the vegetables were often soft or otherwise unappealing. One stated, "The salad bar has beets [but they are] gross and heavily salted. [The lettuce] is iceberg lettuce, so there is no nutritional value to it."

DISCUSSION

The results of this study provide insight into conditions within rural schools and communities that negatively affect children's physical activity and eating habits and may contribute to the high rates of childhood obesity in rural populations. Addressing these conditions is essential, but this will not be an easy task. Just as characteristics of the rural environment create obstacles to healthy behaviors, so too do rural characteristics (such as transportation barriers, limited access to grant funding, low public funding levels for services and programs, and difficulties recruiting staff) present challenges for the delivery of health promotion programs (Phillips & McLeroy, 2004). On the other hand, there are strengths within rural communities upon which health promotion programs might be built. Our study findings suggest several environmental characteristics that could be enhanced or expanded to provide children with increased opportunities to obtain physical activity and healthy foods.

Organized after-school sports may be one resource for promoting physical activity. Similar to other studies (Bilinski, Semchuk, & Chad, 2005; Davis, Boles, James, et al., 2008), we found that involvement in sports is a way that many rural children obtain physical activity, although participation in sports appeared to be more common among boys than girls. Attention should be given to developing after-school activities that appeal to girls. Also, because many traditional sports, such as football and wrestling, are not lifelong activities, offering alternatives, such as dance, would be beneficial.

Another resource that may be especially important in promoting physical activity among rural children is access to the natural environment. A growing body of evidence has documented numerous benefits for children that are associated with spending time outdoors in natural settings, including increased physical activity and improved mental health and cognition (Kuo & Taylor, 2004; Sallis, Prochaska, & Taylor, 2000; Wells & Evans, 2003). Rural communities are fortunate in having ample open spaces. However, efforts may need to be made to improve access and to ensure that children can travel to these areas safely. Also, enhancements to the outdoor spaces, such as trail development, might stimulate increased use.

The culture of gardening and hunting that was identified in this study is an asset that could be further developed to promote healthy eating habits. Potential strategies include developing school gardens, farmers' markets, and venues for sharing produce in churches or community centers; providing information and resources (e.g., pressure canners, community freezers) to families to encourage food preservation; and developing farm-to-school programs, which link farmers with school cafeterias to increase the use of locally grown, fresh produce in the schools.

This study was limited by the use of self-report data, which are subject to error, and by the inclusion of only one rural county. The barriers and assets that we identified might not be the same as those found in other rural areas. For this reason, we recommend that nurses who are interested in developing an obesity prevention program in a rural community begin by conducting a thorough assessment to identify the barriers and strengths that exist in that community. We also recommend that replication of this study be done using a larger and more diverse sample. Finally, the use of objective measures of physical activity and eating patterns would enhance the qualitative findings. Addressing these issues may aid in developing interventions that will be effective in preventing obesity among rural children.

ACKNOWLEDGMENT

This study was funded with a grant from the Northwest Health Foundation, Portland, Oregon.

REFERENCES

Bilinski, H., Semchuk, K. M., & Chad, K. (2005). Understanding physical activity patterns of rural Canadian children. *Online Journal of Rural Nursing and Health Care, 5*, 73–82.

Davis, A. M., Boles, R. E., James, R. L., Sullivan, D. K., Donnelly, J. E., Swirczynski, D. L., et al. (2008). Health behaviors and weight status among urban and rural children. *Rural and Remote Health* (Online), *8*, 1–11.

Joens-Matre, R. R., Welk, G. J., Calabro, M. A., Russel, D. W., Nicklay, E., & Hensley, L. D. (2008). Rural-urban differences in physical activity, physical fitness, and overweight prevalence of children. *Journal of Rural Health, 24*, 49–54.

Kuo, F. E., & Taylor, A. F. (2004). A potential natural treatment for attention-deficit/hyperactivity disorder: Evidence from a national study. *American Journal of Public Health, 94*, 1580–1586.

Lewis, R. C., Meyer, M. C., Lehman, S. C., Trowbridge, F. L., Bason, J. J., Yurman, K. H., et al.(2006). Prevalence and degree of childhood and adolescent overweight in rural, urban, and suburban Georgia. *Journal of School Health, 76*, 126–132.

Liese, A. D., Weis, K. E., Pluto, D., Smith, E., & Lawson, A. (2007). Food store types, availability, and cost of foods in a rural environment. *Journal of the American Dietetic Association, 107*, 1916–1923.

Lutfiyya, M. N., Lipsky, M. S., Wisdom-Behounek, J., & Inpanbutr-Martinkus, M. (2007). Is rural residency a risk factor for overweight and obesity for U.S. children? *Obesity, 15*, 2348–2356.

Miles, M. B., & Huberman, A. M. (1994). *Qualitative data analysis* (2nd ed.). Thousand Oaks, CA: Sage.

Nanney, M. S., Bohner, C., & Friedrichs, M. (2008). Poverty-related factors associated with obesity prevention policies in Utah secondary schools. *Journal of the American Dietetic Association, 108*, 1210–1215.

Ogden, C. L., Carrol, M. D., Curtin, L. R., McDowell, M. A., Tabak, C. J., & Flegal, K. M. (2006). Prevalence of overweight and obesity in the United States, 1999–2004. *Journal of the American Medical Association, 295*, 1549–1555.

Parks, S. E., Housemann, R., & Brownson, R. C. (2003). Differential correlates of physical activity in urban and rural adults of various socioeconomic backgrounds in the United States. *Journal of Epidemiology & Community Health, 57*, 29–35.

Phillips, C. D., & McLeroy, K. R. (2004). Tailoring programs and services to meet rural needs. *American Journal of Public Health, 94*, 1662–1663.

Sallis, J. F., Prochaska, J. J., & Taylor, W. C. (2000). A review of correlates of physical activity of children and adolescents. *Medicine & Science in Sports & Exercise, 32*, 963–975.

Strauss, A., & Corbin, J. (1990). *Basics of qualitative research: Grounded theory procedures and techniques.* Newbury Park, CA: Sage.

Wells, N. M., & Evans, G. W. (2003). Nearby nature: A buffer of life stress among rural children. *Environment and Behavior, 35,* 311–330.

Wilcox, S., Castro, C., King, A. C., Housemann, R., & Brownson, R. C. (2000). Determinants of leisure time physical activity in rural compared with urban older and ethnically diverse women in the United States. *Journal of Epidemiology & Community Health, 54,* 667–672.

Yousefian, A., Ziller, E., Swartz, J., & Hartley, D. (2008). *Active living for rural youth.* Portland: University of Southern Maine, Maine Rural Health Research Center.

Negotiating Three Worlds: Academia, Nursing Science, and Tribal Communities[1]

26

PATRICIA A. HOLKUP, T. KIM CALLAHAN RODEHORST,
SUSAN L. WILHELM, SANDRA W. KUNTZ, CLARANN
WEINERT, MARY BETH FLANDERS STEPANS, EMILY
MATT SALOIS, JACQUELINE LEFT HAND BULL, and
WADE G. HILL

Conducting research in tribal communities requires an approach that is sensitive both to the long history of tribal mistrust of research and to current tribal vulnerabilities associated with the conduct of research in their communities (American Indian Law Center, 1999; Carson & Hand, 1999; Manson, Garroutte, Goins, & Henderson, 2004; Maynard, 1974; Norton & Manson, 1996; Quandt, McDonald, Bell, & Arcury, 1999). Establishing relationships of trust and reciprocity is critical (Rogers & Petereit, 2005). Most research reports focus on the results of studies; there are fewer reports about the process of conducting studies with Native American communities. The purpose of this chapter is to use a cross-cultural model to guide the exploration of common issues and the dynamic interrelationships surrounding entrée to tribal communities as experienced by four nursing research teams. Information in this chapter is expected to be of value to nurse scientists, other members of the academic community, and Native American participants who are engaged in cross-cultural research in Native American communities.

REVIEW OF THE RELATED LITERATURE

In the United States there are more than 561 federally recognized Native American tribes. Although each has a unique culture, there are some commonalities across tribes (Red Horse, 1980a, 1980b; Swinomish Tribal Mental Health Project, 2002; Weaver & White, 1997). These commonalities represent strengths that contribute to the significant resiliency of Native American people over the centuries. Included among these strengths are a strong sense of spirituality, the value placed on family, and the interdependence of members of the tribal community (Red Horse; Swinomish Tribal Mental Health Project; Weaver & White). Those involved in research efforts must be aware of these strengths as well as the challenges that may arise when conducting research with Native American people.

Central to assessing these challenges is understanding of and respect for the traumatic history Native American people have experienced with the colonization of their homelands by western European nations. All tribes share a history of hardships and restrictions, including the loss of land; broken promises and treaties; restrictions of shelter and food; the attempted destruction of language, religion, and culture; stereotyping; and the burden of government interference. Negative sequelae from this history persist in tribal communities today. From the literature reviewed it is evident that Native Americans also have experienced negative results from research practices (American Indian Law Center, 1999; Carson & Hand, 1999; Manson et al., 2004; Maynard, 1974; Norton & Manson, 1996; Quandt et al., 1999). Because of this history of exploitation and abuse by research institutions and the government, mistrust of those who conduct research exists (Mitchell & Baker, 2005).

Increasingly, tribal communities are developing Institutional Review Boards (IRBs) and requiring that researchers apply for project approval prior to conducting research in a community. Tribal members recognize their vulnerabilities associated with research, and wish to maintain decision-making authority regarding which projects are allowed to be conducted in their communities. In addition, in some communities publications and presentations are required to be approved prior to submission, and ownership of the data may be requested to stay at the local level. It is important that researchers and community members discuss the project in relation to community needs to ensure project relevance and obtain permission to conduct the research in any given community. This can be a time-consuming process (Manson et al., 2004), with significant financial expenditures that must be acknowledged when planning grant applications and timelines (Norton & Manson, 1996). Often no financial compensation for either community members or researchers is available for this "up-front" work. Yet, taking the time to develop trusting partnerships, establishing a commitment to the tribal members, and appreciating the sovereignty of tribal communities are foremost in assuring success of research projects (Tom-Orme, 2006).

Entering into tribal communities can be fraught with potential and actual breaches of community protocols (Mitchell & Baker, 2005). Factors that contribute to hesitancy in allowing researchers entry into their communities include distrust of research personnel; researchers' lack of understanding, respect, or both toward cultural practices; and the potential for reporting results that emphasize problems that in turn can demoralize and stigmatize communities while reinforcing negative stereotypes (American Indian Law Center, 1999; Burhansstipanov, Christopher, & Schumacher, 2005; Manson et al., 2004; Mitchell & Baker). Early identification of nuances specific to each tribal community might avert potential breaches that can occur in relation to entry into their communities. It is critical for researchers to reflect upon the ability to establish a working relationship prior to the initiation of a project.

The potential for exploitation and repetition of past abuses might make it difficult for members of tribal communities to perceive many benefits from participating in research relative to the potential risks (Norton & Manson, 1996). Many Native American tribes prefer that a community-based participatory approach be utilized when conducting studies that involve their communities (Burhansstipanov et al., 2005). This approach provides the opportunity for researchers, community members, and agency representatives to have equitable involvement in the research process from its inception to its conclusion. The use of a partnership approach increases the likelihood of conducting research that is relevant to the community and that will make contributions to the scientific literature. Developing a relationship with the community in which representatives from the community and the academic institution both have a role in each step of the research process is essential for success of the project (Burhansstipanov et al.).

Researchers must work diligently with tribal community leaders to ensure that relevant members of the community are involved in all stages of the research process. Acknowledging, valuing, and adapting research based on community members' input is vital for the success of the project. In addition, it is important to provide adequate compensation to community members for their contributions to the research project. Using a community-based participatory approach requires a stance of long-term commitment to the community partnership and begins with taking the necessary time to establish relationships that form the basis for trust to develop and deepen (Norton & Manson, 1996).

Commitment to the community and cultural sensitivity provide the foundation for successful research within tribal communities. Illustrating the importance of research to the community and demonstrating the direct and immediate benefits to the people of the community must be part of the study purpose (Manson et al., 2004). In addition, the process and methodology by which the research is conducted are also noteworthy. Because of the inherent cultural differences of the research team and the community of interest, it is crucial to the success of the project to demonstrate congruency with cultural values and modes of interaction (Dodgson & Struthers, 2005; Red Horse, Johnson, & Weiner, 1989; Stoddard, 1997). Equitable working relationships with Native American communities may include working with tribal leaders in all discussions, having a local office, employing local community members, and providing adequate compensation. Benefit perception may increase as research is translated into meaningful action (Norton & Manson, 1996).

THE *NEGOTIATING THREE WORLDS* MODEL

The impetus for this article emerged from discussions among nurse researchers who were involved with four unrelated projects with several Native American communities. We (the researchers) had been affiliated, at some point in our work, with the Center for Research on Chronic Health Conditions in Rural Dwellers (CRCHC) at Montana State University–Bozeman College of Nursing. We convened at the invitation of the Center's Principal Investigator, who had noticed some similar procedural challenges and successes in our work.

Through discussion of our common experiences with the four projects, we became aware of the ramifications of our involvement with the complex and interrelated activities of three dynamic entities: academic institutions, nursing science, and tribal communities. With this new understanding, we developed a model depicting the interactions of the four research projects with these entities (see Figure 26.1). The cumulative requirements of these three diverse entities, each with their own powerful political and bureaucratic milieus, influenced and directed the research process for all of the projects.

The Venn diagram at the center of the model in Figure 26.1 represents the dynamic, interrelationships of the three entities. The academic institution often serves as a venue through which funds for research

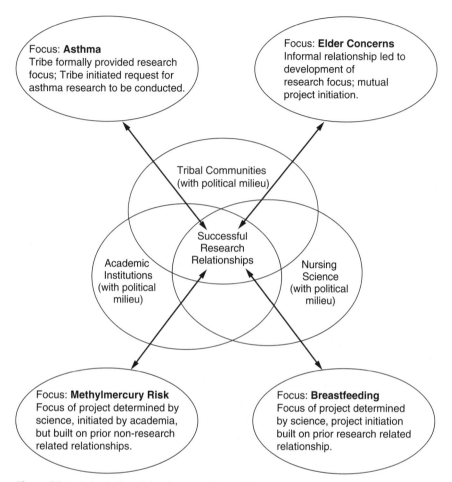

Figure 26.1. A depiction of the three worlds model, representing the interrelationships of the three entities: academia, nursing science, and tribal communities.

projects are secured and administered. As stewards of grant funding, members of academic institutions mandate and monitor requirements that must be followed by those conducting the research. Conflicts can arise when there is dissonance between the requirements of the institution and the cultural needs of the participants.

Nursing science is concerned with the building of a knowledge base to promote the health of individuals, families, and communities. Political pressures in this arena are directly linked to funding sources that have a responsibility to address the integrity of the scientific process. The positivist worldview continues to dominate perceptions of what constitutes good science. Funding sources have been slow to trust research approaches arising from other ontological perspectives. These other perspectives, however, may be more appropriate for conducting relevant research with ethnic minority groups.

Tribal leaders, as mentioned earlier, may have a well-founded and long-standing distrust of the benefits of research endeavors for their communities. Tribal communities, as sovereign nations, have their own agendas which may or may not include the acceptance of various academic research projects conducted within their communities. Finally, the balance among the desires and behaviors of tribal individuals, agencies, and communities constitutes a dynamic political process that outside scientists may find difficult to grasp.

In the second part of the model, we placed each of the projects in proximity to those entities that were involved in the development of the research focus and the initiation of the project. The manner in which the research focus was developed and the project was initiated played a large part in determining the course of the research process.

INTRODUCTION TO THE PROJECTS

The four unrelated projects were conducted in eight separate sites, or communities, involving a total of 11 tribes. All projects received IRB approval from the universities with which they were affiliated. All projects also received approval from their affiliated tribal councils. Two projects received two additional levels of approval from (a) their affiliated tribal health boards, and (b) their Indian Health Service (IHS) IRBs. To acquaint the reader with the four projects, we describe each using the following common categories: (1) impetus and opportunities, (2) emergence of the project in the community, (3) initial steps and negotiations, (4) implementing the project, and (5) evaluating the process.

Project 1: Screening Native American Children for Asthma

Impetus and Opportunities

This project emerged during a meeting between the director of an epidemiology center and a tribal health board, when a concern about the seemingly high rate of asthma in children surfaced. Following this meeting, an announcement was released regarding the opportunity to write a grant proposal as part of the Native American Research Centers for Health (NARCH) initiative, funded through the IHS and the National Institutes of Health. A researcher from the university was selected to write this portion of the grant. The impetus, then, for the asthma screening project was derived from a need identified among the tribal leaders and the availability of a nurse researcher to write a competitive grant proposal and conduct the research with two tribal communities. Please note the upper-left-corner of Figure 26.1.

Emergence of the Project in the Community

The focus of initial discussions regarding the project was on maximizing participation by the two tribal communities. The research protocol allowed the research team to work with the communities to determine how best to conduct asthma screenings in children. A secondary purpose of the grant was to build research capacity in the two tribal communities. Hiring two research assistants, who were members of their respective tribal communities, helped to achieve these goals.

Initial Steps and Negotiations

Successes. Involvement of an academic liaison by the university to facilitate negotiations among the researchers and members of the tribal communities was key to the success of gaining entry into each of the communities. This three-way relationship was characterized by mutual respect. In addition, we followed the steps necessary for conducting research in Indian country. We initially contacted the tribal health director to explain the purpose of the research, to ascertain that the research was something that would be of value for their community, and to ask for support in our efforts. Once support from the tribal health director was garnered, we approached the tribal health board, once again to ensure that we had support and commitment to the project. Finally, the tribal council was approached for support and approval of the research project. Once these steps were completed, we applied for institutional review from the academic institution and from IHS.

Challenges. Major challenges prior to the initial phase of the project involved obtaining resolutions from the tribal communities and institutional reviews from the academic institution and the IHS IRB. There were unexpected changes in personnel at both of the tribal sites which delayed the acquisition of the resolutions needed to seek approval from the IRB. Gentle reminders from the liaison and health directors in both communities spurred the council to pass the resolution. The process from the initial contact with the communities to the point of obtaining the resolution was approximately 6 months.

Obtaining approval from the IRB of the university and the IHS IRB was delayed because of the complex nature of the research proposal. There were three phases to the research project, with each successive phase dependent upon the findings of the preceding phase. The initial phase of the research consisted of conducting focus groups with members of the tribal communities to ascertain ways to develop an asthma screening process that would be most appropriate for their community. The second phase of the research, conducting the asthma screenings, was adapted based on the results of the focus group discussion. The IHS IRB approved the first phase of the study, but indicated they would approve the second phase only after the focus groups had been conducted and appropriate protocol changes made. Though reasonable and understandable, this meant that the researcher needed to resubmit the proposal to the IHS IRB and await approval more than once.

Implementing the Project

Successes. During the focus group discussions, rich data was acquired to be used to shape the asthma screening protocol. A total of 27 community members participated in the focus groups. The research team believes that the high number in attendance was because of the research assistants' ties to and knowledge of each community. There had been some concern raised among participants about how the data would be used and where they would be housed. Participants were reassured that the data would remain with the tribe. Although tribal members did acknowledge that screening children for asthma was important, they also clearly identified that many screenings have been done on the Native American population and they would also like help dealing with the problem of asthma. Members of the research team acknowledged their concern and explained that identifying the prevalence is the necessary first step toward writing a more comprehensive research proposal that could provide an intervention for the children with asthma.

Challenges. Geographic distance of the tribal communities from the university created the major challenge associated with implementation of the research project. Because of the remote location of one community in particular, it has been difficult to secure travel arrangements at reasonable costs. Travel to that community to conduct screenings involved three days at a minimum. In addition, the researcher's teaching responsibilities often had to take precedence over research, making it difficult to arrange a schedule that was compatible for all parties involved.

Evaluating the Process

Because the asthma screening project originated from the administrative level of the epidemiology center and the tribal health board, the bureaucratic barriers have been minimal. The project was initiated from tribal health concerns, so acceptance of the research has not been a major concern. The primary challenges in this project were related to time. The time that it took to go through both the academic as well as the IHS IRBs was problematic. In addition, traveling to each reservation required a major commitment from the university research team. Despite these issues, the timelines delineated in the project proposal were not met. Flexibility, adaptability, and respect have been the elements for success of this project.

Project 2: Caring for Native American Elders

Impetus and Opportunities

The Caring for Native American Elders project was initiated by way of an informal relationship developed through a series of synchronous events between a Native American social worker and a non-Native nurse (see the upper-right-corner of Figure 26.1). The social worker had, in the course of her work, observed with concern the manner in which elders were treated in some of the families she visited. In addition to her own concerns, she knew that members of some of those families also were worried about their elders. The social worker and the nurse joined two additional non-Native nurse scientists to form a formal research partnership.

With concerns about Native American elder abuse as a focus, the research team set about developing a community-based participatory research project. The focus of this project was to collect interview data about the perceived magnitude, causes, and forms of elder abuse. In the spirit of reciprocity, the team also wanted to address families' concerns about elders by offering a culturally congruent family conference intervention (Holkup, Tripp-Reimer, Salois, & Weinert, 2004).

Emergence of the Project in the Community

The team designed a project that combined the collection of data with the delivery of a service. Unfortunately this design is counter to the usual progression of a program of research, which requires documentation of a problem prior to the receipt of funding for piloting an intervention. After some searching, the team received two seed grants from research centers at two colleges of nursing in different states. The simultaneous funding allowed a seamless flow between data collection and piloting the intervention. Subsequently, the team expanded the project to engage two additional communities. The project is at different stages with each of these communities.

Initial Steps and Negotiations

Initially, negotiations began among the research team members in an effort to develop trust and ensure that the equality and unique power of each of the team members would be honored. During this phase, the team discovered the need to build "credibility bridges" (Salois, Holkup, Tripp-Reimer, & Weinert, 2006) between academia and the Native American community and among the members of the research team. It was at this point that the team developed a memorandum of understanding with emphasis on issues such as decision making by consensus, storage and ownership of the data, and cultural review of all project reports (Holkup et al., 2004).

Successes. The Native American research team member has provided insight into respectful cultural norms with regard to community entry. She also made the first contacts with people in the communities. Her negotiations with each of the communities began with a soft entry, through engaging a network of people she has known from various venues: her professional work, former family encounters, and friendships that were forged at boarding schools. After making the initial contacts, the team would request a meeting with community members. Meetings have followed two patterns, with team members as guests or as hosts. As guests, team members often shared in a meal and had a place on the agenda. As hosts, the team members would send a letter of invitation with a brochure describing the project to each prospective participant. Because gracious hospitality requires the sharing of food, the team also made these arrangements. On the day of the meeting, the Native American team member would make a call to each of the invited individuals to check in and see if they were still able to attend. This served as a reminder to the participants in addition to helping the team members understand what currently was happening within the community that might affect the upcoming meeting.

During the initial meeting, the focus of the discussion was on community members' perceptions of need for and their thoughts about the feasibility of the Family Care Conference project in their community. With each of these initial meetings, there has been overwhelming support for the project. Once the team was able to determine there was support for the project, with community guidance, the team requested letters of support from appropriate community members or agency representatives. These letters were necessary for inclusion with applications for funding and most often have come from service providers who are community members with long-term working relationships in the various community agencies.

Challenges. There has always been the need for flexibility in this project. On one occasion it was necessary to reschedule a meeting at the last minute because an unforeseen community need took precedence. Although the team had traveled many miles to attend this meeting, responsibilities for community needs were pressing.

In another situation, the representative from a funding source asked for a letter of support from the tribal chairperson. This request threatened the demise of a portion of the project because the request came in the summer months, just prior to the deadline for funding decisions, and at a time when the tribal chairperson was away from the community. Although the team was able to obtain a letter of support, it is important to note that, during the long process for scientific review, the makeup of the tribal council had changed considerably from the time of first contact with the community, though those people working in the service-providing sectors of the community who had supplied the original letters of support had remained in their positions.

Sensitivity to the current political milieu has been important, as priorities may shift with administrative changes. Progress in one community has halted because the membership of the tribal governing board changed and was no longer supportive of the project. However, because members of the community expressed an interest in the project, the research team hopes there will come a time when the political climate will once again be receptive to the project.

Implementing the Project

Successes. This ongoing program of research at one time involved three communities. In the first community, we hired and trained three community members to serve as facilitators for the Family Care Conference intervention. The project was so well received in this community that at the end of funding one of the tribal human service agencies assumed responsibility for the intervention's continuation. The team provided training for the agency's employees in addition to initial monetary and professional support. The agency director, in turn, agreed to continue to collect data for the project. In the second community, data collection has ended and arrangements are being made to conduct three Family Care Conferences to determine the feasibility of implementing the intervention there. In the third community, as mentioned earlier, progress has stopped.

Challenges. During that portion of the project when three community members served as Family Care Conference facilitators, funding was such that each could be employed for quarter-time for a year. With high rates of poverty and unemployment, community members were happy to receive even part-time work; however, during the course of the project, two trained facilitators left when opportunities for full-time work understandably took precedence over the part-time positions. This loss of personnel slowed the momentum of the project, requiring hiring and training new Family Care Conference facilitators.

Evaluating the Process

Throughout this program of research, the research team has kept careful notes of the processes inherent in working across two cultures. Through analysis of these notes, it became apparent that an essential component of building and maintaining relationships with these Native American communities involved the team's approaching their work from a stance of frequent and thoughtful self-reflection and self-critique in an attempt to guard against cross-cultural misunderstandings, misinterpretations, or both. Working from this perspective has helped to dismantle power imbalances and maintain equitable power dynamics, which has promoted the development of mutually beneficial relationships among members of the scientific and the tribal communities (Holkup et al., 2004; Hunt, 2001; Salois et al., 2006; Tervalon & Murray-Garcia, 1998).

Project 3: Motivational Interviewing to Promote Sustained Breast-Feeding: Native American Women

Impetus and Opportunities

The opportunity for this research project was built on a prior relationship (see lower-right corner of Figure 26.1) that was established through the efforts of the primary investigator of the asthma screening project. The coinvestigator of this project visited the Tribal Epidemiology Center and this provided the occasion to meet with the Healthy Start (HS) program director. The director discussed the HS goals for increasing breast-feeding rates and discussed obstacles to breast-feeding for this population of mothers. She requested further information about strategies to increase breast-feeding initiation.

After this initial encounter, the investigator was asked to provide breast-feeding workshops. Two workshops were conducted in collaboration with HS community coordinators and case managers from all of the midwestern tribal communities. The HS staff members were expected to learn the benefits of breast-feeding babies at the first workshop, and how to assist mothers with problems at the second workshop. The HS mothers encountered barriers to successful breast-feeding, which included lack of expert breast-feeding support in several of the reservations, often a lack of peer support for breast-feeding, concerns about privacy, and stopping breast-feeding because of a perceived insufficient milk supply.

Emergence of the Project in the Community

The university sponsored a competitive minority health opportunity grant and this study was one of the projects selected. Negotiations then began with the HS director about the potential support for this project within the tribal communities. A quasi-experimental design was selected for this study to prevent within-group contamination with one small rural Native American community selected as the primary intervention site. Another site was chosen as the "infant safety attention intervention" site. The HS director expressed concern about members of each community receiving the same opportunities for training, so it was offered at both sites upon completion of study recruitment. The two sites were considered for the study because they would most likely meet the required number of nursing mothers, and all had a high incidence of automobile accidents. Care was taken to identify a site that had high rates of accidents so that the members of the community chosen would benefit greatly from the "attention infant safety intervention." The HS program also wanted to be certain both intervention plans empowered mothers to make their own choices. The Motivational Interviewing intervention was chosen partially because it is a client-centered strategy.

Initial Steps and Negotiations

Once the grant was funded, a project assistant was hired by the research partner; this person was shared with another research project and worked in the partner's central office. However, she happened to be from one of the study communities. This woman, who had breast-fed her children, said she was excited about helping other mothers breast-feed and was helpful in providing feedback about the development of culturally appropriate study materials.

Meeting with tribal health boards was a very positive cultural experience for the university research team members. Food was provided and one of the health board members was invited to say a prayer before the meeting began, as is the custom in this Native American tribal community. Because the university team traveled a long distance to meet at one of the study sites, the chairman gathered a quorum to vote on the resolution to approve the breast-feeding project so the university team members would not have to return a second time for this particular issue. The university research team appreciated this consideration as the breast-feeding project had not been a priority on the tribal council's agenda. Tribal health board members at both sites expressed concern about the protection of the data relative to the study and wanted assurances related to accessing the findings. They also were quite concerned about maintaining confidentiality in publications. The university research team members made a commitment to return to these groups (the tribal health boards and the HS program sites) with a report following the completion of the study. However, time passed and turnover in staffing occurred, so the local team members will be different upon completion of the study.

Implementing the Project

The two tribal communities were selected as either the intervention group or the attention intervention group to prevent within-group contamination as members of tribal communities generally know each other and interact regularly. Because the local research team members (the HS case managers) had not been previously involved in research, they needed to complete the human subject training. The university team members provided support during this training session. Struggles with the technology and the complexity of the material made this session a challenge for the university and local team members. At a later date, the university research team provided training for data collection and interventions both for the local research team members as a whole, and then this training was reinforced at each site. These sessions offered rich opportunities for team building and allowed all members of the research team to get to know each other. The use of humor and university team member vulnerability about past challenges with data collection was essential to relieve tensions as all people strove to do their best.

Evaluating the Process

One of the successes of this study was identifying a project that was important to women who are leaders in promoting the health of infants. Because the HS director and staff had decided that promotion of breast-feeding was important to the success of HS program goals, they were receptive to learning the research protocol. However, the challenge of maintaining continuity in the research project posed difficult problems. There was a change of HS staff (research assistant and one of the HS study site community coordinators) during the implementation of the study, so those two new HS personnel had to be oriented to the study. Therefore, continuity of resources became an issue in terms of limited time and money to orient new personnel. The local research team members diligently recruited mothers to be in the study. However, the study criterion to exclude teen mothers limited their ability to recruit participants in a timely fashion; because of this they had to go outside HS mothers to find study participants.

Their apparent dedication to helping mothers that they cared for in the HS program was very evident and humbling. Both the HS program staff and the university research team learned that even a small study in a tribal community takes a great deal of time for the preliminary approval requirements, and that circumstances beyond the control of anyone, such as the loss of trained staff, can also affect the progress of the study. Mutual trust and respect are essential to unchallenged implementation and outcome reports; so the time and effort spent in building that trust and respect are as important as the adherence to protocols.

Project 4: Methylmercury

Impetus and Opportunities

The development of this academia-initiated study (see lower-left-hand corner of Figure 26.1) resulted from questions raised by researchers regarding the unknowns of methylmercury risk awareness and potential exposure of Native American childbearing women through fish consumption. Efforts to inform the public of methylmercury risks have existed since the early 1990s. However, considerable evidence indicates that fish advisory messages distributed through angler licenses may not have reached vulnerable populations (Anderson, Hanrahan, Smith, et al., 2004). Native Americans fish on home reservations and are exempt from licensing requirements, and therefore may not receive standard fish advisory messages distributed through license brochures.

Initial Steps and Negotiations

Participants for this study were recruited through the Special Supplemental Nutrition Program for the Women, Infant, and Children (WIC) on one reservation. The administrator of the WIC program, a respected tribal member, served as the primary consultant on issues critical to the success of the project. As emissary to the tribal council, the consultant placed the request to conduct the research on the council agenda, monitored the status of the item, and then attended the tribal council meeting to present and advocate for the proposed research study once the agenda item was scheduled. The research team experienced a 2-month delay between repeated agenda-item requests and approval of the research project when more pressing issues were considered by the council. Pacing of this project was shaped in part by a series of tribal events that took precedence over the research approval request.

The course of the study from formulation of the aims through project completion involved partners representing a variety of perspectives and directives. The interdisciplinary research team received funding from the CRCHC. The team consulted with and was advised by state agency representatives from Montana Fish, Wildlife, and Parks; Department of Environmental Quality; and Department of Public Health and Human Services (Environmental Health; Health and Consumer Safety; and the WIC Program). This particular tribal community was chosen based on an existing relationship between research team members and tribal acquaintances. However, established trust can be easily squandered when pressures mount to achieve a research goal. Understanding the urgency embedded in academic culture, often the antithesis of tribal community perspective, requires balancing a respect for pacing differences and finding common ground for initiating, maintaining, and completing a project.

Emergence of the Project in the Community

Investigating health disparities (U.S. Department of Health and Human Services, 2000) on an environmental issue in a tribal community requires knowledge of the people and a specific plan for developing participatory approaches with local community members (Jardine, 2003). In Native American communities, for instance, using a scientific expert, hierarchical scheme that fails to incorporate local knowledge and cultural beliefs, or both is rarely an effective method for assessing risk or implementing change (Arquette, Cole, Cook, et al., 2002; Poupart, Martinez, Red Horse, & Scharnberg, 2000). Indigenous and dominant cultures approach decision making and communication of important messages in strikingly different ways. Risk assessment in tribal communities requires flexibility, collaboration, and respect for points of view that might come from the admonition of an elder rather than the data of a scientific expert (Agency for Toxic Substances and Disease Registry, 2000; Bird, 2002; Cajete, 1994; Colomeda-Lambert, 1999).

Implementing the Project

Project implementation included a review of a fish consumption and advisory awareness tool (Anderson et al., 2004). Reconstruction of this tool was based on recommendations from tribal elders and included deletion of questions, language changes, and inclusion of pictures/ images to enhance survey appropriateness and interest. Once finalized and evaluated for time burden, the computerized survey was placed on a secure Web site using Snap survey software. To overcome reading level and computer skill differences among participants, a tribal research assistant was trained to administer the survey to participant volunteers recruited by WIC personnel during their regularly scheduled visit. After the survey, all participants were thanked for their time, educated regarding safe fish consumption, and given a gift certificate by the research assistant.

Challenges. When research questions emanate from academia, project importance at the community level may hold less significance and urgency. With the tribal community overwhelmed by a variety of pressing health concerns, a slow-motion environmental threat with few outward or immediately apparent sequelae may fail the priority test. Timing of this particular study coincided with a high number of youth alcohol-related deaths on the reservation. Researchers were challenged by the ticking clock that counted down the research window available for conducting the study. Although flexibility, collaboration, and respect are elements critical to a project's success in a tribal community, a collision of academia and tribal cultures related to timing can become a reality and an impediment to success.

Evaluating the Process

Project completion and the successful negotiation of the tribal landscape with the invaluable help of a tribal consultant and local health professionals including the WIC staff, provided an opportunity for reflection. First, suggestions for simplifying the survey language received from tribal elders and tribal members contributed significantly to reducing the complexity of the methylmercury survey. Second, the gift cards not only helped team members demonstrate appreciation to survey participants, but also attracted additional WIC clients who heard about and came to their WIC appointment ready to participate in the survey. Finally, the goal of achieving a mutually balanced and beneficial relationship is reached only when values and beliefs of both the research team and the tribal community are observed. Lessons learned from this academic-initiated project on one reservation may not necessarily apply to another reservation, but the experience of patiently traversing the tribal landscape with respect and humility is irreducible.

LESSONS LEARNED

Through our collective experience with four distinct tribal communities, we have learned valuable lessons to share with others who might have the opportunity to conduct research with Native American people. The lessons we learned are related to the importance of relationship, reciprocity, project relevance, and negotiations of cultural and political differences among the three entities.

Importance of Relationships

As identified in the model and described in the projects' stories, each of the projects had different beginnings depending on which of the three entities (academia, nursing science, and tribal communities) was the source of the project focus and project initiation. Relationships, of varying degrees of formality and informality, played an important role in the inceptions of these projects, as delineated in the project descriptions. Although the beginnings of each project differed considerably, the importance of relationship in these research endeavors was underscored from the beginning (Rogers & Petereit, 2005). Keeping relationships as highest priority maintained the mutual integrity of the research partnership and helped guard against the potential for the research projects to be experienced as fragmented and depersonalizing.

Value of Reciprocity

A key aspect necessary to the establishment of the projects in the communities involved adhering to the value of reciprocity. This is a ubiquitous norm in interdependent Native American communities. Coming from the context that research has sometimes been oppressive to tribal people, it was important for members of the communities who were giving of their time and experiences to the various projects to see how these research projects would directly benefit their communities. Identifying the benefits also was important to the integrity of the nurse scientists who wanted to respect and participate in this norm of reciprocity.

Project Relevance

Related to the value of reciprocity, another critical aspect necessary to the acceptance of each of the projects in the communities was the relevance of the research. With the focus of the research projects coming from different sources, the members of the communities who were to be involved in the projects could perceive the relevance of the projects differently from those who originally conceived the project. Use of a community-based participatory approach allowed for the dialogue necessary to understand what was desired within the communities, how the current projects would be perceived, and what needed to be changed (Burhansstipanov et al., 2005).

It was important to balance articulation of the benefits of the project with sensitivity to the current environment in any community. Events such as a ceremony, the death of a tribal leader, or a community-wide conference could take immediate precedence over any aspect of a project. We recognized and respected this ordering of priorities, such as putting family and community needs first, as a tribal strength.

Negotiations of Political and Cultural Differences

Activities during the beginning stages of each project also focused on negotiation of cultural differences between tribal and academic policies. In addition, working through the bureaucratic structures of the academic IRB, the Tribal Council, and the IHS IRB was a time-consuming process. Challenges related to institutional policies were most apparent in the manner in which they affected issues of time and the window of funding.

Political differences between the academic institution and tribal communities were addressed in a careful negotiation of control over the research project. Questions of ownership of the data were addressed, as were concerns related to the prevention of cross-cultural misinterpretation of the results of the projects. Members of the academic community felt responsible because of the potential for legal ramifications. Tribal leaders felt responsible in allowing the projects to be conducted in their communities because of tribal vulnerabilities. Given the dynamic heritages of academic, scientific, and tribal communities, it was also important for us to recognize and submit that project entrée issues sometimes simply were predicated on personality and current political agendas within the three entities.

SUMMARY

Conducting research with Native American communities involves complexities that are not present when conducting research in the dominant culture. Negotiations must be navigated among three dynamic entities, all with their own powerful political milieus: academia, nursing science, and tribal communities. Challenges may differ, depending on how the focus of the project is derived and who initiates the project. Critical to community entrée is taking the time and making the effort to build rapport and establish trusting relationships between nurse scientists and the community. Honoring the value of reciprocity encourages a mutually beneficial experience for tribal communities and researchers. It is hoped that the lessons learned in these four research projects may be instructive to nurse scientists who wish to conduct research with tribal communities.

ACKNOWLEDGMENTS

This chapter has been reviewed by the Aberdeen Area Tribal Chairman's Health Board and the Aberdeen Area Indian Health Services Institutional Review Board.
We wish to acknowledge the following research projects and research teams:

Screening Native American Children for Asthma

- IHS: U26IHS300002-01/NIH:1S06GM074082-01
- Research Team: T. Kim Callahan Rodehorst, PHD, RNC; Susan L. Wilhelm, PhD, RNC; Mary Beth Flanders Stepans, PhD, RN

Caring for Native American Elders

- NINR P30 NR003979 The Gerontological Nursing Intervention Research Center at the University of Iowa College of Nursing
- NINR P20 NR07790 CRCHC at Montana State University–Bozeman College of Nursing
- NINR R21 NR008528 Caring for Native American Elders: Phase III
- NINR R03 NR09282-A1 Caring for Native American Elders: Grasslands
- John A. Hartford Foundation's Building Academic Geriatric Nursing Capacity Award Program
- Research Team: Patricia A. Holkup, PhD, RN; Emily Matt Salois, MSW, ACSW; Toni Tripp-Reimer, PhD, RN, FAAN; Clarann Weinert, SC, PhD, RN, FAAN

Motivational Interviewing to Promote Sustained Breastfeeding: Native American Women

- Minority Health Research Seed Projects [MIHERO]
- Research Team: Susan L. Wilhelm, PhD, RNC; T. Kim Callahan Rodehorst, PHD, RNC; Mary Beth Flanders Stepans, PhD, RN

Methylmercury Risk Awareness Project

- NINR P20 NR07790 CRCHC at Montana State University–Bozeman College of Nursing
- Research Team: Sandra W. Kuntz, PhD, RN, BC; Wade G. Hill, PhD, RN, BC; Susan King, PhD; Jeff W. Linkenbach, EdD; Gary M. Lande, MD, Montana State University–Bozeman

NOTE

1. This chapter is from *Negotiating three worlds: Academia, nursing science, and tribal communities* by Holkup, P. A., Rodehorst, T. K. C., Wilhelm, S. L., Kuntz, S. W., Weinert, C., Stephans, M. B. F., Salois, E. M., Left Hand Bull, J., & Hill, W. G.. (October 2008), *Journal of Transcultural Nursing, Online First* (Thousand Oaks: Sage). Copyright 2008 Sage. Reprinted by permission.

REFERENCES

Agency for Toxic Substances and Disease Registry. (2000). *Working effectively with tribal governments.* Atlanta, GA: Author.

American Indian Law Center, Inc. (1999). *Model tribal research code* (3rd ed.). Albuquerque, NM: Author.

Anderson, H., Hanrahan, L., Smith, A., Draheim, L., Kanarek, M., & Olsen, J. (2004). The role of sport-fish consumption advisories in mercury risk communication: A 1998–1999 12-state survey of women age 18–45. *Environmental Research, 95,* (315–324).

Arquette, M., Cole, M., Cook, K., LaFrance, B., Peters, M., & Ransom, J. (2002). Holistic risk-based environmental decision making: A Native perspective. *Environmental Health Perspectives, 110* (Suppl. 2), 259–264.

Bird, M. (2002). Health of indigenous people: Recommendations for the next generation. *American Journal of Public Health, 92* (9), 1391–1392.

Burhansstipanov, L., Christopher, S., & Schumacher, A. (2005, November). Lessons learned from community-based participatory research in Indian country. *Cancer Control,* 70–76.

Cajete, G. (1994). *Look to the mountain: An ecology of indigenous education.* Durango, CO: Kivaki Press.

Carson, D. K., & Hand, C. (1999). Dilemmas surrounding elder abuse and neglect in Native American communities. In T. Tatara (Ed.), *Understanding elder abuse in minority populations* (pp. 161–184). Philadelphia: Brunner/Mazel.

Colomeda-Lambert, L. (1999). *Keepers of the central fire: Issues in ecology for indigenous peoples.* Boston: Jones & Bartlett.

Dodgson, J. E., & Struthers, R. (2005). Indigenous women's voices: Marginalization and health. *Journal of Transcultural Nursing, 16,* 339–346.

Holkup, P. A., Tripp-Reimer, T., Salois, E. M., & Weinert, C. (2004). Community based participatory research: An approach to intervention research with a Native American community. *Advances in Nursing Science, 27* (3), 162–175.

Hunt, L. M. (2001). Beyond cultural competence: Applying humility to clinical settings. *The Park Ridge Center Bulletin, 24,* 3–4.

Jardine, C. (2003). Development of a public participation and communication protocol for establishing fish consumption advisories. *Risk Analysis, 23* (3), 461–471.

Manson, S. M., Garroutte, E., Goins, R. T., & Henderson, P. N. (2004). Access, relevance, and control in the research process. *Journal of Aging and Health, 16* (5), 58S–77S.

Maynard, E. (1974). The growing negative image of the anthropologist among American Indians. *Human Organization, 33,* 402–403.

Mitchell, T. L., & Baker, E. (2005). Community-building versus career-building research: The challenges, risks, and responsibilities of conducting research with Aboriginal and Native American communities. *Journal of Cancer Education, 20* (1), 41–46.

Norton, I. M., & Manson, S. M. (1996). Research in American Indian and Alaska Native communities: Navigating the cultural universe of values and process. *Journal of Consulting and Clinical Psychology, 64* (5), 856–860.

Poupart, J., Martinez, C., Red Horse, J., & Scharnberg, D. (2000). *To build a bridge: An introduction to working with American Indian communities.* St. Paul, MN: American Indian Policy Center.

Quandt, S. A., McDonald, J., Bell, R. A., & Arcury, T. A. (1999). Aging research in multiethnic rural communities: Gaining entrée through community involvement. *Journal of Cross-Cultural Gerontology, 14,* 113–130.

Red Horse, J. G. (1980a). American Indian elders: Unifiers of Indian families. *Social Casework: The Journal of Contemporary Social Work, 61* (8), 490–493.

Red Horse, J. G. (1980b). Family structure and value orientation in American Indians. *Social Casework: The Journal of Contemporary Social Work, 61* (8), 462–467.

Red Horse, J. G., Johnson, T., & Weiner, D. (1989). Commentary: Cultural perspectives on research among American Indians. *American Indian Culture and Research Journal, 13* (3/4), 267–271.

Rogers, D., & Petereit, D. G. (2005). Cancer disparities research partnership in Lakota country: Clinical trials, patient services, and community education for Oglala, Rosebud, and Cheyenne River Sioux tribes. *American Journal of Public Health, 95* (12), 2129–2132.

Salois, E. M., Holkup, P. A., Tripp-Reimer, T., & Weinert, C. (2006). Research as spiritual covenant. *Western Journal of Nursing Research, 28* (5), 505–524.

Stoddard, B. (1997). *Breastfeeding management and promotion among Native Americans in Wisconsin.* Paper presented at the Indian Health Service Conference, October 1997, Minneapolis, MN.

Swinomish Tribal Mental Health Project. (2002). *A gathering of wisdoms: Tribal mental health: A cultural perspective* (2nd ed.). LaConner, WA: Swinomish Tribal Community.

Tervalon, M., & Murray-Garcia, J. (1998). Cultural humility versus cultural competence: A critical distinction in defining physician training outcomes in multicultural education. *Journal of Health Care for the Poor and Underserved, 9* (2), 117–125.

Tom-Orme, L. (2006). Research and American Indian/Alaska native health: A nursing perspective. *Journal of Transcultural Nursing, 17* (3), 261–265.

U.S. Department of Health and Human Services. (2000). *Healthy people 2010: Understanding and improving health.* Washington, DC: U.S. Department of Health and Human Services, Government Printing Office.

Weaver, H. N., & White, B. W. (1997). The Native American family circle: Roots of resiliency. *Journal of Family Social Work, 2* (1), 67–79.

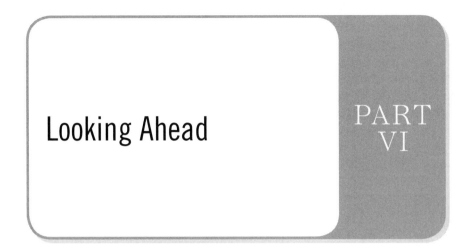

Looking Ahead

PART
VI

27

Implications for Education, Practice, and Policy

JEAN SHREFFLER-GRANT and MARLENE A. REIMER

As an applied discipline, nursing has traditionally measured the relevance of theory by the extent to which it can inform practice, education, and health care policy. Our purpose in this chapter was to make more explicit the relevance of key elements of the rural theory base. We discuss selected educational, practice, and health care policy implications of the key concepts and theoretical statements as reported by Long and Weinert (1989) and Lee and McDonagh (2006). We explore how these implications may need to change as rural nursing theory is revised and extended. We also present exemplars from the United States, Canada, and Australia to illustrate how the key concepts and theoretical statements can inform education, practice, and health care policy that address rural populations and their health across international borders.

IMPLICATIONS OF THE FIRST THEORETICAL STATEMENT

How a group of citizens perceive health, manage their health, and seek health care has broad implications for education, practice, and policy that transcend national borders. The first theoretical statement is "[R]ural dwellers define health primarily as the ability to work, to be productive, to do usual tasks" (Long & Weinert, 1989, p. 120). The interrelated concepts associated with this statement are work beliefs and health beliefs;

health is defined in relation to work, and health needs are secondary to work needs.

Education

On the basis of the original rural nursing theory work, the first theoretical statement suggests that nursing programs should include the concept of role performance as health in curricula so that nurses include actual or potential effects of a health problem on the ability to work and to do usual tasks in their assessments and plans of care. Nursing educators should also offer opportunities for students to learn how clients' definitions of health influence their health and illness management behaviors.

Practice

In the practice arena, the first theoretical statement suggests that rural health services should be oriented, structured, and timed to fit with the rhythm of work and role performance. In addition, the benefits of preventive care may be better communicated by framing them according to what will assist rural dwellers to continue to work and do their usual tasks. Data from both Canada and the United States demonstrate the need to find new ways to approach preventive care among rural dwellers based on trends in health indicators such as obesity, hypertension, smoking, and having regular health care visits (Fried, Prager, MacKay, & Xia, 2003; Mitura & Bollman, 2003).

Policy

Policy implications of the original work include establishing funding mechanisms whereby health services can be offered near where people work and scheduled around the cycle of rural work. Rural residents may not seek timely health services if work must be delayed or disrupted to seek care (Sellers, Poduska, Propp, & White, 1999).

The original theory development work on definitions of health, as well as beliefs about work and health was conducted in the United States. Research participants were principally Caucasian rural dwellers, the majority population in the Rocky Mountain and High Plains area in which this work was conducted (90.8% of Montana population, U.S. Bureau of the Census, 2006). It was not intended to characterize these concepts for American Indians, the primary minority population in the same rural areas (6.4% of the Montana population, U.S. Census). Canadian research on health beliefs of rural dwellers, as reported by Winters, Thomlinson, O'Lynn, et al. (2006), was also drawn primarily from Caucasians living in the western part of the country. Further research is warranted to explore how Native American and Aboriginal people living in rural areas define health and how their conception of health is the same or different from the dominant population. In any case, it is unlikely that one definition of health or one set of health beliefs would emerge that would characterize health beliefs among different Aboriginal communities or tribes, any more than it is likely among Caucasian groups of different cultures.

As discussed by Lee and McDonagh (2006), rural dwellers' views of health may now be more diverse across different geographic areas, age and ethnic groups, and occupations than when the original theory development work began and may require a reconceptualization of definitions of health, work beliefs, and health beliefs. Of particular note are the subpopulations among rural dwellers.

Discussion

Martin (1997) pointed out that farming and ranching are now experienced more as a lifestyle than as an occupation, thus calling for different approaches to affect behavior change than simply appealing to individual's motivations to continue working. Another example of a potential need to reframe rural dwellers definition of health can be found within rural subpopulations where unemployment has now persisted for multiple generations. Defining health based on ability to work may not be relevant for those who have never had regular work (Long, 1993). Some rural areas are now more racially and ethnically diverse than in the past. Culturally based beliefs about what it means to be healthy are likely to result in different definitions of health among racial and ethnic groups. Migration of urban residents to rural areas has resulted in a subpopulation of exurban rural dwellers who bring their urban values and expectations about health and health care with them (Troughton, 1999). The "graying" of rural areas is well documented in the literature, as people age in place and younger people migrate out for employment and other opportunities (McLaughlin & Jensen, 1998; Ricketts, Johnson-Webb, & Randolph, 1999). With improved health care and healthier lifestyles, people are living many more years postretirement than they once did. How health is defined among this rural population may well have nothing to do with what we traditionally think of as work, but instead may be more consistent with the concept of health as role performance or ability to do usual tasks. Healthy elders may define health as the ability to actively participate in leisure, voluntary activities, and travel. Elders in poor health may define health as nothing more than the ability to complete their activities of daily living. Further research and exploration is warranted to refine the definitions of health for these multiple rural subpopulations.

IMPLICATIONS OF THE SECOND THEORETICAL STATEMENT

The second theoretical statement is "[R]ural dwellers are self-reliant and resist accepting help or services from those seen as 'outsiders' or from agencies seen as national or regional 'welfare' programs" (Long & Weinert, 1989, p. 120). Related key concepts are self-reliance, outsider, insider, old-timer, and newcomer.

Education

The second theoretical statement underlines the importance of a participative, community development approach in which rural dwellers identify and design health initiatives to fit with their own needs and resources. This approach is consistent with the second theoretical statement as originally conceptualized, as well as the proposed newer subtheme of symptom-action-time-line (SATL) and the new theme involving choices discussed by Lee and McDonagh (2006). The importance of working in partnership with rural dwellers and communities is essential content for nursing curricula so that graduates can and will apply the principles of community development and participatory action in rural practice. Skills essential for partnership development and maintenance should also be included in nursing curricula. As a middle-range theory of rural health-seeking behavior evolves, this theory should be derived and validated in partnership with rural residents themselves so that it is consistent with their local needs and beliefs.

Practice

Goeppinger (1993) advocated partnership as a core intervention strategy in health promotion with rural populations at both individual and aggregate levels. Considering the rural tendency to "make do" and what

Weissert, Knott, and Stieber (1994) referred to as the "asymmetry of information between citizens and health professionals . . . about what constitutes good care" (p. 366) in traditional care models, empirical testing of the partnership model in promoting the health of rural residents is needed. A Canadian example of a tool to support participative community development for rural citizens is a workbook that was tested in Manitoba, Canada (Ryan-Nicholls, 2004). The workbook was designed to help rural citizens assess the health of their communities, and identify goals and strategies to improve the sustainability of rural communities. In the United States, Findholt (2004) studied how rurality influenced community participation in health promotion initiatives. She found that having a structured process for the initiative appeared to compensate for some of the resource and experiential limitations in rural communities. Communities, for example, that had limited experience and success with previous planning efforts were not hindered in their current efforts because they had structured support and resources from a state level Office of Rural Health.

Policy

The question of what health care resources are necessary and sufficient in rural and remote areas, given the distance to other sources of care, continues as a focus of debate and policy shifts for which evidence for decision making is scarce. The major constraint is the lack of sufficient population to justify a full mix of acute care, long-term care, and supported residential and home care services (Keyzer, 1995). In a study of home care resources for rural families with cancer, Buehler and Lee (1992) found that the more rural the family, the more limited and inadequate the formal resources available to assist them. These investigators also found that the longer the dying trajectory and the greater the deterioration of the person's health, the more resources became inadequate and the greater the caregiver burden. These findings illustrate one of many policy questions that has emerged: the relationship between length of illness and sustainability of resources through the trajectory of illness in rural versus urban environments. It would seem that a mix of formal and informal resources and the resiliency of each to prolonged illness vary but few studies have systematically addressed this phenomenon.

The Australian Rural Health Strategy adopted in 1994 (Keyzer, 1995) called for "relocation of resources away from services based on existing facilities towards services based on expressed demand" (p. 28).

The strategy included changes that would shift power bases from traditional rural primary and hospital care delivery to a system that relied much more on nurse practitioners and interdisciplinary collaboration. However, more than 10 years later tension still exists in Australia and elsewhere between the economic arguments for downsizing and closure of rural facilities versus advocacy for aging in place, new life-saving treatments that require pretransfer interventions at local health care facilities, and other new technologies such as telehealth that minimize the need for travel to urban locations for health care (Mueller, 2001; Ricketts, 2000).

In the United States, the Critical Access Hospital (CAH) has gained broad support as an alternative to closure of local rural hospitals and is being implemented in rural areas across the nation. CAHs must be located in remote areas and are limited to short-stay lower-intensity services in exchange for more flexibility in staffing and other licensure requirements and more favorable Medicare reimbursement as compared with traditional rural hospitals. The underlying goal is to shift the facility's emphasis from inpatient and surgical services to emergency, out-patient, primary, and long-term care, which are services that may be more sustainable in remote rural areas because they better match the needs of area residents (Shreffler, Capalbo, Flaherty, & Heggem, 1999). One of the prototypes for this national model of care was a grass-roots effort initiated by a partnership of rural citizens and legislators in a remote rural area in Montana. There are currently 45 CAHs in Montana (Montana Hospital Association, 2008) and 1,294 certified CAHs nationwide (Rural Assistance Center, 2008).

IMPLICATIONS OF THE THIRD THEORETICAL STATEMENT

Finally, the third theoretical statement is "[H]ealth care providers in rural areas must deal with a lack of anonymity and much greater role diffusion than providers in urban or suburban settings" (Long & Weinert, 1989, p. 120). A related theme mentioned by Long and Weinert that characterizes rural nursing is "a sense of isolation from professional peers" (p. 120).

Education

Implicit in the third theoretical statement is that students planning or potentially interested in rural practice should be given opportunities to develop skills to function in a generalist role or what McLeod, Browne, and Leipert (1998) refer to as a multispecialist role that is characteristic of rural nursing practice. Offering undergraduate students a rural elective experience is one such strategy, particularly when it not only involves placement in a rural site but also seminars on rural health and practice issues. Students with an interest in rural practice should have opportunities to develop strategies to cope with or overcome practice isolation, such as skill development in the use of mentors, consultants, and telehealth applications. Through full engagement with their communities, nurses who are newcomers in rural areas may begin to appreciate the familiarity of life in a rural community and gradually be seen as insiders rather than outsiders which may mediate the negative aspects of lack of anonymity and practice isolation. Some nurses, of course, are already insiders having come from the particular community. The sense of practice isolation may be less acute for them, but the practical issues of limited access to educational opportunities and ready consultation are nevertheless present to varying degrees.

Practice and Policy

Dealing with lack of anonymity, role diffusion, and practice isolation may contribute to recruitment difficulties and high turnover of rural health care professionals that contribute to shortages of providers in rural practice settings. Here too, policy makers can look to innovative approaches and exchange of best practices. For example, the Rural Physician Action Plan in Alberta recognized that (a) medical students from rural areas were more likely to go into rural practice, but (b) rural applicants were often disadvantaged in the interview and selection processes for medical school because of lack of sophistication in interviewing and preparation of materials (I. Pfeiffer, personal communication, March 4, 2004). An experienced recruiter was hired to help rural applicants prepare for admission interviews. Thus, they went to a root cause with what appear to be positive results.

Another innovative strategy for addressing shortages of nurses and other health care providers in rural areas can be seen in the growth of educational outreach efforts via distance technology to rural areas. Rural residents or insiders who are more likely to select rural practice upon graduation can access all or part of educational programs without leaving their rural communities for significant periods of time. Another successful approach for recruitment of health professionals in rural areas has been educational scholarships for rural residents or "grow your own" programs (Hagopian, Johnson, Fordyce, Blades, & Hart, 2003).

CONCLUSIONS

The radical changes necessary to shift education, practice, and policy for rural health require a strong theory base and depth of understanding of rural health and practice that can emanate only through experience and research. Those who focus on rural health are used to thinking in terms of local contextual factors and the unique nature of a single rural area, region, or nation. Through engagement in across-border collaborative research and scholarly work on rural nursing theory, we and our respective teams have deepened our understanding of the extent to which larger issues of health care reform are also shifting. At the end of the day, the relevance of rural nursing theory and concepts as described in this book will likely be measured by its ability to evolve and change as new knowledge shapes it and to positively influence education, practice, and health care policy—and thereby improve the health of rural citizens on both sides of the border.

REFERENCES

Buehler, J. A., & Lee, H. J. (1992). Exploration of home care resources for rural families with cancer. *Cancer Nursing, 15*, 299–308.

Findholt, N. (2004). *The influence of rurality on community participation in a community health development initiative.* (Unpublished doctoral dissertation, Oregon Health & Science University, Portland).

Fried, V. M., Prager, K., MacKay, A. P., & Xia, H. (2003). *Chartbook on trends in the health of Americans. Health, United States, 2003.* Hyattsville, MD: National Center for Health Statistics.

Goeppinger, J. (1993). Health promotion for rural populations: Partnership interventions. *Family and Community Health, 16* (1), 1–10.

Hagopian, A., Johnson, K., Fordyce, M., Blades, S., & Hart, L. G. (2003). Health workforce recruitment and retention in critical access hospitals. *CAH/FLEX National Tracking Project, 3* (5). Retrieved April 9, 2004, from http://rupri.org/rhfp–track/results/vol3num5.pdf

Keyzer, D. M. (1995). Health policy and rural nurses: A time for reflection. *Collegian, 2* (1), 28–35.

Lee, H. J., & McDonagh, M. K. (2006). Further development of the rural nursing base. In H. J. Lee, & C. A. Winters (Eds.). *Rural nursing: Concepts, theory, and practice* (2nd ed., pp. 313–321). New York: Springer.

Long, K. A. (1993). The concept of health: Rural perspectives. *Nursing Clinics of North America, 28* (1), 123–130.

Long, K. A., & Weinert, C. (1989). Rural nursing: Developing the theory base. *Scholarly Inquiry for Nursing Practice: An International Journal, 3*, 113–127.

Martin, S. R. (1997). Agricultural safety and health: Principles and possibilities for nursing education. *Journal of Nursing Education, 36* (2), 74–78.

McLaughlin, D. K., & Jensen, L. (1998). The rural elderly: A demographic portrait. In R. T. Coward & J. A. Krout (Eds.), *Aging in rural settings: Life circumstances & distinctive features* (pp. 15–43). New York: Springer.

McLeod, M., Browne, A. J., & Leipert, B. (1998). Issues for nurses in rural and remote Canada. *Australian Journal of Rural Health, 6,* 72–78.

Mitura, V., & Bollman, R. D. (2003). The health of rural Canadians: A rural–urban comparison of health indicators. *Rural and Small Town Canada Analysis Bulletin, 4* (6), 1–21. (Available from the Agriculture Division, Statistics Canada, Ottawa).

Montana Hospital Association. (2008). *Critical Access Hospital List.* Retrieved December 22, 2008, from http://www.mtha.org/mhref4.htm

Mueller, K. J. (2001). Rural health policy: Past as prelude to the future. In S. Loue & B. E. Quill (Eds.), Handbook of rural health (pp. 1–23). New York: Kluwer Academic/Plenum.

Ricketts, T. C. (2000). The changing nature of rural health care. *Annual Review of Public Health, 21,* 639–657.

Ricketts, T. C., Johnson-Webb, K. D., & Randolph, R. K. (1999). Populations and places in rural America. In T. C. Ricketts (Ed.), *Rural health in the United States* (pp. 7–24). New York: Oxford University Press.

Rural Assistance Center. (2008). CAH frequently asked questions. Retrieved December 26, 2008, from http://www.raconline.org/info_guides/hospitals/cahfaq.php

Ryan-Nicholls, K. (2004). Rural Canadian community health and quality of life: Testing of a workbook to determine priorities and move to action. (Preliminary Report). *Rural and Remote Health, 4* (278), 1–10. Retrieved June 23, 2004, from http://rrh.deakin.edu.au

Sellers, S. C., Poduska, M. D., Propp, L. H., & White, S. I. (1999). The health care meanings, values, and practices of Anglo-American males in the rural Midwest. *Journal of Transcultural Nursing, 10,* 320–330.

Shreffler, M. J., Capalbo, S. M., Flaherty, R. J., & Heggem, C. (1999). Community decision-making about Critical Access Hospitals: Lessons learned from Montana's Medical Assistance Facility program. *The Journal of Rural Health, 15* (2), 180–188.

Troughton, M. J. (1999). Redefining "rural" for the twenty-first century. In W. Rampy, J. Kulig, I. Townshend, & V. McGowan (Eds.), *Health in rural settings: Contexts for action* (pp. 21–38). Lethbridge, AB: University of Lethbridge.

U.S. Bureau of the Census. 2006. Retrieved December 22, 2008, from http://quickfacts.census.gov/qfd/states/30000.html

Weissert, C. S., Knott, J. H., & Stieber, B. E. (1994). Education and the health professions: Explaining policy choices among the states. *Journal of Health Politics, Policy and Law, 19,* 361–392.

Winters, C. A., Thomlinson, E. H., O'Lynn, C., Lee, H. J., McDonagh, M. K., Edge, D. S., et al. (2006). Examining rural nursing theory across borders. In H. J. Lee, & C. A. Winters (Eds.). *Rural Nursing: Concepts, Theory, and Pactice* (2nd ed., pp. 27–39). New York: Springer.

An Analysis of Key Concepts for Rural Nursing

28

HELEN J. LEE, CHARLENE A. WINTERS,
ROBIN L. BOLAND, SUSAN J. RAPH,
and JANICE A. BUEHLER

Long and Weinert (1989) noted that during the initial "process of data organization . . . some concepts appeared repeatedly in the ethnographic data collected in several different areas of the state" (p. 118). Following the initial publication of their article in 1989, faculty in the Rural Nursing Theory Special Committee within the Montana State University–Bozeman College of Nursing embarked on a plan to analyze identified concepts. The committee's efforts were enhanced through course work involvement of graduate nursing students enrolled in Montana State University College of Nursing's rural generalist program. The purpose of this chapter is to summarize the analyzed concepts contained in the first edition of *Conceptual Basis of Rural Nursing* (Lee, 1998) along with any conducted relevant research. The summary provides a quick reference of the analyzed concepts and allows for easy identification of areas needing further work.

The concepts are organized according to the framework provided in the rural nursing theory base. Following each theoretical statement are concept summaries pertinent to that particular statement. Each concept summary is presented using the analysis framework selected by the chapter authors from *Conceptual Basis of Rural Nursing* (Lee, 1998). Elements of the framework, whether explicit and implicit, contained in the chapters are presented; elements not evident are indicated by statements such as "none given" or "not identified."

FIRST STATEMENT: HOW RURAL DWELLERS DEFINE HEALTH

The first statement indicates that " . . . rural dwellers define health primarily as the ability to work, to be productive, to do usual tasks" (Long & Weinert, 1989, p. 120). Work beliefs and health beliefs were key concepts while isolation and distance were identified as related concepts. Health beliefs, isolation, and distance were three of the four concepts analyzed.

Health Beliefs (Long, 1993)

Method of analysis: Smith's (1983) four models of health—clinical, role performance, adaptive, eudemonistic.

Definition: Rural dwellers often conceptualize health within the role performance model (Long).

Defining attributes:

1. "[A]bility to work . . . [and] perform one's daily activities" (p. 124).
2. "[D]etermine health needs primarily in relation to work activities" (p. 124).
3. "[A]s a result of their environment, rural dwellers are more frequently called upon to be independent and self-reliant" (p. 124).

Antecedents: Beliefs held will affect "health-promotion behaviors, health care seeking, and acceptance of preventive and treatment interventions" (p. 123).

Consequences: Knowledge of client's concept of health is important for development of relevant and acceptable assessment approaches and intervention strategies (p. 123).

Empirical referents: none identified.

Isolation (Lee, Hollis, & McClain, 1998)

Method of analysis: Wilson's method (Walker & Avant, 1995).

Definition: None given.

Essential attributes:

1. Separation—"[B]eing divided from the rest" (Lee et al., p. 69).
2. Relativeness—"[S]omething dependent on external conditions for its specific nature . . . existing or having its specific nature only by relation to something else; not absolute or independent" (p. 69).
3. Perception—"[C]onsciousness or awareness" (p. 69).

Antecedents: "[P]resence of an indicator directing attention to the condition of isolation (geographical terrain, distance, changes imposed by weather, economic costs, time or personal preference)" (p. 69).

Consequences: "[D]ecreased communication or interaction with other individuals that results in social or professional isolation" (p. 70).

Empirical referents: None identified.

Distance (Henson, Sadler, & Walton, 1998)

Method of analysis: Wilson's method (Walker & Avant, 1988).

Definition: "[I]mplies a degree of separation between two or more entities. . . . The nature of separation may be in space, time or behavior" (Henson et al., p. 51).

Essential attributes:

1. Mileage—"[T]otal number of miles traveled" (p. 56).
2. Time—"[M]easurement in minutes it takes to travel from one place to another" (p. 56).
3. Perception—"[V]ariation in awareness of data that is different from others' awareness" (p. 56).

Antecedent: "[A]ccess to health care" (p. 58).
Consequence: "[P]otential for compromised health care" (p. 58).
Empirical referents:

1. Objective:
   a. "[D]istance" (miles, kilometers) (p. 58).
   b. "[T]ravel time" (p. 58).
   c. MSU Rurality Index (county of residence population, distance to emergency care) (Weinert & Boik, 1995).
2. Subjective:
   a. "[P]erception" (Henson et al., p. 58).

SECOND STATEMENT: SELF-RELIANCE

The second statement is " . . . rural dwellers are self-reliant and resist accepting help or services from those seen as 'outsiders' or from agencies seen as national or regional 'welfare' programs. A corollary to this statement is that help, including needed health care, is usually sought through an informal rather than a formal system" (Long & Weinert, 1989 p. 120). Key concepts analyzed were self-reliance, outsider, insider, old-timer, newcomer, resources, informal networks, and lay care network.

Self-Reliance (Chafey, Sullivan, & Shannon, 1998)

Method of analysis: Qualitative research inquiry (Morse, 1995). Definition:

1. "[T]he capacity to provide for one's own needs" (Agich, 1993, as cited in Chafey et al., 1998, p. 158).
2. "[T]he desire to do for oneself and care for oneself" (Long & Weinert, 1989, p. 119).

Sample: Cohort of nine women between 70–85 years of age living in small rural towns.

Data collection: Interview using structured guide developed to elicit participants' perceptions of self-reliance (Chafey et al., p. 160). Characteristics:

1. Primary
   a. Learned—"A skill emanating from previous learning events that started in their youth (family chores & assumption of responsibilities), continued into adulthood, and was reinforced by later life events (retirement, death of a parent or spouse)" (p. 162).
   b. Decisional choice—"[M]aking one's own decisions and choices" (p. 164).
   c. Independence—"[I]ndependence or dependence on self, dependence of others, self-assertion or freedom of action, and self-identity" (p. 166).
2. Secondary—Embodied an aspect of their self-reliance experience.
   a. Self-confidence (p. 170).
   b. Self-competence (pp. 170–171).

Outsider (Bailey, 1998)

Method of analysis: Wilson's method (Walker & Avant, 1988).

Definition: "[B]eing exterior to the group, matter, or boundary in question" (Bailey, p. 140).

Defining attributes:

1. Differentness—"[I]n terms of cultural orientation, standards, lifestyle, education, religion, occupation, social status, worldview, interests, or experience;" "the quality or state of being different" (pp. 143–144).
2. Unfamiliarity—With the matter in question (p. 144).
3. Unconnectedness—"[H]aving no family of personal ties" (p. 144).

Antecedents: "[L]acking understanding or knowledge of the social context, beliefs, rituals, customs and history of the community" (p. 144).

Consequences: "[O]ne may be excluded from access to knowledge and information, not be accepted, not be recognized, be isolated, and be distrusted" (p. 144).

Empirical referents: None identified.

Insider (Myers, 1998)

Method of analysis: Wilson's method (Walker & Avant, 1995).

Definition: "[S]omeone who is a member of a group and has access to special or privileged information" (Myers, p. 127).

Defining attributes:

1. "[M]ember of a group" (p. 132).
2. "[H]aving access to privileged information" (p. 132).
3. "[A]n awareness of implicit assumptions and social context" (p. 132).
4. "[A] long-time occupant" (p. 132).

Antecedents: "[A]cceptance by the group" (p. 135).

Consequences:

1. "[P]ower . . . because of having information that others lack" (p. 135).

2. "[R]eserved social position . . . that is unavailable to others" (p. 135).
3. "[L]ack of objectivity" (p. 135).
4. "[C]ommitted to the group" (p. 135).

Empirical referents: None identified.

Old-Timer (Caniparoli, 1998)

Method of analysis: Wilson's method (Walker & Avant, 1995).
Definition:

1. "[O]ne who is long established in a place or position" (Caniparoli, p. 103).
2. "A man who has lived in the county a long time" (American slang, 1968, as cited in Caniparoli, 1998, p. 103).

Defining attributes:

1. "[A]ge" (p. 108).
2. "[L]ength of time spent in a community" (p. 108).
3. "[E]stablishment of a relationship within the community" (p. 108).

Antecedents: "[I]dentification as an old-timer" (p. 110).
Consequences: "[E]stablishes a relationship within the community . . . [that] can be viewed as positive or negative depending on the role of the viewer" (p. 110).
Empirical referents: None identified.

Concept Verification Research

Boland conducted a qualitative study with a convenience sample of nine participants living in small rural communities in central Montana (Boland & Lee, 2006). The study findings confirmed the three defining attributes for old-timer and identified land ownership as the key element of the third attribute. The old-timers spoke of their functions within the community as working together for survival, holding social events to accomplish work and play, to share traditions, and act as historians.

Most participants identified themselves as "old-timers" despite earlier historical literature describing "old-timers" as persons who were "mysterious, unusual and fiercely independent" (Caniparoli, p. 106). These study participants expressed doubt about their level of influence within the communities as was originally attributed in the earlier rural nursing theory development. Loss of influence was attributed to changing times (fewer farms and ranches, increased identification with the nearby larger towns and cities) and "the loss of respect for elderly people in today's society" (Boland & Lee, p. 50).

Newcomer (Sutermaster, 1998)

Method of analysis: Wilson's method (Walker & Avant, 1995).
Definition: "[O]ne tha[t] has recently arrived" (Sutermaster, p. 113).
Defining attributes:

1. "[N]ewly arrived" (p. 120).
2. "[U]naware of the history of the area/institution" (p. 120).
3. "[T]heir existence may result in change" (p. 120).

Antecedents: "Individuals or families would have had a need or desire to move" (p. 121).
Consequences: "There is a new individual or family living in the community" (p. 121).
Empirical referents: None identified.

Resources (Ballantyne, 1998)

Method of analysis: Wilson's method (Walker & Avant, 1995).
Definition: "Resources are properties, resorts, or assets that are finite by nature and are made available for use by populations through an allocation process. Resources are accessed and used in response to a population's or individual's motivation for need satisfaction. . . . Furthermore, these three elements can be visualized in a circle with the flow of energy between the allocated resource, accessibility of the resource, and use of the resource" (Ballantyne, p. 181).
Defining attributes:

1. Property—"[R]esource is a property or an asset that has value for consumption by populations in need of that property" (p. 181).

2. Expedient—"[C]ontinuance or plan for solution of a particular problem" (p. 181).
3. Resort—"[T]urning inward to one's resources" (p. 181).

Antecedents: Knowledge of "local, regional, and national availability" (p. 187).
Consequences: "[A]llocation, accessibility, and use" (p. 187).
Empirical referents: None identified.

Informal Networks (Grossman & McNerney, 1998)

Method of analysis: Wilson's method (Walker & Avant, 1995).
Definition: "[N]etworks are interconnected relationships, durable patterns of interactions, and interpersonal threads that comprise a social fabric" (Grossman & McNerney, pp. 201–202).
Defining attributes:

1. Volunteer; includes family members, coworkers, and neighbors who offer assistance free of charge (p. 204).
2. Information exchange (p. 204).
3. Support; has two components: Emotional component (being a friend, listening) and physical (assistance with daily living, health promotion, and maintenance activities) (p. 204).
4. Guidance; "may be given as advice, consultation (availability of resources, referral to health care providers, sources of alternative treatments), and information" (p. 204).

Antecedents:

1. "[A] bond . . . the tie that exists among . . . the core of the informal network (family, friends, neighbors, and coworkers)" (p. 206).
2 "[A]re generated in response to a perceived need" (p. 206).

Consequences: "[T]he perceived need is met or not met" (p. 206).
Empirical referents: None identified.

Lay Care Network (Turnbull, 1998)

Method of analysis: Wilson's method (Walker & Avant, 1988).
Definition: None given.

Defining attributes:

1. Interconnection or net—"An interconnection is the means by which one thing connects with another, whereas a net consists of fibers woven together for catching something" (Turnbull, p. 195).
2. Of the people—"[B]elonging to, concerned with, or performed by the 'people' in a nonprofessional capacity" (p. 195).
3. Sense of concern—"[T]he idea that one develops or maintains an interest in the well-being of a person or object, to oversee with the intent to protect" (Oxford, 1989 as cited in Turnbull, p. 195).

Antecedents: None identified.
Consequences: None identified.
Empirical referents: None identified.
Conclusion: Turnbull recommended "further refinement of the concept, 'lay care provider,' and suggests a change in the wording of the concept itself" (p. 198). The literature review clearly delineates between *lay providers* and *informal care providers*, whereas the wording *lay care providers* combines two different concepts.

THIRD STATEMENT: LACK OF ANONYMITY AND ROLE DIFFUSION

The third statement is "health care providers in rural areas must deal with a lack of anonymity and much greater role diffusion than providers in urban or suburban settings" (Long & Weinert, 1989, p. 120). The key concepts are lack of anonymity and role diffusion. Related concepts are familiarity and professional isolation. Analyzed were anonymity, familiarity, and professional isolation.

Lack of Anonymity (Lee, 1998)

Method of analysis: Wilson's method (Walker & Avant, 1995).
Definition: "[A] condition in which one cannot remain nameless or unknown" (Lee, p. 77).

Defining attributes:

1. Visible—"[T]hat which can be seen, is apparent or obvious" (p. 83).
2. Identifiable—"[B]eing able to recognize or establish; the condition or character of a person" (p. 83).
3. Diminished personal/professional boundaries: "[B]orders or perimeters through which one functions are smaller, more circumscribed" (p. 83).

Antecedents: "Lack of anonymity occurs in an environmental context characterized by a low level of stimulation. It contains fewer number of individuals and/or objects (e.g., automobiles, buildings) needing to be considered in the normal deliberation of one's activities" (pp. 83–84).

Consequences: "[A] relationship [in which] one's actions are visible and readily observed" (p. 84). Greater difficulty in maintaining personal and professional privacy exists because of the relationship.

Empirical referents: None identified.

Concept Verification Research

Raph conducted a pilot study focusing on the phenomenon "lack of anonymity" with four informants employed in a western rural "frontier" county health department (Raph & Buelher, 2006). Using grounded theory technique, four differing interactive categories emerged through the data analysis: (a) Personally affirming interactions were defined as "friendly encounters that did not place the informant in a professional role" (p. 199); (b) Professional affirming interactions were these seeking clarification on "general information about vaccines, appointments, or needed after-hour services . . . usually (taking place in) public places in the community" (pp. 199–200); (c) Professionally threatening interactions "placed them in a position of potentially doing harm if not handled correctly" (p. 200); and, (d) Personally threatening encounters were those that "provoked fear and anger" (p. 201). The four categories, placed in a continuum from positive to negative, extend the second and third defining attributes of the lack of anonymity (see above) and verify the consequences of the "greater difficulty in maintaining personal and professional privacy" (Lee, p. 84).

Familiarity (McNeely & Shreffler, 1998)

Method of analysis: Wilson's method (Walker & Avant, 1995).

Definition: "[A]n antithetical concept that includes the positive ideas of thorough knowledge of or an acquaintance with and closeness and intimacy, such as one would find in a family or deep friendship, and the contrasting perspective of offensive, unwarranted, intimate conduct that might include behaviors such as flirting, sexual harassment, domestic violence, abusive relationships, or incest" (McNeely & Shreffler, p. 91).

Defining attributes:

1. "[F]riendly relationship or close acquaintance" (p. 98).
2. "[I]ntimacy" (p. 98).
3. "[I]nformality" (p. 98).
4. "[T]he exhibited familiarity is welcome or unwelcome depending on the perceptions of the receiver" (p. 98).

Antecedents: None identified.
Consequences: None identified.
Empirical referents: None identified.

Professional Isolation (Shreffler, 1998)

Method of analysis: Wilson's method (Walker & Avant, 1988).
Definition: None given.
Defining attributes: "[A]n actual separation from or a deficiency in a resource needed to fulfill one's professional responsibilities or needs (objective component)" (Shreffler, p. 426); "professional need is perceived as partially or wholly unmet (subjective component)" (p. 426); "the actual separation or deficiency is on a continuum" (p. 426); "the individual is not voluntarily separating her/himself from an available professional resource" (p. 426); and "the objective component is more likely to be present in rural areas" (p. 426).

Antecedents: The individuals experience "separation from or deficiency in resources needed to fulfill professional responsibilities" and have "needs for resources to fulfill their professional responsibilities," "can make choices about the use of available resources," and "are able to perceive whether professional needs are met" (p. 429).

Consequences: "[A]re specific to the need that is unmet and the vulnerabilities of the individual in the occupation or job position" (p. 429).

Empirical referents:

1. "[T]he availability of the needed resource is measured and found deficient" (p. 429).
2. "[I]ndividuals . . . express awareness of an unmet need or exhibit signs of the consequence of the unmet need" (pp. 429–430).

CONCLUSION

In this chapter, we summarized the concepts found in *Conceptual Basis of Rural Nursing* (Lee, 1998). Most of the analyses were conducted using the Wilson method (Walker & Avant, 1988, 1995). However, some of the elements (e.g., definitions, antecedents, consequences, empirical referents) were not addressed. Furthermore, some key concepts were not analyzed (e.g., work beliefs, role diffusion). Further development of the concepts is needed. Paramount is the need for validation of concepts with rural dwellers.

REFERENCES

Bailey, M. C. (1998). Outsider. In H. J. Lee (Ed.), *Conceptual basis for rural nursing* (pp. 139–148). New York: Springer.

Ballantyne, J. (1998). Health resources and the rural client. In H. J. Lee (Ed.), *Conceptual basis for rural nursing* (pp. 178–198). New York: Springer.

Boland, R., & Lee, H. (2006). Old-timers. In H. J. Lee & C. A. Winters (Eds.), *Rural nursing: Concepts, theory, and practice* (2nd ed., pp. 43–52). New York: Springer.

Caniparoli, C. D. (1998). Old-timer. In H. J. Lee (Ed.), *Conceptual basis for rural nursing* (pp. 102–112). New York: Springer.

Chafey, K., Sullivan, T., & Shannon, A. (1998). Self-reliance: Characteristics of their own autonomy by elderly rural women. In H. J. Lee (Ed.), *Conceptual basis for rural nursing* (pp. 156–177). New York: Springer.

Grossman, L. L., & McNerney, S. (1998). Informal networks. In H. J. Lee (Ed.), *Conceptual basis for rural nursing* (pp. 200–208). New York: Springer.

Henson, D., Sadler, T., & Walton, S. (1998). Distance. In H. J. Lee (Ed.), *Conceptual basis for rural nursing* (pp. 51–60). New York: Springer.

Lee, H. J. (1998). Lack of anonymity. In H. J. Lee (Ed.), *Conceptual basis for rural nursing* (pp. 76–88). New York: Springer.

Lee, H. J., Hollis, B. R., & McClain, K. A. (1998). Isolation. In H. J. Lee (Ed.), *Conceptual basis for rural nursing* (pp. 139–148). New York: Springer.

Long, K. A. (1993). The concept of health: Rural perspectives. *Nursing Clinics of North America, 28,* 123–130. Philadelphia, PA: Saunders.

Long, K A., & Weinert, C. (1989). Rural nursing: Developing the theory base. *Scholarly Inquiry for Nursing Practice: An International Journal, 3* (2) 113–132.

McNeely, A. G., & Shreffler, M. J. (1998). Familiarity. In H. J. Lee (Ed.), *Conceptual basis for rural nursing* (pp. 89–101). New York: Springer.

Morse, M. J. (1995). Exploring the theoretical basis of nursing using advanced techniques of concept analysis. *Advances in Nursing Science, 17* (3), 31–46.

Myers, D. D. (1998). Insider. In H. J. Lee (Ed.), *Conceptual basis for rural nursing* (pp. 125–138). New York: Springer.

Raph, S., & Buehler, J. A. (2006). Rural Health Professionals' Perceptions of Lack of Anonymity. In H. J. Lee & C. A. Winters (Eds.), *Rural nursing: Concepts, theory, & practice* (2nd ed., pp. 197–204). New York: Springer.

Shreffler, M. J. (1998). Professional isolation: A concept analysis. In H. J. Lee (Ed.), *Conceptual basis for rural nursing* (pp. 420–432). New York: Springer.

Smith, J. A. (1983). *The idea of health: Implications for the nursing profession.* New York: Teachers College Press.

Sutermaster, D. J. (1998). Newcomer. In H. J. Lee (Ed.), *Conceptual basis for rural nursing* (pp. 113–124). New York: Springer.

Turnbull, T. S. (1998). Lay care network. In H. J. Lee (Ed.), *Conceptual basis for rural nursing* (pp. 189–199). New York: Springer.

Walker, L., & Avant, K. (1988). *Strategies for theory construction in nursing* (2nd ed.). Norwalk, CT: Appleton-Century-Crofts.

Walker, L., & Avant, K. (1995). *Strategies for theory construction in nursing* (3rd ed.). Norwalk, CT: Appleton-Century-Crofts.

Weinert, C., & Boik, R. (1995). MSU rurality index: Development and evaluation. *Research in Nursing and Health, 18,* 453–464.

Index

Special discounts on bulk quantities of our books are available to corporations, professional associations, pharmaceutical companies, health care organizations, and other qualified groups.
If you are interested in a custom book, including chapters from more than one of our titles, we can provide that service as well.

For details, please contact:
Special Sales Department, Springer Publishing Company, LLC
11 West 42nd Street, 15th Floor, New York, NY 10036-8002
Phone: 877-687-7476 or 212-431-4370; Fax: 212-941-7842
Email: sales@springerpub.com